THE Mind Body Bible

THE Mind Body Bible

Your Personalised Prescription for Total Health

DR MARK ATKINSON

PIATKUS

Copyright © 2007 by Dr Mark Atkinson

First published in Great Britain in 2007 by
Piatkus Books Ltd
5 Windmill Street, London W1T 2JA
email: info@piatkus.co.uk

The moral right of the author has been asserted

A catalogue record for this book is available from the British Library

ISBN 978 0 7499 2768 4

Copy-edited by Jan Cutler
Text design by Paul Saunders

This book has been printed on paper manufactured with respect for the environment using wood from managed sustainable resources

Typeset by Palimpsest Book Production Limited,
Grangemouth, Stirlingshire
Printed and bound in Great Britain by
MPG Books, Bodmin, Cornwall

Dedication

This book is dedicated to my wife Serena, and daughter Annabelle.

Serena, your love, support and commitment to our
growth through our relationship has enriched my life and inspired
me in so many ways.

Annabelle, the way you make people light up and the
joy that you bring into their hearts is truly incredible. I am so
proud to be your dad.

Contents

About Dr Mark

Dr Mark Atkinson is an integrated medical doctor and one of the UK'S leading authorities on mind–body medicine. His passion for helping his patients live life fully, and his ability to get to the heart of the issues that underlie his patients' symptoms, have earned him a reputation as an authority in helping people recover from health challenges using innovative mind–body approaches.

After graduating in medicine from St Mary's Hospital Medical School in London, and having spent a number of years working as a hospital doctor, he took the decision to broaden and deepen his understanding of complementary and alternative approaches to healing. What followed was a period of intensive research and training within the field of mind–body medicine. This included training in energy psychology, mindfulness meditation, hypnotherapy, brief therapy, nutrition and guided imagery.

Today, Dr Mark has a busy private practice in which he provides personalised, integrated mind–body programmes to his patients. Rather than focusing just on symptom eradication, his unique approach is designed to provide his patients with the knowledge and skills to help them experience their highest potential for physical, emotional and psychological health.

In addition to his clinical work, Dr Mark is the founder of the British College of Integrated Medicine – a post-graduate training college for health professionals. He is also an award-winning writer, a lecturer and an experienced workshop facilitator.

Dr Mark is a fellow of the Royal Society of Medicine and Royal Institute of Public Health, and a member of the British Society of Integrated Medicine, the British Holistic Medical Association and the British Medical Association.

Acknowledgements

I want to start by acknowledging and thanking my own father. Your open mindedness, unwavering enthusiasm for my work and curiosity for all things alternative have instilled in me the ability to see the big picture and think outside the box. It is because of you that I had the confidence to trust my intuition and take those first steps to becoming an integrated medical doctor. To my mother, I thank you for being you. Your unconditional love, and desire for me to be happy and fulfilled in what I do, has been a source of comfort and support to me, particularly when times have been challenging. And to my brother Carl, your humour and enthusiasm have reminded me, on numerous occasions, to take life a little less seriously and to believe in myself – thank you bro.

Thanks also to my agent David Riding at MBA Literary Agents. I thank you for bringing me together with my publishers Piatkus and for the support and encouragement that you have provided during the creation of this book. Jo Brooks and Gill Bailey, my editors at Piatkus, you have been an absolute joy to work with. You've made my transition from novice writer to author (relatively) painless and your encouragement and direction have been spot on. And to my copy editor Jan Cutler, a big thank you for all of your hard work; your suggestions have enriched the book.

Introduction

This book has been written to provide you with the best current information on how to maximise your potential for total health – the positive and vibrant state of physical, emotional and psychological health that emerges from within when the major barriers to healing are overcome. It is the culmination of my own insights and experience from advising thousands of people in my capacity as an integrated medical doctor, and over 15 years of studying and researching the healing relationship between the mind and body.

I am going to be sharing with you in simple, clear language the discoveries of the world's leading mind–body pioneers, the scientific research that shows how your emotions interact with your body, and the latest insights relating to 14 of the most important influences and contributors to your physical, emotional and psychological health. I will be providing step-by-step instructions on how to create your own personalised healthy-eating plan, and how to heal emotional pain and heartbreak rapidly, increase your energy, transform and lift your mood, create better relationships, enhance your resistance to stress, improve your physical health, raise your self-esteem and confidence, and prevent disease. That's a lot of promises and a lot of information. But is it achievable?

My experience as an integrated medical doctor has taught me that if you are committed to your health, and are given enough time, these goals are not only very possible but also realistic. The majority of people that I have assisted to overcome the barriers to total health have used a personalised combination of the exact same approaches that I will be sharing with you here. Indeed, the catalyst for writing this book was the numerous requests from patients and attendees at my lectures and workshops for me to produce a book that summarised succinctly everything to do with the mind–body and integrated approaches that I advocate. The message that I have been hearing for quite some time now is that many people feel the advice they had read in books or have received in consultations didn't go deep enough into the core issues, didn't fulfil their need for information and somehow seemed incomplete. This is such a widespread and common problem. So what's going on? And why, when there are so many books on health, is there a request for one more?

In a nutshell, the advice that many healthcare practitioners provide is incomplete, for two reasons. Firstly, it fails to embrace mind–body–soul–environment as a reality. Secondly, it fails to address the unique and complex social, emotional, environmental and psychological challenges that each of us are facing on a daily basis. Let's take a look at each of these in more detail.

Mind–body–soul–environment

Back in the 17th century a philosopher by the name of Descartes (1596–1650) proposed the idea that the mind and body were separate entities. Although this was not uniquely his idea, it did set in motion a cascade of assumptions and beliefs that were to result in science, medicine and some religions being structured around the idea that human beings consist of three separate entities: the body, the mind and the soul, plus the environment within which they live. You just have to look at how the delivery of healthcare is set up today to see the impact of this idea. If you have a problem of the soul you go to a priest, a spiritual teacher or mystic; a problem of the mind you go to a psychiatrist, hypnotherapist or counsellor; a problem of the body you go to a doctor, nutritional therapist or osteopath; and a problem with the environment within which you live you go to a doctor specialising in environmental medicine or even a feng shui consultant. Each of these specialists sees problems relating to health and life through their body, mind, soul or environment filter and perspective. Once they have identified what they think the problem is according to their own belief systems, they'll respond to the issues with the tools of their trade: soul tools – love, prayer, forgiveness and compassion; mind tools – affirmation, visualisation, relaxation; body tools – medications, surgery, supplements or physical manipulation; environmental tools – avoidance, desensitisation and detoxification. For some people it will work well, they'll resolve the issues and move on with their life. However, I'm meeting a lot of people who do not experience sustainable positive change from addressing just one level – mind, body, soul or environment – and do feel that their programme of treatment is incomplete because of this. What I am proposing, therefore, and what my own professional experience bears out, is that you can potentially increase the probability of overcoming many of the health and life challenges in your life by embracing the largest possible perspective: that body, mind, soul and environment are not separate but a unity, and that each is a gateway into this unity.

This is not a pie-in-the-sky proposition, but one grounded in good science and thousands of years of Eastern wisdom. By embracing this perspective, my intention is for this book to meet the need for completeness of information. For more detailed information on the mind–body connection please see Appendix 1.

New challenges

One of the most compelling reasons to make health advice more comprehensive and more tailored to addressing the physical, environmental, emotional, social and psychological influences on disease and quality of life is the fact that the health and lives of millions of people are deteriorating, not improving. That's evident when you take a look at some sobering health statistics: for example, the prevalence of depression is soaring, an estimated 2.3 million people in Britain (5 per cent of the population) at any one time are affected by clinical depression;[1] 110,000 people die each year in England because of coronary heart disease;[2] obesity levels in England have tripled in the past two decades, almost 24 million adults are now overweight or obese.[3] Furthermore, in the last 30 years, the incidence of functional illnesses, such as chronic fatigue syndrome, fibromyalgia, irritable bowel syndrome, migraines, attention deficit disorder, unexplained chest pain, post-traumatic stress disorder and dyspepsia have rocketed. So what's behind all of this?

In a nutshell, it's happening because of the mismatch between the way we live our lives and the way we are genetically programmed to live our lives. Our genetic makeup has changed in the last 30,000 to 40,000 years – we are still hardwired to eat fresh produce, keep physically active and be socially connected through community-orientated living.[4] That's a far cry from today's reality of nutrient-depleted, processed diets, physical inactivity, social isolation, increasing levels of stress, sleep deprivation, high job anxiety, resistant microbes and overburdening chemical and electromagnetic pollution. The fact is our social, chemical, physical, emotional and psychological environment has changed so dramatically that many millions of people are simply failing to cope. That failure to adapt is, I believe, at the heart of the tidal wave of illnesses that we are seeing in the UK. So what is the solution? My personal and professional opinion is that we need to face the full reality of this situation, and bring a 21st-century integrated strategy to it, one that explores and provides solutions to these issues. This is what is offered in *The Mind–Body Bible*. Rather than providing a one-size-fits-all solution to disease recovery and health improvement, it champions a truly holistic total-health approach built around three core principles.

1 Identify the core issues

Firstly, the root causes and contributors underlying a given challenge/disease must be identified and addressed. For example, let's take the case of depression; if you've been given a label of depression, the 'cause' of your depression will often depend on the formal training and belief systems of the person who diagnosed you – a doctor will probably say its due to a biochemical imbalance, a psychologist might tell you that it's due to your childhood or because of a failure to get your emotional needs met, a nutritional therapist may say it's due to food allergies or nutrient deficiencies, and a spiritual teacher might tell you that the depressive experience is an invitation to surrender to 'what is' – in doing so you can reconnect more fully with your soul. So who is correct? Well the answer is all of them, and none of them. They will be right for some people with depression but not for others; it depends on the person who is being discussed. One person's depression might result from allergies, another from nutritional imbalances, another from failing to have certain emotional needs met, and another from the toxic build-up of repressed emotional charge. Any effective approach to true healing and lasting personal change must therefore identify and resolve the barriers to total health in the person that is being treated. This is why treating the person, is *more* important than treating the disease.

2 Select the right tools, tailor the advice

Secondly, blanket advice such as getting in touch with your emotions, taking supplements, meditating, eating a low-fat diet or using guided imagery just isn't appropriate and relevant for everyone. In order for any personal change or healing system to be complete and comprehensive it must, of course, address the underlying barriers, but it must also take into account the preferences and reality of the person the advice is recommended for. If you absolutely know there's no way you are going to be able to remember to take your supplements every day, then using an energy psychology technique, such as emotional freedom technique (EFT), to change this habit to one in which you do take your supplements would be your first priority. If meditation is recommended, but you are tired all of the time and find it hard to concentrate, then focusing on increasing energy through supplements, exercise and diet first would be a better strategy. Once your energy levels are higher and your ability to concentrate better, then you could start meditation. The message is simple: you need to know your own unique requirements, and take into account your circumstances, before deciding which health approaches and tools you should use.

3 Embrace the wake-up call

Thirdly, the experience of any illness or significant life challenge can be a gateway to a whole new level of awareness and understanding. Many of my patients reflect on their disease experience and pronounce it as being one of, if not the most, significant turning point in their lives. Disease, when embraced for what it can be – a wake-up call – is an invitation to transform the way we live, and how we prioritise our life. The consequence of facing and embracing challenges can be stunning, it can dissolve many of our deepest fears, allow unique talents, gifts and insights to emerge, and help us fulfil our innate and unique emotional, psychological and spiritual potentials.

And that's the beauty of the total health approach – it helps you to get to the heart of the issues you are facing, it tailors information and recommendations to your exact needs and circumstances, and helps you to liberate your physical, emotional, psychological and spiritual potential. Here's how I have structured this book to help you make this happen in your life:

Part one, Chapter 1 looks at the psychology of change, and what steps you can take to maximise the benefits of reading this book and stay committed to your programme.

Chapters 2 and 3 provide you with two ways of discovering which of the pieces of information in this book is of most use to you. The first involves filling in the same self-assessment questionnaires that my patients complete prior to their consultation with me. And the second makes recommendations based on the specific health challenge that you are currently facing. Both will tell you which of the 14 barriers and mind–body tools you should focus on. This way the information you get is personalised to you and your situation.

Part 2 explores 14 of the most common barriers or obstacles to you experiencing your potential for total health. For each I have provided a comprehensive explanation, plus a step-by-step programme of the nutritional, mind–body and self-help approaches that will allow you to address that particular barrier.

Part 3 offers you access to my Mind–Body Toolbox. These are the 16 tools and self-help techniques that I use in my clinic and workshops to help people overcome the health and life challenges that they face. Don't worry, you won't need to use or learn them all!

It's my intention that by the time you have finished reading *The Mind–Body Bible*, you will have identified the areas of your life and health that are holding you back. Also, even more importantly, that you are inspired to follow the suggestions and make the necessary changes so that you can live an even healthier, happier and more fulfilling life. I wish you every success.

Yours in health,

Dr Mark Atkinson

PART ONE

The quest for
total health

chapter 1

Taking charge of your health

The first step in overcoming any health challenge is to take charge of your health. I'll explain why.

Justine had suffered from a variety of illnesses for 25 of her 32 years of life. She was fed up. She had been passed from doctor to doctor, visited numerous nutritional therapists, seen a psychologist and spiritual counsellor, and received diagnoses ranging from chronic fatigue syndrome, depression and emotional repression, to candida, syndrome X (insulin imbalance) and irritable bowel syndrome (IBS). When she looked to her future all she saw was loneliness, pain, suffering and fatigue. She had lost faith in practitioners and had (almost) resigned herself to being this way for the rest of her life. Her inner light was fading fast.

So what was the solution? When someone like Justine, who appears to have tried everything, comes to me for advice I take a step back and try to look at the bigger picture. At face value, Justine should be enjoying better health. She had seen some renowned practitioners, been prescribed the right supplements, and even explored the underlying spiritual and psychological issues. She had a lot of awareness as to what was causing her to feel so unwell, and she knew a lot about diet and how to manage her emotions, so why wasn't she experiencing any benefit? As I spoke with her, it became apparent. Whereas Justine had been told what to do and told what was wrong with her, she hadn't translated her knowledge into action. For some reason, she wasn't doing what she knew she should do, and to add to that she had become so exhausted and overwhelmed by her circumstances that she had lost sight of what she was trying to achieve. Does this ring true for you?

The reason I'm sharing Justine's story with you is because her experience encapsulates two common challenges faced by anyone who wants to improve their health:

Challenge 1 – **How can you translate information into transformation?**

Challenge 2 – **How can you take a list of things that will benefit your health and make them part of your new way of life?**

Finding answers to these questions greatly increases the likelihood of using information for change. Justine's challenge was not so much *what* should she do (the remainder of this book will focus on that for you), but identifying what it was that was stopping her from *implementing* what she knew she should do. The solution for Justine, and the process that I invite you to use before reading the remainder of the book, involves the following two steps.

Step 1 • **Taking charge**

Who is in control of your health and your life? Is it you, or is it the desires and expectations of your parents, society, the media, your doctor, your peers or your partner? How much are you *really* committed to your health and happiness? Is the way you are living your life testament to your commitment, or not?

OK, these are direct questions, but they are there for a good reason. When I meet my patients for the first time I want to know whether they are committed to their health, or not. If they are, that's great; they will usually make a lot of progress quickly. However if the aren't, and I would estimate at least 40 per cent aren't, I know that the single most important contribution I can make to their health is to help them tap into their power to change. I am absolutely convinced that the most important predictor of someone's future health and quality of life is not what they eat, not the supplements they take or even how much exercise they do, but how committed they are to improving their health and life. Commitment provides the fuel and foundations for making all change happen. If that building block is in place, the rest – diet, exercise, and so on – tends to follow. The words of the Scottish mountaineer, W. H. Murray, have inspired me in my own work, and they are very appropriate here:

> Until one is committed, there is hesitancy, the chance to draw back, always ineffectiveness. Concerning all acts of initiative (and creation), there is one elementary truth the ignorance of which kills countless ideas and splendid plans: that the moment one definitely commits oneself then providence moves too. A whole stream of events issues from the decision, rising in one's favour all manner of unforeseen incidents, meetings and material assistance, which no man could have dreamt would have come his way.[1]

In other words, taking charge of those areas of our life that we have control over allows us to tap into the power that can change them.

Step 2 • Taking action and making change

If you sense any resistance to making changes in your life, or you know from past experience that it's unlikely that you will stick to the suggestions in this book, then I would invite you to try the following exercise. This is the process that I use with my own patients, to help them transform the knowledge of what to do (from the recommendations that I and others have made) to taking action to implement what they now know. It involves asking two questions:

1. What might stop you from making a change to your life?

2. How can you overcome the barriers to change?

What might stop you from making a change to your life?

Here are some questions to help you work out which issues and factors might potentially stop you from making positive changes to your lifestyle:

1. Is it lack of energy, or motivation?

2. Do you enjoy staying in the comfort zone?

3. Are you OK with the way things are?

4. Do you get bored easily?

5. Do you prefer talking more about change than implementing change?

6. Do you live for the moment, and don't really worry about the future?

7. Are you too busy?

8. Do you get distracted easily?

9. Are you not really committed?

10. Do you lack support?

11. Do you believe nothing can help you?

12. Are there any practical issues such as finances, family or work that are a factor?

13. Are you sceptical about integrated and alternative approaches?

14. Is there a part of you that doesn't want you to succeed?

15. Is there anything else?

Once you have identified the specific factors that might stop you from making changes to your life, the next step is to decide how you are going to overcome these potential barriers.

How to overcome the barriers to change

There are four strategies that appear to work well for most of my patients. You can use any combination of the four. Take a look at them and see which one appeals most to you.

1. **Create a clear and precise goal and vision of what it is you want to achieve.** This is really important. Having a target to aim for helps keep you on track by reminding you why you are doing what you are doing. This is very useful during those inevitable times when you feel like giving up on your diet or exercise. The mind–body tool, goal setting (page 362), will show you how to get clear on creating goals.

2. **Find a compelling reason to change some aspect of your lifestyle.** This one is easier said than done. What you are looking for is a reason that evokes a strong shift in the way you feel. It must carry meaning and be important to you. For example, stopping smoking because your doctor told you to usually doesn't work. Stopping smoking because you and your partner are going to have a baby, might work, however. The most compelling reasons to change often involve other people.

3. **Resolve the underlying beliefs that are preventing change from happening.** Anyone who works with people facing health challenges will be very familiar with the idea that our beliefs can hold us back in life. Beliefs are silent assumptions that we have about ourselves and the world. They hold incredible power over us, as they shape the majority of our behaviours and influence the decisions we make. If you look to your past, and can identify repeating patterns – for example you tend to stop exercising after a week, you always give up on diet, or you forget to take your supplements – then beliefs are probably playing a part. The mind–body tool, emotional freedom technique (EFT) (page 332), is a very simple and effective way to overcome these self-limiting beliefs.

4. **Find practical solutions to address the specific barriers that you identified.** For example if 'being distracted' or 'lack of support', are potential barriers for you, one solution, for example, would be to employ a life coach to support and motivate you. If time is an issue,

why not sit down for an hour or two and rearrange your schedule? The most important thing is to put in place strategies to deal with these potential barriers before they happen.

Being clear about your goals, having strategies to deal with the potential barriers, and feeling emotionally committed to improving your health and life provides the best possible mental climate for making the most of the information in this book. Now it's time to move on to the next stage and find out what is holding you back from experiencing your potential for total health.

TAKING CHARGE OF YOUR HEALTH

- Total health is the positive and vibrant state of physical, emotional, psychological and spiritual health that emerges from within when all major barriers to healing are overcome.

- Resolving any health challenge involves the three steps of identifying the underlying issue, selecting the right tools for you and embracing the wake-up call.

- However, in order for lasting change to take place and for you to benefit from what you are about to read, you need to translate knowledge into action.

- The process of change starts by taking responsibility for your health, and being honest about the factors and barriers that might come in the way of you making change in your life.

- Four of the most effective ways to make change happen are: to create a goal, to find a compelling reason to change, to overcome any self-limiting beliefs, and to find practical solutions to the barriers that you have identified.

chapter 2

What are your barriers to total health?

Now you are hopefully feeling motivated and more committed, it's time to work out what is standing between you and an improved level of health.

To do this effectively I want to introduce an idea that might be new to you. I mentioned in my introduction that the delivery of healthcare within the Western world is based around the notion that mind and body are separate entities. So if you have a particular health challenge that appeared to originate from the body (for example, back pain) you see a doctor, and if you have a problem that appeared to relate to your mind (such as depression or addictions) you would see a psychiatrist or psychologist. Everything appears to be clear and straightforward. But there is a problem with this approach. It goes against the grain of two lines of emerging evidence. The first, that the body and mind are not separate but the same entity – a bodymind so to speak – and the second, that a problem affecting the body often has its roots within, and is influenced by the mind, and vice versa. Let's look at these in a little more detail.

The bodymind

Research dating back to the 1970s has discovered that the activities of our mind (thoughts, emotions, beliefs, images and attitudes) have very real, measurable physical equivalents called neuropeptides.[1] Just as a signal from a particular broadcasting station is converted by your television set into pictures and sound, so the tissues and cells of the body convert this mind activity into neuropeptides. The type of neuropeptide produced (there are over a hundred), is determined by the tone or flavour of emotions that you are experiencing. So if you feel happy, your body will produce 'happy' neuropeptide equivalents, if you are sad, it will produce 'sad' equivalents. Your psychology, via neuropeptides, literally becomes your biology. They mirror one another.

Once produced, these messenger substances flood the body with information, and that information influences the way your body works, and feeds back to the mind, affecting how you feel and even what you think. Your body and mind is in fact one giant conversation! What's more, these neuropeptides are produced not only in response to emotions but also to the food we eat, the way we breathe, and even the way we move and hold our body. In fact any disease process or physical body imbalance will interfere with the production and flow of neuropeptides (emotions) around the body. This blurring of the boundaries between mind and body is in fact so considerable that I, along with many others, have been forced to re-evaluate the nature of the mind–body connection. Rather than seeing mind and body as separate entities, Western science has brought us to the same realisation held by many of the Eastern healing traditions, that body and mind are in fact two gateways into a unified field of intelligence and information called the bodymind. To read more about this take a look at Appendix I.

Healing the bodymind

Given that there are no real boundaries between mind and body, we can start to see how it is possible that some health challenges, in some people, might have their origins in places that we would not expect; for example, back pain. At the physical level it can usually be put down to muscle sprain, or problems with the various joints in and around the back. This is a very common problem and can usually be treated effectively with a combination of light exercise, anti-inflammatory supplements or medications and/or manipulation by an osteopath or chiropractor.

But what if the back pain is long-standing and doesn't readily respond to these treatments? What are the possible causes then? My own work with such patients, and that of mind–body pioneers, such as Dr John Sarno, has lead me and a number of integrated practitioners to believe that the root cause of a significant number of health problems within people originate at the level of the mind. In fact Dr John Sarno has coined the phrase 'tension myositis syndrome' to describe a group of emotionally induced painful conditions.[2] This includes chronic pain relating to the back, neck, shoulders and limbs, fibromyalgia (widespread bodily pain and fatigue) and carpal tunnel syndrome. His belief is that the mind creates pain as a means of distracting us from the accumulated emotional upset and pain contained within our psyche. This distraction technique is designed to protect us from being overwhelmed by negative emotions. By encouraging people to acknowledge and accept the emotional origins of their pain fully he has helped thousands of people free themselves of their pain. I have seen this with my own patients as well, and to be quite honest with you I am in awe of how this works.

And then there is the reciprocal relationship in which problems of the mind, such as anxiety or depression, can have their roots in the physical body. Allergies to food, nutritional deficiencies, toxins, medications and hormonal imbalances, for example, can all make a person feel depressed.[3] People with schizophrenia can have their symptoms worsened by nutritional deficiencies, allergies, blood-sugar imbalances and a condition called pyroluria, in which they produce an abnormal amount of chemicals called pyrroles; these in turn make them deficient in zinc and vitamin B_6.[4] Replacement of these two, using supplementation, can transform the quality of life for some people with schizophrenia.

Often people's symptoms result from a combination of bodymind factors. This is by far the most common situation. I'll illustrate this with a case study.

Emma came to me for help with losing weight. She was 25kg (4 stone/56lb) overweight. She had a good track record of keeping to diets and was usually successful at achieving her

target weight. However, once she got there, her willpower
almost instantly ran out and she started binge eating again.
Within two months her weight would be back on.

In Emma's case treating the body would be straightforward – I would
start her on a healthy-eating and exercise programme, and give her
some supplements to stabilise her blood sugar and balance her hormones. But it was obvious to me (and to her as well) that this wasn't
going to be enough; her past history of yo-yo dieting told me that we
also needed to address the mind – the emotional and psychological
factors – as well.

The questions I asked of myself and Emma included: why did
Emma really want to lose weight? What was stopping her from maintaining her programme? How was she managing her feelings? What
were her beliefs about herself? Does she accept and value herself? Is
she fulfilled and happy with her life? It turns out that the reason
Emma put weight back on was because she used food to manage her
emotions. While focused on losing weight, she temporarily overrode
this because of her strong willpower, but by the time she arrived at
her target weight she was mentally exhausted and once again at the
mercy of her feelings. So, in addition to the body-based approaches,
my work with Emma focused on managing her emotions (Barrier
13), meeting her emotional needs (Barrier 8) and lifting her low self-
esteem (Barrier 14). Because she was courageous enough to do this
emotional work as well as change her diet and exercise, Emma was
able to achieve her target weight and, more importantly, maintain it
for the first time in her life.

This case study for me represents the essence of the total-health
approach that I am going to be sharing with you. To overcome a
health challenge you've got to identify the underlying physical and
emotional/psychological imbalances and then resolve those imbalances from all directions: mind, body and environment. In the next
chapter I explain how to create your own total-health programme.

Now it's over to you!

chapter 3

Creating your own total-health programme

If you are currently experiencing any significant health or life challenges, or if you are committed to discovering a better quality of health, then I would encourage you to create your own total-health programme. A total-health programme provides you with a personalised prescription for helping you achieve your health and life goals.

The best way of creating your own programme, and the method I use with my own patients, is for you to fill in a series of mini-questionnaires, each of which is designed to identify the specific barrier or issue that is preventing you from improving your health and overcoming health challenges. I have identified 14 potential barriers, seven of which influence the health of the bodymind via the body (unhealthy diet, body acidification, digestive health imbalance, toxicity, chronic inflammation, hormonal imbalances, and candida and parasites), and seven through the mind (unmet emotional needs, stress, addictions, disconnection, denial of reality, emotional mismanagement and low self-esteem). These are by no means all of the possible obstacles to total health, but they are, in my own clinical experience, some of the most common ones.

The second and alternative way is to use my Health Condition Guide on page 33. This is particularly useful if you already have a diagnosis. I've listed the top 40 most common health conditions, and for each of these I have provided three groups of information:

(1) The four barriers to total health that are most likely to be relevant to you; (2) The four mind–body tools that will probably be of most use to you; and (3) Suggestions as to which supplements you can take. But please do bear in mind that this second approach is not as accurate as the first in the sense that the recommendations are based on my experience, rather than what is true for you. So, if you have the time, I would encourage you to use a combination of the two.

OPTION 1

Identify your barriers to total health

As you go through the questionnaires, take your time and make sure that the response you give feels right. When you have finished, add up the scores and enter it into the score chart at the end of this chapter. This questionnaire takes 20 to 30 minutes to complete. This might feel like a long time but in the context of improving your health I guarantee it will be worth it.

QUESTIONNAIRE

For each question score 0 for no; 1 for occasionally; 3 for yes, then total up each section.

1 Unhealthy diet

Do you:

1. Feel that your diet is in any way negatively affecting your health and energy levels? ☐

2. Get confused as to what you should and shouldn't be eating? ☐

3. Have any problems with your digestion? ☐

▶

4. Feel unsure as to what constitutes unhealthy food? ☐

5. Want to know which foods promote good health? ☐

6. Have a disease or health concern of any kind? ☐

7. Want to change your eating habits? ☐

8. Feel as though you could do with more energy? ☐

9. Want to lose weight? ☐

10. Want to learn about the secrets of healthy eating (score yourself 10)? ☐

Total score ☐

2 Body acidification

Do you:

1. Have any chronic health problems? ☐

2. Eat convenience, microwave, and/or fast foods more than three times a week? ☐

3. Rarely eat your five fruit and vegetables a day? ☐

4. Have a tendency to be angry, get frustrated or hold resentment? ☐

5. Have any problems with your liver or intestines? ☐

6. Experience low energy levels? ☐

7. Rarely exercise or make time to relax deeply? ☐

8. Experience moderate to high levels of stress? ☐

9. Find it hard to recover from infections, or suspect your immune system is under-functioning? ☐

▶

10. Want to learn about the secrets to pH balancing your body (score yourself 10)?

Total score

3 Digestive health imbalance

Do you:

1. Have irritable bowel syndrome or inflammatory bowel disease?

2. Get intermittent or continuous diarrhoea or constipation?

3. Have a yeast infection, such as thrush?

4. Experience foggy-headedness?

5. Have abdominal bloating, burping, indigestion or abdominal distension?

6. Experience tiredness or chronic fatigue?

7. Suspect that you might have problems absorbing nutrients?

8. Have any allergies and/or food intolerances?

9. Want to learn about the secrets to improving your digestive health (score yourself 10)?

Total score

4 Toxicity

Do you:

1. Have any mercury amalgam fillings in your mouth?

2. Get headaches or migraines?

►

3. Have a diagnosis of an unexplained neurological disease?

4. Experience itchy ears, frequent ear infections or ringing in the ears?

5. Have a history of amalgam filling removal?

6. Have a weakened immune system or history of candida and/or parasites?

7. Have short-term memory loss?

8. Have any unexplained physical or psychological symptoms?

9. Have watery, itchy eyes, red eyelids or dark circles under the eyes?

10. Want to learn about the secrets to detoxifying your body and environment (score yourself 10)?

Total score

5 Chronic inflammation

Do you:

1. Have any inflammatory health conditions (score yourself 10)?

2. Have presently or have had previously a history of diabetes, cancer, heart disease, or lupus?

3. Have a waist size greater than 86cm (34in) for women/102cm (40in) for men?

4. Eat convenience, microwave, and/or fast foods more than three times a week?

5. Have bleeding gums?

▶

6. Have diabetes or syndrome X? ☐

7. Experience morning stiffness? ☐

8. Exercise vigorously and regularly? ☐

9. Experience moderate to high levels of stress? ☐

10. Want to learn about the secrets to treating chronic inflammation (score yourself 10)? ☐

Total score ☐

6 Hormonal imbalance

Do you:

1. Feel stressed, restless, overwhelmed and/or exhausted? ☐

2. Suffer from interrupted sleep, insomnia or low libido? ☐

3. Experience anxiety, depression, nervousness, phobias or panic attacks? ☐

4. Get absent-minded or feel that your short-term memory lets you down? ☐

5. Keep yourself going on sugar, caffeine and/or snacks? ☐

6. Get easily chilled (especially your hands and feet)? ☐

7. Gain weight easily despite eating little, or find it hard to lose excess weight? ☐

8. Experience low energy levels? ☐

9. Experience peri- or post-menopausal discomfort, period problems or have been known to have PMS or PCOS? ☐

10. Want to learn about the secrets to balancing your hormones (score yourself 10)? ☐

Total score ☐

▶

7 Candida and parasites

Do you:

1. Experience repeated yeast infections, such as thrush? ☐

2. Get foggy-headedness or find it hard to concentrate? ☐

3. Use antibiotics extensively (at any time in your life)? ☐

4. Have chronic fungus on your nails, skin or athletes foot? ☐

5. Experience restless sleep? ☐

6. Have any skin problems – such as rashes or itches? ☐

7. Feel tired most of the time? ☐

8. Experience constipation or diarrhoea? ☐

9. Have foul-smelling stools? ☐

10. Want to learn about the secrets to treating candida and parasites (score yourself 10)? ☐

Total score ☐

8 Unmet emotional needs

Do you:

1. Have depression, anxiety or any type of mental illness? ☐

2. Feel disconnected from others and/or yourself? ☐

3. Find it difficult to receive positive comments and attention? ☐

4. Feel insecure and/or unsafe? ☐

5. Have low self-esteem and/or confidence? ☐

6. Wish to feel more happy and fulfilled? ☐

▶

7. Have any addictions, compulsive or obsessive behaviours? ☐

8. Lack respect and positive attention from those around you? ☐

9. Want to know what emotional needs are necessary in order to experience total health? ☐

10. Want to learn about the secrets to fulfilling your emotional needs (score yourself 10)? ☐

Total score ☐

9 Psychological stress

Do you:

1. Feel stressed most of the time? ☐

2. Find it hard to cope with stressful situations? ☐

3. Live a stressful life? ☐

4. Find it hard not to worry about things? ☐

5. Struggle to manage your stress? ☐

6. Find it difficult to relax and enjoy life? ☐

7. Think/know that stress is negatively affecting your health/life? ☐

8. Manage stress through the use of food, drink, smoking, gambling, drugs or sex? ☐

9. Get easily irritated, depressed, upset and/or anxious? ☐

10. Want to learn about the secrets to managing stress (score yourself 10)? ☐

Total score ☐

▶

10 Addictions

Do you:

1. Have an addiction (score yourself 10)? ☐

2. Find that your tolerance for a particular substance or substances (food/drink/drug/smoking/activity) is increasing? ☐

3. Get unsettled at the thought of not being able to have the substance(s), if I told you that you could not have it/them? ☐

4. Find yourself giving up or reducing important social, occupational, or recreational activities because of this substance? ☐

5. Continue with the substance(s) despite the knowledge of having a persistent or recurrent physical or psychological problem that is likely to have been caused or exacerbated by the substance? ☐

6. Have a persistent desire or a history of unsuccessful attempts to cut down or to control a particular substance? ☐

7. Get jittery or anxious without a coffee, cigarette or something sweet? ☐

8. Smoke cigarettes? ☐

9. Experience withdrawal symptoms from the substance(s)? ☐

10. Want to learn about the secrets to overcoming addictions (score yourself 10)? ☐

Total score ☐

►

11 Disconnection

Do you:

1. Have few friends? ☐

2. Lack someone that you can share everything with? ☐

3. Feel disconnected from yourself and others? ☐

4. Deliberately avoid or feel uncomfortable in social situations? ☐

5. Struggle to receive and experience compliments and love? ☐

6. Tend to keep your guard up and reveal little about yourself to people you know? ☐

7. Have any hurt or upset relating to a member of your family? ☐

8. Think that your relationship with your partner could be better? ☐

9. Feel uncomfortable talking about issues to do with intimacy and love? ☐

10. Want to learn about the secrets to connecting with others (score yourself 10)? ☐

Total score ☐

12 Denial of reality

Do you:

1. Ignore certain aspects of reality? ☐

2. Pretend something hasn't happened, even though you know it has happened/is happening? ☐

▶

3. Keep yourself busy or distracted as a means of not addressing a particular issue? ☐

4. Feel uncomfortable when someone challenges or argues against your world view? ☐

5. Turn a blind eye to certain aspects of your relationships (personal and professional)? ☐

6. Know that there is some aspect of your life that needs addressing, but you are not doing anything about it? ☐

7. Justify or defend your lack of action in relation to certain aspects of your life or health? ☐

8. Feel particularly fearful towards certain things or issues? ☐

9. Have certain topics or issues that you simply do not want to discuss or think about? ☐

10. Want to learn about the secrets to opening your eyes and facing reality (score yourself 10)? ☐

Total score ☐

13 Emotional mismanagement

Do you:

1. Find it difficult to empathise and connect to other people? ☐

2. Feel unsure of, or uncomfortable with, your own emotions or the emotions of others? ☐

3. Get stuck in self-limiting habits and beliefs? ☐

4. Struggle to manage and express your emotions? ☐

5. Have difficulty in developing intimate relationships? ☐

6. Find it hard to be vulnerable? ☐

▶

7. Find it hard to identify which emotions you are feeling? ☐

8. Disregard your intuition? ☐

9. Get overwhelmed by your emotions? ☐

10. Want to learn about the secrets to managing your emotions (score yourself 10)? ☐

Total score ☐

14 Low self-esteem

Do you:

1. Have low self-esteem (score yourself 10)? ☐

2. Find it difficult to be honest with yourself and others? ☐

3. Hold back because of lack of self-belief and confidence? ☐

4. Rely on people and events outside you to feel good about yourself? ☐

5. Find it hard to accept yourself? ☐

6. Feel inferior to other people? ☐

7. Put on an act or brave front to distract people from knowing how you feel? ☐

8. Have a feeling of emptiness, or a sense of lack within? ☐

9. Have any addictions or patterns of behaviour that stop you from achieving your goals? ☐

10. Want to learn about the secrets to lifting your self-esteem (score yourself 10)? ☐

Total score ☐

Score chart

Well done on completing the questionnaires. The next step is to transfer your scores to the chart below. A score of 10 or more on any of the questionnaires suggests you would benefit from reading the relevant chapter; however, if you intuitively feel drawn to a chapter that you scored low on, trust your intuition.

Chapter	Your score	Tick if you scored 10 or more
Unhealthy diet		
Body acidification		
Digestive health imbalance		
Toxicity		
Chronic inflammation		
Hormonal imbalance		
Candida and parasites		
Unmet emotional needs		
Psychological stress		
Addictions		
Disconnection		
Denial of reality		
Emotional mismanagement		
Low self-esteem		

Those you have ticked indicate the chapters that are relevant to you now. My advice is to prioritise these chapters, by starting with the highest-scoring ones. As you go through them, jot down on a piece of paper any pieces of advice that are relevant to you. Good luck!

OPTION 2

Health condition guide

If you already know what specific health condition you have, you can use this chart to identify which chapters of the book will help you most. Let's say, for example, you often feel angry. The Barrier column tells you which of the four barriers to total health are most likely to be contributing to your anger. In this case it's emotional mis-management, hormonal imbalance, unmet emotional needs and low self-esteem. To work out which of these are relevant to you (often there's a combination of two or three) just quickly do the relevant questionnaires in Option 1. If you score more than 10, then that's the chapter you need to read. The next column gives you a list of the four most helpful tools from my Mind–Body Toolbox. These are the ones that you should focus on initially, as I've found them to be of most use. In the final column, I've provided a list of supplements that can be taken to help treat the underlying causes and symptoms relating to that particular health condition. So if you have anger, you can take omega-3 fish oil and l-theanine. I've included this column because quite a lot of people like to take supplements to help with their health condition; however, there are two things to bear in mind. Firstly, in an ideal world the supplements would be individualised to you, i.e. the type and dose of supplements required to help individuals with the same health challenge will vary. What may work for one, may not work for another. Secondly, because the supplements have the potential to interact with other medications and supplements, you must check with a nutritional therapist or doctor before using them. The reference section of the website www.wholehealthmd.com has a list of drug–nutrient interactions that you might also find useful.

Health Condition Guide

Condition	Barriers	Mind–body tools	Supplements
Acne	Body acidification Unhealthy diet Hormonal imbalance Low self-esteem	Bach Flower Remedies Creative visualisation Exercise Emotional freedom technique	**Zinc** (30-90mg), reduce to 30mg after 3 months **Vitamin C** (1,000mg daily) and **B-100 vitamin** (1 a day) If related to PMS, add **agnus castus** (follow manufacturer's directions) If cystic-type acne, add **guggul** (follow manufacturer's directions)

Anger	Emotional
	   mismanagement
	Hormonal imbalance
	Unmet emotional
	   needs
	Low self-esteem
		Emotional freedom
		   technique
		Instant stress release
		Exercise
		Conscious breathing
			Fish oil (3,000–10,000
			mg daily)
			L-theanine (100–300mg
			daily)

Angina	Unhealthy diet Body acidification Psychological stress Disconnection	Exercise Meditation Sleep Emotional freedom technique	**L-carnitine** (3,000mg daily) **Coenzyme** Q10 (100–300mg daily) **L-arginine*** (1,000–2,000 mg daily) *take with an amino-acid complex **Hawthorn** (follow manufacturer's directions)

Anxiety	Unmet emotional
	   needs
	Emotional
	   mismanagement
	Psychological stress
	Body acidification
		Emotional freedom
		   technique
		Relaxation
		Bach Flower Remedies
		Emotional trauma
		   release
			L-theanine
			(100–300mg daily)
			or **inositol** (12g daily)
			or **stabilium** (200mg
			daily)
			or **valerian** (100–200mg

Condition	Barriers	Mind–body tools	Supplements
			daily) often taken with **passionflower** or **hops**
Arthritis	Body acidification Chronic inflammation Psychological stress Food allergies	Exercise Meditation Conscious breathing Emotional freedom technique	**Glucosamine sulphate** (1,500mg daily) or **hydrochloride** (1,200mg daily) **Litozin** (rosehip extract) – (follow manufacturer's directions) **Omega-3 fish oil** (3,000mg daily) and **evening primrose oil** (3,000mg daily) For pain: **DLPA Complex** (1 capsule 3 times daily)

Asthma	Toxicity
	Unhealthy diet
	Psychological stress
	Food allergies
		Relaxation
		Emotional trauma
		  release
		Conscious breathing
		Emotional freedom
		  technique
			Oralmat (rye grass extract, 9 drops daily)
			Lyprinol (green-lipped mussel extract, 2 a day)
			Vitamin C (1,000mg daily)
			Magnesium (400mg daily)

Chronic fatigue syndrome	Body acidification
	Hormonal imbalance
	Toxicity
	Psychological stress
		Relaxation
		Goal setting and
		  manifestation
		Sleep
		Emotional freedom
		  technique
			D-ribose (2–10g daily)
			L-carnitine (3g daily)
			Magnesium (400mg daily)
			Coenzyme Q10 (100–200mg daily)

Chronic pain	Body acidification Chronic inflammation Psychological stress Unhealthy diet	Creative visualisation Focusing Journaling Emotional freedom technique	**DLPA Complex** (1 capsule 3 times daily) **Ginger** (300mg daily) If accompanied with depression/anxiety, try **St John's Wort** (900mg daily)

Condition	Barriers	Mind–body tools	Supplements

Colds/flu	Body acidification
	Psychological stress
	Unhealthy diet
	Digestive health
	  imbalance
		Relaxation
		Creative visualisation
		Conscious breathing
		Emotional freedom
		  technique
			Vitamin C (2,000–8,000 mg daily)
			Echinacea (follow manufacturer's directions)
			Black elderberry (follow manufacturer's directions)
			Sublingual zinc (60mg daily) or **zinc** lozenges (60mg daily)

Colitis	Chronic inflammation
	Digestive health
	  imbalance
	Psychological stress
	Candida and parasites
		Creative visualisation
		Symptom dialogue
		Relaxation
		Emotional freedom
		  technique
			Seacure (6 capsules a day)
			Acidophilus probiotic (follow manufacturer's directions)
			Omega-3 fish oil (3,000mg daily) and **evening primrose oil** (3,000mg daily)
			Take 800mcg **folic acid** to reduce risk of colon cancer

Constipation	Unhealthy diet
	Digestive health
	  imbalance
	Psychological stress
	Candida and parasites
		Exercise
		Relaxation
		Creative visualisation
		Emotional freedom
		  technique
			Psyllium (3–5g daily)
			Magnesium (400–800mg daily)
			Vitamin C (1,000mg daily)
			Acidophilus probiotic (follow manufacturer's directions)

COPD (chronic obstructive pulmonary disease)	Body acidification Chronic inflammation Psychological stress Toxicity	Conscious breathing Symptom dialogue Creative visualisation Emotional freedom technique	**N-acetyl cysteine** (600mg daily) **L-carnitine** (4g daily) **Vitamin C** (1,000mg daily) **Omega-3 fish oil** (3,000mg daily) and **evening primrose oil** (3,000mg daily)

Condition	Barriers	Mind–body tools	Supplements

Cystitis	Body acidification
	Unhealthy diet
	Psychological stress
	Digestive health
	  imbalance
		Creative visualisation
		Emotional freedom
		  technique
		Symptom dialogue
		Emotional trauma
		  release
			D-mannose (follow
			manufacturer's directions)
			Cranberry extract
			(800mg daily)
			Vitamin C (1,000mg daily)

Dysmennor-rhoea (painful periods)	Hormonal imbalances Body acidification Psychological stress Toxicity	Relaxation Meditation Conscious breathing Emotional freedom technique	**Magnesium** (400mg daily) **Vitamin E** (600IU) for 5 days, starting 2 days before period **Vitamin C** (1,000mg daily)

Depression	Unmet emotional
	  needs
	Hormonal imbalances
	Unhealthy diet
	Low self-esteem
		Exercise
		Meditation
		Emotional freedom
		  technique
		Tame the inner critic
			Fish oil (3,000–10,000 mg
			daily) and **B-100 vitamin
			complex** (1 a day)
			Chromium (600mcg) if
			associated with cravings,
			weight gain, and
			oversleeping
			Folic acid (800mcg)
			may help improve
			response to standard
			antidepressants
			If not on antidepressants
			try **5-HTP** (50–200mg
			daily) or **St John's Wort**
			(900mg)

Diabetes	Unhealthy diet Body acidification Psychological stress Denial of reality	Emotional freedom technique Exercise Creative visualisation Symptom dialogue	**Chromium*** (200–1,000mcg daily) *make sure you monitor your sugar levels **Gymnema*** sylvestre (400mg daily) *make sure you monitor your sugar levels **Alpha-lipoic acid** (600–1,200mg daily)

Condition	Barriers	Mind–body tools	Supplements
			Evening primrose oil (3,000mg) and **B-100 vitamin** complex (1 a day)
Eating disorders	Low self-esteem Emotional mismanagement Unhealthy diet Body acidification	Emotional freedom technique Bach Flower Remedies Exercise Emotional trauma release	**Zinc** (50mg daily) – preferably taken as a liquid **5-HTP** (50–100mg daily) **B-100 vitamin** complex (1 a day)
Eczema	Digestive health imbalance Body acidification Unhealthy diet Candida and parasites	Creative visualisation Symptom dialogue Exercise Emotional freedom technique	**Zinc** (50mg daily) – preferably taken as a liquid **Chlorophyll** (100mg–200mg daily) **Omega-3 fish oil** (3,000mg daily) and **evening primrose oil** (3,000mg daily) **Liquid aloe vera** (follow manufacturer's directions)
Fibroids	Hormonal imbalance Unhealthy diet Toxicity Unmet emotional needs	Creative visualisation Symptom dialogue Emotional freedom technique Emotional trauma release	**Natural progesterone** (under medical supervision) **Agnus castus** – follow manufacturers' instructions (do not take if on the contraceptive pill) **Omega-3 fish oil** (3,000mg daily) and **evening primrose oil** (3,000mg daily) **Indole-3-carbinol** (300mg daily)

Condition	Barriers	Mind–body tools	Supplements
Hair loss	Body acidification Unhealthy diet Hormonal imbalance Low self-esteem	Emotional freedom technique Creative visualisation Exercise Relaxation	Nourkin (2 tablets daily), plus Nourkin Shampoo Omega-3 fish oil (3,000mg) and evening primrose oil (3,000mg) Zinc (50mg daily) and B-100 vitamin complex (1 a day) For male-pattern baldness, try saw palmetto (160mg a day)

High blood
pressure
	Unhealthy diet
	Hormonal imbalance
	Psychological stress
	Emotional
	  mismanagement
		Relaxation
		Creative visualisation
		Sleep
		Emotional freedom
		  technique
			Coenzyme Q10
			(100–200mg daily)
			Omega-3 fish oil
			(3,000–10,000mg daily)
			Garlic (900mg daily)
			Vitamin C (1,000mg
			daily)

High cholesterol	Unhealthy diet Body acidification Digestive health imbalance Chronic inflammation	Creative visualisation Exercise Sleep Relaxation	Guggul (follow manufacturer's directions) Lestrin (follow manufacturer's directions)
High homo- cysteine[a]	Unhealthy diet Psychological stress Digestive health imbalance Hormonal imbalance	Creative visualisation Meditation Relaxation Sleep	Folic acid (1,200mcg), Vitamin B_{12} (1,000mcg) Vitamin B_6 (50mg), Vitamin B_2 (20mg) Trimethyl glycine (1–6g daily) Choline (2g daily)
Infertility (male)	Unhealthy diet Body acidification Psychological stress	Emotional freedom technique Symptom dialogue	Zinc (60mg daily) L-carnitine (3g daily) Vitamin C

Condition	Barriers	Mind–body tools	Supplements
	Toxicity	Creative visualisation Emotional trauma release	(1,000–3,000mg daily) **Fish oil** (3,000mg daily)
Infertility (female)	Unhealthy diet Hormonal imbalance Psychological stress Toxicity	Emotional freedom technique Symptom dialogue Creative visualisation Emotional trauma release	If known luteal-phase defect – **agnus castus** (60mg daily) If known endometriosis – **propolis** (1,000mg daily) **Zinc** (40mg), and **B-50** **vitamin** complex (1 a day) **Omega-3 fish oil** (3,000mg daily) and **evening primrose oil** (3,000mg daily)
Irritable bowel syndrome	Digestive health imbalance Unhealthy diet Psychological stress Emotional mismanagement	Symptom dialogue Emotional freedom technique Emotional trauma release Relaxation	**Psyllium** (5–10 g daily) **Peppermint oil** (1–2 capsules) **Acidophilus probiotic** (follow manufacturer's directions) **Aloe vera** (follow manufacturer's directions)
Lupus	Chronic inflammation Unhealthy diet Hormonal imbalance Digestive health imbalance	Creative visualisation Relaxation Symptom dialogue Emotional freedom technique	**DLPA Complex** (3 tablets daily) **Omega-3 fish oil** (3,000mg) and **evening** **primrose oil** (3,000mg) **Vitamin C** (1,000mg daily) **Chlorophyll** (100–200mg daily)
Macular degeneration[b]	Body acidification Chronic inflammation Psychological stress Unhealthy diet	Emotional freedom technique Creative visualisation Symptom dialogue Meditation	**Lutein** (6mg daily) **Bilberry** (240mg daily) **Ginkgo biloba** (240–600mg daily) **Zinc** (40mg daily)

Condition	Barriers	Mind–body tools	Supplements
Menopausal symptoms	Unhealthy diet Hormonal imbalance Digestive imbalance Disconnection	Creative visualisation Relaxation Symptom dialogue Emotional freedom technique	**True Food Soyagen** (3–6 tablets a day) **Black cohosh** (40mg daily) **Omega-3 fish oil** (3,000mg) and **evening primrose oil** (3,000mg) **Natural progesterone cream** (under doctor's supervision)

Migraine	Body acidification
	Digestive health
	   imbalance
	Psychological stress
	Emotional
	   mismanagement
		Relaxation
		Symptom dialogue
		Emotional freedom
		   technique
		Meditation
			Butterbur or **feverfew** (follow manufacturer's directions)
			Magnesium (400mg daily)
			Vitamin C (1,000mg daily)
			5-HTP (50–200mg daily)

Multiple sclerosis	Unhealthy diet Body acidification Toxicity Psychological stress	Emotional freedom technique Meditation Exercise Symptom dialogue	**Calcium AEP** (2–3g daily), **magnesium** (400mg daily) Sublingual **vitamin B$_{12}$** (1,000mcg) and **B-100 vitamin complex** (1 a day) **Alpha lipoic acid** (100mg daily) and **vitamin C** (1,000mg daily) **Omega-3 fish oil** (3,000mg daily) and **evening primrose oil** (3,000mg daily)

Obesity	Unhealthy diet
	Body acidification
	Hormonal imbalance
	Psychological stress
		Exercise
		Emotional freedom
		   technique
		Emotional trauma
		   release
		Symptom dialogue
			Chromium (600mcg)
			Vitamin C (1,000mg daily), and **B-50 vitamin complex** (1 a day)
			Omega-3 fish oil (3,000mg daily) and **evening primrose oil** (3,000mg daily)

Condition	Barriers	Mind–body tools	Supplements

Osteo-porosis	Body acidification
	Digestive health
	  imbalance
	Psychological stress
	Hormonal imbalance
		Exercise
		Creative visualisation
		Relaxation
		Emotional freedom
		  technique
			Calcium (1,200mg),
			magnesium (1,200mg),
			vitamin D (800IU),
			boron (6mg)
			Omega-3 fish oil
			(3,000mg daily) and
			evening primrose oil
			(3,000mg daily)
			Vitamin C (1,000mg daily)
			and **B-50 vitamin**
			complex (1 a day)
			Natural progesterone
			cream under doctor's
			supervision

Parkinson's disease	Unhealthy diet Body acidification Toxicity Psychological stress	Emotional freedom technique Meditation Exercise Symptom dialogue	Sustained-release **lipoic acid** (800mg daily) **L-theanine** (100–300mg daily) **Coenzyme** Q10 –200mg daily) **NADH** (5–10mg daily)

Premenstrual syndrome (PMS)	Unhealthy diet
	Body acidification
	Psychological stress
	Digestive health
		Creative visualisation
		Emotional freedom
		  technique
		Relaxation
		Symptom dialogue
		  imbalance
			Vitamin B6 (200mg
			daily)
			Calcium (1200mg)
			and **Magnesium** (400mg
			daily)
			Agnus castus (20mg daily)
			Evening primrose oil
			(3,000mg daily)

Prostate enlargement	Body acidification Unhealthy diet Psychological stress Hormonal imbalance	Emotional freedom technique Creative visualisation Exercise Symptom dialogue	**Saw palmetto** (320mg daily) **Nettle** (500mg daily) **Zinc** (60mg daily) **Omega-3 fish oil** (3,000mg daily)

Condition	Barriers	Mind–body tools	Supplements

Psoriasis	Body acidification
	Chronic inflammation
	Psychological stress
	Digestive health
	  imbalance
		Creative visualisation
		Emotional freedom
		  technique
		Symptom dialogue
		Emotional trauma
		  release
			Saw palmetto (320mg daily)
			Omega-3 fish oil (3,000mg daily) and **evening primrose oil** (3,000mg daily)
			Liquid aloe vera (follow manufacturer's directions)

Raynaud's syndrome	Body acidification
	Chronic inflammation
	Psychological stress
	Addictions
	  (if smoker)
		Relaxation
		Meditation
		Creative visualisation
		Emotional freedom
		  technique
			Inositol hexaniacinate* (1.5–3g daily) *only under a doctor's or nutritional therapist's supervision
			Omega-3 fish oil (3,000mg daily) and **evening primrose oil** (3,000mg daily)
			Magnesium (400mg daily)
			Ginkgo biloba (120mg daily)

Sinusitis	Body acidification
	Addictions
	  (if smoker)
	Digestive health
	  imbalance
	Candida and
	  parasites
		Creative visualisation
		Symptom dialogue
		Exercise
		Emotional freedom
		  technique
			Vitamin C (1,000mg daily)
			DLPA Complex (3 tablets daily)
			N-acetylcysteine (600mg daily)

Syndrome X	Body acidification
	Unhealthy diet
	Digestive health
	  imbalance
	Emotional
	  mismanagement
		Emotional freedom
		  technique
		Symptom dialogue
		Creative visualisation
		Exercise
			Chromium (600mcg)
			Alpha-lipoic acid (600–1200mg daily)
			Fish oil (3,000mg daily)

[a] High levels of this amino-acid breakdown product are known to be toxic to the body.

[b] A leading cause of blindness and reduced central vision.

By now you have the secrets to taking charge of your health and the knowledge as to which of the 14 barriers are preventing you from experiencing your total-health potential. Now it's time to discover exactly how you can overcome those barriers.

PART TWO

The 14 barriers to total health

Unhealthy diet

Annie couldn't understand why she felt tired all of the time and was putting on weight – despite eating a healthy vegetarian diet. She would start each day with a home-made vegetable juice, two slices of wholemeal bread and a small bowl of muesli with milk. Lunchtimes tended to be soup and a salad, dinner times three different veggies, with either rice or a piece of fish. In between she would snack on fruit and rice cakes. In theory she should be the picture of health. She was getting her five fruit and veg a day, eating mainly organic produce, and she exercised and meditated regularly – so what was going on?

Annie's case is a real reminder of the importance of not immediately labelling the way you feel (in her case low mood and mood swings) as a psychological problem. It's all too easy to put someone's antisocial behaviour, irritability, lack of attention or even depression down to 'their mind' or 'their upbringing'. Whereas these do have a role to play, in some people the problems have their roots firmly in the body. And how do we know? Because their mood and behaviour transforms when they start eating an optimum healthy diet.

At least half of the people who come to see me for advice are faced with the same dilemma as Annie. Despite eating what they consider to be a healthy diet, their body is sending back the clear message that all is not well. Tiredness, mood swings, immune-system problems, weight gain are just a handful of the signs – and clues – that they, like Annie, are eating the wrong kind of diet.

The optimum diet depends on you

Research spanning nearly one century has come to validate the famous declaration of Lucretius (c.99–55BC), the Roman scientist and philosopher, who said, 'What is food to one, is to others bitter poison.' What he meant by this is that the determinant of whether a diet is healthy or not is not just the types of food eaten but, as importantly, the genetically programmed requirements and sensitivities of the person who is eating the food. It is not just what we eat, but the ratios of carbohydrates, protein and fat that we eat that play a significant role in determining our health, mood and vitality.

More recent research has come to find that one-third of us are genetically hardwired to thrive on a high-protein, high-fat and low-carbohydrate diet (similar to the Atkins diet), another third on a high-carbohydrate, low-fat and low-protein diet, and another third something in between. Get the ratio wrong – for example, by eating a high-carb vegetarian diet when you are programmed for a high-protein diet (which was the case with Annie) – and the body-mind struggles to fulfil its total health potential. Get it right and you'll feel great and energised.

That's one half of the story. Even when you do get to grips with the types of foods you should be eating through a process called metabolic typing (which I'm going to talk about in a moment), you've then got to make sure that your body isn't adversely reacting to those individual foods. According to the British Allergy Foundation, 45 per cent of people have an intolerance or sensitivity to one or more different types of food.[1] Tucking into a cheese and tomato pizza might pose no problem for one person, yet for another person who is sensitive to wheat and cow's milk produce, it might trigger diarrhoea, fatigue and even depression. Eating a handful of salted peanuts for one person might be an enjoyable experience, but for another person who is allergic to peanuts it might mean death.

When designing a healthy diet, therefore, it is essential to make sure that you are eating the right kinds of foods that are compatible with your genetically programmed needs, and that your diet does not include foods to which you are sensitive. In a nutshell, a healthy diet *needs* to be personalised.

Food and mood

One of the barometers with which you can measure whether you are providing your bodymind with the right kind of food and nutrients is your mood. Indeed, every aspect of you – mood, body, health, libido, appearance, behaviour, thoughts, sleep, vitality, and even IQ – is influenced by the food that you eat. Getting your diet wrong, by eating the wrong ratios of macronutrients (carbs, proteins and fats), or by eating foods that are known to adversely affect mood (such as sugar, refined foods, caffeine and trans-fatty acids) is a major contributor to mental ill health. In fact the research is so strong in this area that I believe the majority of people facing any emotional or psychological challenge, such as depression, anxiety, ADHD (attention deficit hyperactivity disorder) or learning difficulties would benefit from a change in their diet. Here's a brief overview of how nutrients influence mood:

- **Glucose from carbohydrates** provides the brain with its fuel. A fluctuating and inconsistent supply of glucose leads to tiredness, irritability and difficulty in concentration.[2]

- **Amino acids from proteins** provides the building blocks for neuro-peptides and neurotransmitters, the molecules of emotion that allow the cells and systems of the body to communicate. A lack of these is known to contribute to depression, loss of motivation, anxiety and poor memory.[3]

- **Essential fatty acids** (EFAs) Omega-3 and omega-6 from fats are used to make up part of the myelin sheath (the fatty insulating layer that surrounds nerve cells). As importantly, both are converted into biologically active hormone-like substances called prostaglandins. These are involved in pretty much everything you can imagine, from hormonal balance and controlling inflammation to maintaining blood pressure and regulating neurotransmitters. A lack of these EFAs is associated with depression, schizophrenia, attention deficit hyperactivity disorder, learning difficulties and behavioural problems.[4]

- **Vitamins and minerals** These are essential to all of the above working properly and functioning efficiently. Deficiencies are associated with numerous problems including poor concentration and attention, depression, irritability, confusion, lack of motivation, anxiety and even anorexia.[5]

- **Phospholipids** Phosphatidyl choline and phosphatidyl serine make up the bulk of the myelin sheath that insulates the body's nerve cells. They allow the cells and systems of the body to communicate efficiently. Deficiencies are associated with poor memory, slow learning, difficulty concentrating, forgetfulness and declining memory.[6]

- **Food allergies**, toxins, sugar, excess alcohol, caffeine and transfatty acids are all associated with mood imbalances and behavioural problems. We'll be looking at these in a minute.[7]

So, as you can see, food for your body is also food for your mind! To experience total health, to help our bodies overcome disease, we really do need to eat a personalised healthy diet.

How to create your personalised healthy-eating plan

Step 1 Work out your metabolic type

Step 2 Identify which foods to eat and not to eat

Step 3 Fine-tune your diet

Step 4 Transform the way you eat

Step 5 Supplement your diet

Step 1 • **Work out your metabolic type**

Why do some people's health and energy levels thrive on a vegetarian diet, whereas others eating exactly the same foods experience deterioration in their health and feel exhausted? How is it that choline (one of the B vitamins) can help alleviate memory problems in one person and yet the same dose causes a deterioration of mental functioning in another person? Why does a low-fat diet for some people raise cholesterol levels? Why do so many diet books have conflicting messages?

These are the questions that used to baffle me in my early days of working as an integrated medical doctor. However, fortunately I was introduced to a system called metabolic typing that provided answers to all of these. Here's what I learnt, and what I consider to be the key to healthy eating.

Genetic programming

Just as your genes influence your height, your temperament, the efficiency of your immune system and rate of chemical reactions within your body (plus a lot more), so your genes also have a strong influence on the nutrients that you need in order to experience health and well-being. Any food or nutrient can have virtually opposite biochemical influences in different people. So, for example, giving a high carb diet containing loads of fruits and veggies to someone who is genetically designed to thrive on a high protein diet will probably cause that person to feel tired, hungry and, at worst, contribute to a more serious disease, such as heart disease or cancer. To work out what a healthy diet is for you, you need to determine your own metabolic type.

Metabolic typing

Metabolic typing is an accurate and precise way of creating a customised diet and nutritional programme.[8] Rather than guessing which foods are best for you, it uses a questionnaire to identify your particular metabolic type: carb-type, mixed-type or protein-type. Each 'type' reflects a dominant pattern of metabolic processing, which in turn determines how food is dealt with by the body and the effect that food has on the body's homeostatic (maintenance) systems. Among many other things, it tells you what ratio of macronutrients (carbohydrates, protein and fat) you are designed to run on. Generally a *carb-type* thrives on a high-carbohydrate, low-protein, low-fat diet; a *protein-type* thrives on a high-protein, high-fat, low-carbohydrate diet; and a *mixed-type*, as the name suggests, thrives on a mixture of the three.

Knowing your metabolic type, and refining it to take into account other influences on your metabolism, such as your level of activity, stress, age and nutritional imbalances, is a simple way of identifying the specific foods and food combinations that you require for optimum health. I'm not going to overcomplicate things by going into the detail of all of the influences that determine your metabolic type, but I would encourage you to get yourself a copy of the two main books on the subject: *The Metabolic Typing Diet* by William Wolcott and Trish Fahey, and *The Nutrition Solution: A Guide To Your Metabolic Type* by Harold Kristal and James Haig.

What are the advantages of eating a metabolically typed diet?

These are just some of the benefits that I've witnessed with my own patients:

Short term	Long term
Increased energy	Improved skin
Enhanced mood	Increased libido
Improved clarity of thinking	Enhanced immunity
Reduced food cravings	Fat loss
Improved concentration	Improved digestive health

How to identify your metabolic type

There are three main ways to identify your metabolic type. Firstly, you can use my oxidative typing questionnaire (see page 52) to assess your oxidation status (the speed at which tissues of the body convert food into energy). I have found a close correlation between this (in

80 per cent of cases) and an individual's metabolic type. A slow oxidiser is usually a carb-type, a mixed oxidiser group is a mixed-type, and a fast oxidiser tends to be a protein-type. This is sufficiently helpful, in my experience, to be of use to the majority of people who use it. However, for a more accurate assessment, you can go the website www.metabolictypingonline.com. The originators of the metabolic typing concept have pooled all of their experience and knowledge into a detailed and comprehensive questionnaire that can be accessed online for a small fee. You will receive your personal metabolic type, a customised dietary programme and meal plan, advice on supplements, and access to a metabolic typing adviser. As a third option you can purchase one of the two books mentioned previously, which both have a self-assessment questionnaire. If you have a serious health condition, however, I would strongly recommend that you go straight to the online questionnaire for a fully accurate assessment.

The oxidative-typing questionnaire

This mini-questionnaire is a tool to help you assign yourself to one of the three oxidative-typing groups. Choose one answer for each question and total up your answers A, B or C at the end. All of the parts of a particular answer don't have to be true in order for you to select that answer.

QUESTIONNAIRE: oxidative typing

1. If I presented you with something sweet, such as chocolate, a piece of cake or candy, would you:

☐ **A** Eat it and be satisfied?

☐ **B** Eat it, but possibly be tempted to ask for more?

☐ **C** Eat it, but almost certainly start craving for more?

▶

2. How often do you need to snack in between meals?

☐ **A** Rarely, if ever.

☐ **B** Occasionally, it varies.

☐ **C** Quite often.

3. If I gave you just a tall glass of orange or apple juice for breakfast, what effect would it have on you?

☐ **A** Good – it would keep me going until lunchtime.

☐ **B** OK – I would probably start to get hungry after a few hours.

☐ **C** Couldn't cope – I would get very hungry quickly, it would make me feel uneasy, tired and a little jittery.

4. How easy do you find it to go without food?

☐ **A** Easy – I can go for at least six to eight hours quite comfortably.

☐ **B** Varies – I would probably get hungry about my usual mealtimes.

☐ **C** Couldn't cope – would get really tired, irritable, I'd have to eat something.

5. How would you describe your appetite?

☐ **A** Low, weak or poor.

☐ **B** Normal or average.

☐ **C** Strong or excessive.

Results

Count how many As, Bs and Cs you have circled. If you have circled three or more of any one group, A, B or C, you can comfortably assign yourself to that group.

- Three or more As: carb-type (slow oxidiser).

- Three or more Bs: mixed-type (mixed oxidiser).

- Three or more Cs: protein-type (fast oxidiser).

If you scored less than three, then you are probably going to be a mixed-type. My recommendation is for you to follow the mixed-type diet recommendations to start off with, and then adjust your foods (I'll show you how in a moment) if need be.

Step 2 • Identify which foods to eat and not to eat

Once you have identified which metabolic typing group you belong to you can start to work out which foods are ideally suited to your genetic requirements.

General advice

Regardless of your metabolic type, there are certain types of food and food ingredients that you would be well advised to avoid, or at least limit in your diet. I'm sure that the majority won't come as a surprise to you.

TRANS-FATTY ACIDS – *try to avoid or limit your consumption of these*

As found in crisps, biscuits, crackers, doughnuts, margarine, vegetable shortening, baked goods, French fries, fried food, snack foods and most processed foods. Trans-fatty acids are damaged fats that are linked to heart disease, insulin resistance and Alzheimer's disease.[9]

SATURATED FATS – *maximum of 20g (¾oz) a day*

As found in meat, dairy, eggs and seafood products. While there is no doubt that excessive consumption of saturated fats can increase

▶

your risk of developing heart disease, you do need some to maintain good health. As with most things it's best to eat them in moderation.[10]

REFINED CARBOHYDRATES – *maximum of three products a week*

As found in white bread, white pasta, rolls, pastry, cakes, biscuits, confectionery, carbonated drinks, juice drinks and certain breakfast cereals. There is a lot of evidence linking the consumption of refined carbohydrates with obesity, heart disease, certain cancers, stroke, non-insulin dependent diabetes, atherosclerosis and a lower life expectancy.[11]

SUGAR – *maximum 10 teaspoons, 40g (1½oz) of sugar a day*

As found in table sugar, processed foods, soda, baked beans, sausages, cheese and cornflakes, beefburgers and cereals. The regular consumption of sugar has been associated with a considerable number of health problems including attention deficit disorder, suppression of the immune system, obesity, tooth decay, osteoporosis, heart disease, diabetes, increased inflammation and cancer.[12]

SWEETENERS – *avoid*

As found in Nutrasweet, Equal and Spoonful. There is an increasing body of evidence linking the regular consumption of sweeteners to mental agitation, headaches, depression, lowered seizure threshold and even cancer. Consider sugar substitutes such as xylitol (also shown to reduce tooth decay and risk of middle-ear infections), agave nectar, stevia, molasses (which is also rich in iron), manuka honey, date juice, amasake (from fermented rice), fruit juice, raisins and maple syrup.[13]

REFINED SOYA PRODUCTS – *avoid*

The subject of soya and whether it is good or bad for your health tends to divide the world of nutritional therapists into two camps, each passionately fighting for or against it. On the one side soya is touted as nature's answer to anything from alleviating menopausal symptoms, lowering your cholesterol to improving your memory; on the other side it stands accused of blocking the absorption of key

▶

minerals, negatively interfering with thyroid function and possibly increasing the risk of breast cancer. Having spent some considerable time reviewing the research, my own conclusion is that if you are not allergic to soya, the following can be eaten in moderation most days of the week without any detriment to your health: fermented forms of soya, such as miso, tempeh, tamari, natto and shoyu soya sauce, and some unfermented whole soya forms, such as organic non-genetically modified soya milk derived from whole soya, roasted soy nuts, edamame (soy beans) and organic tofu fermented with nigari (a curdling agent found in seawater). In fact, overall, the research shows that the regular consumption of traditional whole soya products does have some health benefits, but probably not of the magnitude proclaimed by the companies that produce them. My concern, however, which is shared by many others within the field of integrated medicine, is not with traditional forms of soya, but with the processed forms. My advice is to avoid any products containing any of the following: textured vegetable protein (TVP), soya protein isolate (SPI), soya lecithin, soya oil, soya flour, hydrolysed vegetable protein or hydrolysed soya protein. My suspicion is that these adulterated and unnatural forms of soya, when eaten in significant quantities (as many people do) are having a yet-to-be-conclusively-proven negative effect on our health. Until I see evidence to the contrary I cannot recommend them.

SALT – *maximum 6g (⅛oz) a day*

As found in table salt, and many processed and refined foods. Salt has been linked in some salt-sensitive people to high blood pressure, stroke, stomach cancer, heart disease and osteoporosis.[14] If you know how much sodium is in a food, you can work out roughly the amount of salt it contains by multiplying the sodium by 2.5. So if a portion of food contains 1g sodium then it contains about 2.5g of salt. Try Solo salt instead.

MERCURY-LADEN FISH – *avoid or limit*

Coldwater fish are naturally rich in omega-3 fatty acids and excellent sources of protein. However, because most fish is now contaminated

►

with toxins such as mercury, polychlorinated biphenyl (PCBs) and dioxins, fish really does, regrettably, need to be eaten in moderation. Some types of fish, such as tuna, halibut and swordfish, have such high levels of mercury they should be avoided all together or eaten very infrequently.[15]

There are a couple of other important guidelines that I share with most of my patients, they include to:

Eat protein at each meal

Protein helps to stabilise the fluctuations in blood sugar that normally occur following the consumption of carbohydrates (see Barrier 6). So, regardless of which type you scored yourself to be, you should try to eat some protein at every main meal; however, the amount you will eat is determined by your type. Protein-types need to eat quite a lot of protein, carb-types a little, and mixed-types a moderate amount.

Follow the 80/20 rule

If you are fairly fit and well and you are following most of the healthy-eating suggestions outlined here, you can ease up on your eating plan from time to time. Eat healthily 80 per cent of the time and enjoy less healthy alternatives 20 per cent of the time. Eating out, getting a take-away or eating processed food to a maximum of three times a week is OK. If you are facing any health challenges, this needs to be reduced to once or twice a week.

Eat at least five portions of fruit and veg a day

Fresh fruits and vegetables are packed with nutrients, plant chemicals and fibre – all of which are necessary for total health. Regardless of which oxidative type group you found yourself to be in, you need to eat, as baseline minimum at least five portions of fruit and veg a day. If you are a carb-type, you should try and eat eight or nine!

Go organic

Switch to organic if you can afford it. On average, organic food contains higher levels of vitamin C and essential minerals such as calcium, magnesium, iron and chromium as well as cancer-fighting antioxidants.[16] Organic food tends to taste better and it has much lower levels of pesticides. Most people have pesticide residues in their body – we still don't know the health consequences of this. My advice is to play safe and go organic. If your budget is limited, my advice is to spend your money on organic meat. This way you avoid eating meat laden with the hormones, steroids and antibiotics from animals that have been raised in the difficult living conditions that non-organically raised animals can endure.

Keep hydrated

We need water more than any other nutrient, which makes sense when you consider that 75 per cent of the body is water! Although the benefits of drinking six to eight glasses of water a day have never been proven, I've personally seen the health of many of my own patients improve considerably when they have increased their water intake to between one and three litres (1¾ and 5¼ pints) a day. Rehydrating the body can lift fatigue and a depressed mood, alleviate water retention, prevent the skin sagging and even help metabolise fat more efficiently. Tap water contains a lot of impurities and chemicals such as chlorine and fluoride – some research shows that these might have a detrimental effect on our body, so play safe and invest in either a wellness filter system or a reverse osmosis system (see Resources, page 424); both will provide you with clean water, free from contaminants.

Specific guidelines

These are the recommendations for each of the three metabolic types.

The protein-type diet

As a protein-type your bodymind is designed to eat a diet relatively high in proteins and fat, and lower in carbohydrates, as this will help to balance your metabolism. The number one golden rule for you is to eat protein with every meal and with every snack. A good way to remember to do this is to ask yourself, 'what protein am I going to have?' Then add your carbohydrates and fat-rich foods around that. Here are the specific recommendations for the three main food groups:

Proteins

Foods that are high in protein should account for about 40 per cent of the foods you consume each day. The best sources of protein for you are:

- **Meat** such as beef, kidney, bacon, pate, liver, duck, lamb, veal, pheasant, dark chicken, dark turkey, rabbit and pork chops in preference to white chicken or white turkey.

- **Seafood** such as mussels, sardines, herring, anchovies, salmon, shrimp, crab, mackerel, and dark tuna (the latter should only be eaten a maximum of once a month because of its high mercury content).

- **Dairy** such as whole fat milk, cheeses (such as Brie, Cheddar, blue cheese, goat's cheese, Edam, mozzarella, Parmesan, feta), yogurt, cottage cheese, and cream. You should avoid these if you are known to be, or suspect that you are, intolerant to dairy produce.

- **Eggs** – don't be afraid to eat these highly nutritious foods (unless you are allergic to them). They are rich in protein, vitamins, minerals and amino acids. Just make sure they are free range or organic. Consider having them raw (unless you are pregnant).

- **Other good protein sources** include hummus, nut butters (almond, hazelnut and sugar-free peanut butter), quinoa, organic tofu, nuts and seeds.

Carbohydrates

Too many carbs will make you feel tired and probably cause cravings (often for sweet things or caffeine), so try and limit your carb-rich foods to no more than 30 per cent of your diet. My advice is to:

- **Eat 3 to 4 portions of vegetables** and 1 to 2 pieces of fruit a day. Eat vegetables with a relatively high protein content. These include: spinach, cauliflower, spring greens, asparagus, fresh green beans, carrots, artichokes, celery and mushrooms. Cooked spinach is particularly well suited to protein-types.

- **Steer clear of white potatoes** (use sweet potatoes instead).

- **Limit your intake of grains** to the occasional serving of oats, rye, spelt, buckwheat, kamut, and wild rice. Quinoa is relatively high in protein and can therefore be eaten in moderation. Avoid plain white rice. If you do have the occasional slice of bread, put butter on it.

- **Fruit** – the best fruits for you are avocados, olives, coconut, bananas, apples and pears. The occasional serving of berries is okay. Always eat fruit with protein, such as nuts and/or seeds.

- **Legumes (beans, peas and lentils) are okay in moderation,** they should include aduki, green, lima, black, mung and red beans. Lentils and green peas are also fine.

Fats

These can be used generously:

- Butter, cream, ghee, almond oil, coconut oil, olive oil, peanut oil and flax oil are all good.

- Nuts such as red-skinned peanuts, walnuts, almonds, cashews and brazil nuts.

- Seeds such as pumpkin, flax, sunflower and sesame.

- Whenever you can, have butter, coconut oil or olive oil on your vegetables.

- Nuts and seeds are good for mid-morning and mid-afternoon snacks.

For some suggested meal and snack combinations see Appendix 2, page 411–12.

The carb-type diet

As a carb-type your bodymind is most likely to benefit from eating a diet relatively high in carbohydrates, and lower in fats and protein, as this will help balance your metabolism. A vegetarian diet is particularly well suited to people who are carb-types. Here are the specific recommendations for the three main food groups:

Carbohydrates

These should form the bulk of your diet (60–70 per cent):

- **All vegetables and fruits** are good for you. Try eating different ones each day – that way you get to benefit from the unique nutritional content of each.

- **One great way to enjoy your veggies** is to juice them.

- **Most grains** in moderation, with the exception of white rice, are good for you. Examples of grains include: buckwheat, millet, couscous, oats, quinoa, rice (basmati, brown and wild), rye and spelt.

- **Salads** are great for you.

- **Legumes in moderation** – this includes all types of beans, peas and lentils.

Proteins

Although you only want to be eating small amounts of protein it's a good idea to eat a little with each meal. This will help to prevent swings in your blood sugar and mood. The best sources of protein for you are:

- **Light meats** such as chicken breast (no skin), turkey breast, pork, ham and, only occasionally, red meat.

- **Light fish** such as cod, trout, bass, haddock, halibut and light tuna. (The latter should only be eaten a maximum of once a month because of its high mercury content.)

- **Low-fat dairy,** such as cottage cheese, cheese, milk, yogurt and eggs.

- **Other good protein sources** include hummus, nut butters (almond, hazelnut and sugar-free peanut butter), beans, chick peas, lentils, quinoa, tempeh, tofu, nuts and seeds.

Fats
These are to be used sparingly

- The occasional handful of nuts and seeds, such as cashews, almonds, pine nuts, sesame and sunflower seeds.

- Occasional use of butter (unsalted), olive oil, coconut oil, flax oil and fish oil.

For some suggested meal and snack combinations see Appendix 2, page 412.

The mixed-type diet

As a mixed-type you have a metabolic tendency to metabolise your food at a steady rate and therefore require relatively equal amounts of proteins (30 per cent), fats (20 per cent) and carbohydrates (50 per cent) to optimise your physical health and emotional wellbeing. Your diet recommendations involve a mixture of the protein- and carb-type diets. So for example, in an average week you might have mackerel with a salad for lunch and then cod with steamed vegetables for dinner the following night. One night you might have chicken breast, then, on the weekend, beef. The key for you is to monitor your body's response to what you are eating. Take a look at Appendix 2 on page 411–12 and use the two suggested menu choices to create a menu that combines both.

Now you know what types of foods you should ideally be eating, and avoiding, the next step is to fine tune your diet.

Step 3 • **Fine-tune your diet**

Once you've started your new healthy-eating plan, it's important to keep reviewing how the changes are impacting on your health. The two main areas that tend to stop you from feeling well on your food are the ratios of carbs, fats and proteins, and potential allergies to the foods that you are eating.

Watch your ratios

If you are experiencing any problems with your energy or mood within a couple of hours after finishing a meal, it usually indicates that a fine-tuning of the carbohydrate/protein/fat ratio of your meals is required.

- Cravings for fat, protein or sweets, continuing hunger, and nervous or jittery energy usually indicate that you might be eating too much carbohydrate. Try increasing the amount of protein (such as fish, meat, hummus, dairy, nuts or seeds), fat (olives and avocados) and lowering the amount of carbohydrate (for example, by eating fewer grains).

- If you are experiencing lethargy, a depressed mood or mental sluggishness it usually indicates that you are eating too much protein and fat. Try adding more complex carbohydrates (such as steamed vegetables or whole grains) to your meals.

Reassess every couple of weeks, until you feel happy, satisfied and energised by your food. If at anytime you get confused over which foods are best suited to you, then I would recommend you use the services provided by the website www.metabolictyping.com.

Food allergies and intolerances

This is covered in some detail in Barrier 3 (see page 107), but as a general rule if you know you have a food allergy, you suspect you have a food allergy or you suffer from any of the allergy-related symptoms, such as headaches, skin rashes, fatigue, cravings, fluid retention or facial puffiness, it is worthwhile arranging a food-allergy blood test (see page 109). The most common food allergies are to cow's milk, wheat, gluten (found in wheat, rye, spelt, oats and barley), eggs, soya and yeast.

Using these guidelines, the considerable majority of my patients will find the right diet for them in less than three weeks. There are occasions, however, when having a particular disease or health problem will necessitate an alteration in the foods that you are selecting. For example, someone with candida will need initially to avoid all sugar and yeast products. If this applies to you, my advice once again is to do the online metabolic-typing questionnaire, as it gives you an option to note the condition you have so that it can modify its recommendations to you.

Step 4 • Transform the way you eat

Knowing what types of food are ideally suited to you is just one half of the equation for total health. The other half is about eating smart. By that I mean making a conscious effort to be in the optimum mental state that will maximise the nutritional benefit and amount of pleasure that you derive from the food you eat. Here are a few suggestions:

Slow down and relax

Stress reduces the efficiency with which your digestive system works. Research shows that when your bodymind is in a state of stress, worry or anxiety, blood diverts away from the gut and in doing so reduces the amount of nutrients that are absorbed from the food you are eating.[17] If you are prone to eating on the go, rushing your food or eating while being stressed, try the following suggestions:

- Take a couple of deep belly breaths before eating your food. This will help your bodymind to relax.

- Add five minutes on to your usual eating time. For example, if you normally eat breakfast in five minutes, give yourself ten minutes; if you give yourself 15 minutes for lunch, make it 20 minutes. Giving yourself more time to eat will automatically reduce the stress you are under.

- Make relaxed eating a priority. Build your other activities and chores around meal times, so that you are guaranteed enough time to eat.

Bring awareness to your plate

When you eat are you fully engaged in the experience of eating or is your focus on something else? Are you aware of the full spectrum of smells, tastes, feelings and sensations evoked by each piece of food that you place into your mouth, or is it a case of shove it in, swallow and eat more? If you are like most people (including myself on occasions), the chances are that your default way of eating will be to eat your food as quickly as possible without really paying any attention to your internal experience when you are eating. This is called unconscious eating. Conscious eating, on the other hand, is about becoming present to each aspect of the eating experience as it happens. Doing this not only enlivens your eating experience it also has numerous direct benefits to your health.

One study, for example, estimated that 30 to 40 per cent of our total digestive response to any meal is triggered by our awareness of the sight, smell and pleasure associated with eating.[18] Digestion literally begins with awareness. So if this is missing, if we are not allowing ourselves to embody the experience of the food that we eat, our digestive efficiency is reduced to between 60 and 70 per cent of its potential. This can lead to indigestion, bloating and even possible nutrient deficiencies. Awareness also prevents overeating. Have you ever kept eating and eating, come to the end of your plate and realised how full and stuffed you were feeling? Conscious eating prevents this from happening. By being aware of your body's sensations as you eat you can choose to stop eating when you sense that your body has become satisfied. If you are an unconscious eater, who wants to become a conscious eater, try the following:

- For the next two days, make an effort to practise conscious eating at every mealtime.

- When you cook food (if you cook food!), really take time to enjoy the experience of preparing it.

- When you sit down to eat, focus completely on what you are eating. Become aware of how your body is feeling. When you put food into your mouth, chew on it for much longer than you would normally do – at least ten times per mouthful is good. This will also help with the process of digestion.

- When you eat, eat slowly and allow yourself to enjoy each mouthful. When you feel satisfied or you feel that your energy levels are at their highest, stop eating. Spend a moment enjoying the pleasurable sensations inside you.

- Once conscious eating becomes a habit – it usually takes a couple of weeks – try to use it whenever you remember to, especially if you are feeling stressed.

Nurture your gut brain

Your gut brain is a centre of intelligence that controls events in your digestive tract and influences the way you feel and even what you think via its connections to the head brain (we will be explaining this in further detail in Barrier 3). Well, just like the head brain, it also stores information and accumulates wisdom, and it knows which foods do and don't work for you – if you listen! It also serves as a powerful and immediate emotional barometer. Have you ever had a sense in the pit of your stomach that a situation wasn't right and then found that it was true? If so, that was your gut brain trying to speak to you. Therefore, nurturing and listening to your gut brain is an important part of creating total health. Here are a few ideas to get you started.

- Before selecting which foods you eat, take a couple of deep breaths in and out through your belly and get a real sense of which of the food choices will bring you the greatest health benefit.

- Take care of your gut health – see Barrier 3.

- Practise abdominal breathing whenever you can – see Conscious breathing (page 314).

- Gently massage your stomach area at least once a day – we tend to hold a lot of stress in the stomach area, this helps to release it.

- Develop and strengthen your stomach and back muscles through yoga or Pilates.

The next step is to create a supplement programme for you.

Step 5 • **Supplement your diet**

In the UK we spend over £400 million each year on supplements and an estimated one in three adults takes them. The most popular of which are multivitamin–minerals and fish oils, which are mainly taken to make up for deficiencies in the diet. In addition to these, specific supplements are taken to treat certain disease conditions; for example, glucosamine sulphate for osteoarthritis, chromium for insulin resistance, St John's Wort for depression, and black cohosh for the menopause.

Why you need to supplement your diet

If you believed some health professionals you'd think we could get all of the nutrients we need for health from eating a balanced diet, but is this true? In an ideal world, of course, everyone would eat a minimum of five portions a day of nutrient-loaded veggies and fruits. If this happened then it is feasible that those people who were otherwise well and healthy would get all of their nutrients, but:

- The National Diet & Nutrition Survey (the largest dietary survey of its kind in the UK) showed that only 14 per cent of people are eating the recommended five portions of fruit and vegetables each day. In addition, the majority, especially those aged between 19 and 24, are not meeting the Reference Nutrient Intake (RNI) of key essential nutrients. (RNI is the amount of a nutrient that is adequate to prevent deficiencies in 97.5 per cent of the population – it takes into account age and sex.)[19]

- The study found that women are particularly lacking in essential minerals with more than 91 per cent not getting their RNI of iron (14.8mg), more than 74 per cent not getting their RNI of magnesium (270mg), and almost 50 per cent not getting their RNI of calcium (700mg). Furthermore, nearly half of men are not getting their RNI of magnesium, and one in three men are not getting their RNI of zinc, which is considered to play an important role in male fertility.[20]

- According to the Malnutrition Advisory Group, over 2 million people in the UK are malnourished, with the most vulnerable groups being those people with chronic disease, the elderly, those recently discharged from hospital and those who are socially isolated or on a low income. Statistics show that up to 50 per cent of patients in care or residential homes as well as up to 30 per cent of patients attending outpatient clinics and GP surgeries, and up to 14 per cent of elderly people not in hospital or in care, are either mal-nourished or at risk of malnourishment. To the list of at-risk groups I would add children, especially young children, adolescents, preg-nant and breastfeeding women, vegans and some vegetarians, smokers, heavy alcohol drinkers, those taking long-term medica-tions, and dieters.[21]

- The fruit and vegetables that we do eat have only a fraction of the nutrient content compared with equivalents some 50 years ago. A report published by the Food Commission concluded that if you were eating the same foods today as you were in 1940, you would be consuming between 10 and 70 per cent less essential minerals with each meal.[22]

In a nutshell, to help our bodies reach their total health potential, we all need to supplement our diets.

Do multivitamin–mineral supplements work?

Here's just some of the research suggesting that they can work:[23]

- A study of nearly 3,000 men and women by researchers at the Karolinska Institute in Sweden found that men and women who take a daily multivitamin have fewer heart attacks than those who don't. Women had a 33 per cent less chance and men a 22 per cent less chance of experiencing a non-fatal heart attack, when com-pared with patients who did not take a multivitamin–mineral.[24]

- Researchers at the Harvard School of Public Health found that women who took a multivitamin containing at least 400 units of vitamin D were 40 per cent less likely to develop multiple sclerosis (MS) than those who didn't take supplements.[25]

- Women who take folic acid supplementation have a significantly reduced risk of having a baby with a neural tube defect such as spina bifida. The Council for Responsible Nutrition in America states that if all women of childbearing age used multivitamins with folic acid the current incidence of neural tube birth defects could be reduced by as much as 70 per cent.[26]

- One study found that individuals who took a multivitamin that contained vitamin C or E for more than ten years had a 60 per cent lower risk of developing a cataract regardless of other risk factors.[27]

- A study of 145,260 men and women found that people who took multivitamins regularly for a period of ten years following the commencement of the study had an approximately 30 per cent lower risk of developing colorectal cancer.[28]

What supplements do you need to take?

Well you are definitely not short on choice! Supplements are a very personal thing, and it really does depend on you, your health, age, budget, level of physical activity, preferences, goals of supplementation, and metabolism etc, as to what constitutes the optimum supplement for you. However, as a general rule of thumb and as a foundation nutritional programme I recommend most of my patients to take:

- A multivitamin–mineral–antioxidant supplement

- A whole food supplement

- Omega-3 fish oils

- +/- additional minerals

Multivitamin–mineral–antioxidant supplement

Because most people have one or more nutritional deficiencies, I recommend taking a multivitamin–mineral–antioxidant supplement to prevent deficiencies and to provide the body with optimum levels of nutrients. There are generally two options available to you.

Option one

The optimum dose really does depend on you and your circumstances, however as an adult, you should consider taking supplements that provide a daily dosage in the region of: vitamin A (2500–10,000iu), beta-carotene (2500–15,000iu), vitamin D (100–400iu), vitamin C (200–2000mg), vitamin E (100–500iu), vitamin B1 (25-100mg), B2

(25–100mg), B3 (25–100mg), B5 (25–100mg), B6 (25–100mg), B12 (10–100mcg), Biotin (50–300mcg), Choline (20–100mg), Folic Acid (400–800mcg), Inositol (20–200mg), Calcium (150–1500mg), Magnesium (150–750mg), Chromium (200–400mcg), Boron (0.5–5mg), Copper (1–5mg), Manganese (1–10mg), Selenium (25–100mcg), Zinc (10–20mg) and possibly others such as vanadium, molybdenum, iodine, potassium, and vitamin K. Iron as a general rule of thumb only needs to be included if you are you known to be deficient in it or at risk of deficiency. Because calcium and magnesium are bulky minerals, the amount of calcium and magnesium in multivitamin/mineral supplements is often limited; an additional calcium/magnesium supplement might therefore be required. Antioxidants – substances that neutralise damaging chemicals called free radicals – should also be considered. They include: glutathione, bilberry extract, alpha lipoic acid, grape seed extract, green tea extract, astaxanthin, and pycnogenol.

Obviously these dosages and recommendations are not written in stone, and you will need to adapt them as you progress through various lifestyle and health challenges. If in doubt, seek guidance from a nutritional therapist or integrated medical doctor.

Recommended products include:

- Solgar's Formula VM-75 Tablets

- Nature's Plus Source of Life

- Higher Nature's Superphyte (antioxidant formula)

Option two

The nutritional company Higher Nature have developed a range of products called True Food. These are made by feeding vitamin and mineral ingredients to yeast, which is then allowed to ferment, so that the nutrients become incorporated into its nutrient matrix. The yeast cells are then killed off; leaving a highly absorbable food form supplement that is as close to nature as possible. According to some of the research that has been carried out using True Food products, the component nutrients are between two and 12 times more potent than the equivalent synthetic nutrient. Because of this, smaller dosages are needed. For more information visit the Higher Nature website (see Resources).

Recommended products include:

- Higher Nature's True Food Wise Women, or True Food All Man

- True Food C (contains food form vitamin C)

Whole food supplements

Whole food supplements, as their name suggests, are made from concentrated whole foods, such as tomatoes, broccoli sprouts, berries and apples. These whole foods are dried, ground up, put into powders and then drunk, sprinkled on food or taken in capsule form. The considerable advantage of using whole food supplements, versus the isolated nutrients found in most multivitamin–minerals, is that they contain everything that makes up the whole food – this includes enzymes, coenzymes, phytonutrients, antioxidants, trace elements, activators and many other unknown or undiscovered factors. Whole food supplements are not, however, an alternative to fruit and vegetables. Nothing can match the health benefits of real, whole, natural foods – these are just to supplement your diet!

Recommended whole food supplements:

- Higher Nature's Liquid Health (which also contains added vitamins and minerals)

- NSA's Juice Plus from www.juiceplus.com

Omega-3 fish oils

Essential fatty acids (EFAs) are fats that cannot be manufactured by the body, but are required by the body to maintain optimum health. The two main types – omega-3 (alpha-linolenic) and omega-6 (linoleic) – are required for almost every body function including growth and repair, mood and memory, healthy cell membranes, immune function, hormonal balance, energy production, cardiovascular health and maintaining the health of skin, hair and nails, brain and nervous system. Omega-3 and omega-6 work optimally together when taken in roughly equal amounts. The challenge faced by most people in the Western world is that the ideal 1:1 ratio of omega-3 to omega-6 is nearer 1:6 and even 1:20 in some people. The excessive consumption of vegetable oils found in processed foods combined with a 34 per cent decline in vegetable consumption and a 59 per cent drop in fish intake in the last 60 years (both sources of omega-3) has led to this imbalance, and this is thought to be a critical factor in the epidemic of inflammation-related diseases, such as heart disease, asthma, arthritis and cancer.[29] I go into this in much further detail in Barrier 5.

My advice, therefore, particularly if you have any of the classic symptoms of omega-3 deficiency – which include fatigue, dry and/or itchy skin (including a goose-bump rash on the upper arms and/or upper thighs), excessive thirst, sweating, or urination, brittle hair and nails, constipation, frequent infections, PMS, depression, poor concentration or memory, lack of physical endurance, and/or joint pain – is to start taking an omega-3 fish oil supplement.

Recommended omega-3 supplements:

- Nutri Eskimo 3 fish oil

- Biocare Mega EPA

- Higher Nature's lemon fish oil

- Solgar fish oil

- Flaxseed oil (if vegetarian)

After three months (which should be long enough to make up for any deficiencies) you could then add in evening primrose oil (an omega-6 rich oil) or switch to hemp seed oil (contains omega-3 and 6) to get a balance of both.

+/- minerals

While a healthy metabolically typed diet and a multivitamin–mineral supplement will ensure that you receive most of the vitamins and minerals that you need, I tend to find that a number of my patients, especially those with a chronic health challenge, need additional minerals as well. Deficiencies in many of the essential minerals, such as calcium, zinc and magnesium, are more common than deficiencies of vitamins, because our body doesn't manufacture minerals. Many of the soils within which our fruits and vegetables grow are depleted in minerals, which in turn make for mineral-depleted produce. And whereas organic produce does tend to have higher levels, they are fairly modest increases in the range of 5 to 15 per cent.

To work out which minerals you need to take, you can either have a blood test, which can be expensive and obviously invasive, or you can use a mineral test kit. Although the research relating to the use of mineral test kits is limited, the exception being the zinc taste test[30], my patients have found the kit to be a very useful way of personalising and adjusting the types and levels of minerals that they take.

Using the mineral test kit

Ordering one of these kits (see Resources, page 421) can help you work out which minerals you need to be taking, and also help monitor your progress. The test kit consists of eight bottles, each containing a mineral in liquid form. The eight minerals tested for are: potassium, zinc, magnesium, copper, chromium, manganese, molybdenum and selenium.

Starting with bottle 1, you pour a small amount into a glass, taste it and record the number that best fits how that mineral tastes to you.

1 = sweet; 2 = pleasant; 3 = no taste; 4 = hmm, taste something; 5 = so, so; 6 = don't like; 7 = pretty bad

You then repeat the exercise for the remaining seven minerals. On completion, review your scores. Any mineral solution that you gave a score of 1, 2 or 3 would indicate that you would benefit from taking that mineral. A score of 4–7 indicates that you don't need to take it.

You then order the relevant liquid minerals, start taking them, and every week repeat the test to monitor your progress. Most people need to take the replacement minerals for at least a couple of months.

The great thing with this test is that the results have been found to be comparable to blood tests. I also like it because it allows you to become your own detective and to monitor your response to treatment.

Golden rules for taking supplements

When buying and taking supplements, there are a few principles that are worth following, so that you get the most out of them:

1. As a general rule of thumb you get what you pay for.

2. If you are vegetarian, choose products whose capsules are made from vegetable cellulose.

3. Most supplements are best taken with food; the exceptions are amino acids, such as tyrosine and 5-HTP, and vitamin C ascorbate.

4. The best-absorbed forms of minerals are those that are bound to amino acid chelates, ascorbates and citrates.

5. Supplements generally take much longer to work than medications – you should wait at least six weeks before coming to a conclusion about their effectiveness.

6. It is normal for the urine to go yellow when taking supplements containing vitamin B_2 (riboflavin).

7. Avoid taking supplements with tea, coffee or alcohol as these can block the absorption of key nutrients.

8. Reassess the need for a supplement every three months, particularly if it contains herbs.

9. You only benefit from what you absorb; it's essential to make sure your digestive-system health is good before taking supplements (see Barrier 3 for more information).

10. Listen to your body for feedback on the supplements you are taking. If you develop any nausea, a rash, abdominal discomforts or any concerns, contact the company who produced the product for advice.

11. People can be allergic to supplements, particularly to the fillers and binders that pack out tablets. If you are in any doubt or are known to be sensitive, choose a hypoallergenic form or capsule.

12. To benefit from supplements you need to take them every day. Although it is preferable to spread them throughout the day, most people forget to do this, so my advice is to make a habit of taking them every morning without exception.

Now that you have reached the end of this chapter, my advice is to re-read it one more time. While doing so highlight those sentences (using a highlighter pen) that you feel are important to you. Once you've done this write down at least five steps or actions that you are going to take, and spend a moment visualising yourself implementing them. Once you have completed this, move on to your next barrier.

MIND–BODY ESSENTIALS

- Your health and mood is intimately linked to the food choices that you make.

- A healthy diet is one that meets all your genetically programmed nutritional needs, and fits in with your life circumstances.

- To experience total health we have to supplement our diet with high-quality nutritional supplements.

- Recommended mind–body tools to accompany this chapter are: emotional freedom technique (page 332), goal setting (page 362), creative visualisation (page 319), relaxation (page 380).

- For recommended reading see Resources, page 425.

Body acidification

Doris was scheduled to have her leg amputated. A large, deep ulcer had been progressively growing on her left leg, and, despite her doctor's drugs and the wound care provided by her district nurse, it was getting worse. She had been told by her doctor that the only real solution for her was to have the leg removed. Their fear was that if the wound became infected, her advancing age and her poor state of health would provide little resistance to the infection spreading. This would almost certainly result in her premature death.

I was invited to meet with Doris. My challenge was to see if I could come up with an alternative solution, one that would provide her body with everything it needed so that it could overcome the barriers to the healing of her ulcer. As I looked at Doris, I knew that one of my priorties was to support her body's attempt to heal and repair itself by pH-balancing it. I'll explain what I mean by that in a moment. I started her on a diet and nutritional programme, which included large quantities of chlorophyll and aloe vera, and I prescribed twice-daily treatments of the ulcer using a hand-held electromagnetic device. Within one month the ulcer had started to heal, and within six months it had improved considerably. Doris no longer needed to lose her leg.

In Doris's case I would have also welcomed the opportunity to have explored the extent to which her emotional world was contributing to, and could be harnessed to improve, her body's state of health. In Part One, Chapter 2 I talked about how our biology mirrors our psychology. The tissues surrounding her ulcer were breaking down, so what was going on at the emotional level – what was breaking down inside? How strong was her will to live? Those are the questions I asked myself when I met Doris, but she didn't want to talk about these issues and I respected that. I have learnt through experience that it is more important to respect the wishes of the person I am helping than attempt to force them to go somewhere they don't want to go! Having said that, my advice to you as you proceed through this chapter, is to keep reflecting on the emotional and life situation factors that might be contributing to this particular health challenge.

pH balancing

The pH-balancing approach that I used with Doris was in part inspired by an American microbiologist, Robert Young. I had met with him in London, following the launch of his book, *The pH Miracle*.[1] His theories of what causes disease, and how to treat it, were quite unlike anything I had ever come across before. The essence of his message was this:

Over-acidification of the body's tissues is the root cause of disease. Correction of this by adopting a pH-balancing lifestyle is the key to optimal health.

Put another way, he is saying that the consequence of eating a poor diet, failing to exercise, being stressed etc. is that some parts of the body become acidic, and that this acidic environment leads to disease. Now I do not agree with this, as I think it's an over-simplification. Whilst acidity might contribute to disease there are many other factors – emotional, psychological, environmental, biochemical, physical, spiritual and social – which are also important. However, like Dr Young, I do believe that the acid–alkaline balance of the fluids within and surrounding our cells is an important influencing factor in whether we experience disease or health. Here's an analogy to help explain this.

The Stagnant Pond

Imagine a large fish tank, with a couple of fish swimming around. Now, any fish lover will tell you that to maintain the health of those fish, you need to feed them, but also you need to keep the water (the environment) in the best possible health. Temperature, oxygen levels and pH all need to be monitored and adjusted in order to keep the fish well and alive. But what would happen if we neglected to do this? Eventually the oxygen levels would fall, the water's acidity would rise and you can pretty much guarantee that those fish would will become unwell, probably with an infection.

To help the fish we have two choices. The first would be to treat the fish with antibiotics in the hope that this would clear up any infection. The second is to change the water, to pump in oxygenated, pH-balanced water. Both approaches will probably result in an improvement in the fishes' health in the short term, but here is the crucial difference. Because the first would have failed to address the underlying cause (the toxic environment), the fish would soon get ill again, and eventually die. The second approach, however, deals with the underlying problem, and because of that it's reasonable to expect that the fish would return to good health.

This analogy is a good example of what happens in the human body and the choices that we can make. We can chase after the disease and try to fix it, or we can focus on changing the factors that caused the environment to become toxic in the first place. The total health-approach does both.

Body acidification

So what Robert Young is claiming is that the primary trigger and contributor to many of today's diseases, such as arthritis, fatigue, heart disease, and possibly even cancer, is a disturbance in the pH of the body's tissues – a process called body acidification. As I mentioned earlier I don't think it is as black and white as this and I am yet to see any absolute scientific proof of this theory. However, I have witnessed the considerable benefits of correcting acid problems within the bodies of my own patients, and it is for that reason I am writing about it.

Before we go any further I need to explain a bit about acid–alkaline balance and pH, as this holds the key to understanding the process of body acidification.

What is pH?

pH is a measure of how acidic or alkaline something is. It comes from the French phrase *pouvoir hydrogene*, and is a measure of the concentration of hydrogen ions within a particular solution. It is measured on a scale of 0 to 14 – a pH of 7 is neutral, a pH lower than 7 is acidic, and a pH above 7 is alkaline. Because the pH scale is logarithmic, a difference of one pH unit represents a tenfold, or ten-times change; for example, the acidity of a sample with a pH of 4 is ten times greater than that of a sample with a pH of 5. A difference of 2 units, from 5 to 3, would mean that the acidity is 100 times greater.

Body pH

You might be familiar with the idea that some parts of the body are more acidic or alkaline than other parts. For example the pH of stomach juices is usually between 1 and 3 (acidic), and that of the pancreatic juices between 8 and 9 (alkaline). While it's essential to keep these juices operating in their optimum range, what I am interested in is the acid–alkaline balance of the fluids within and surrounding your cells. This is the key to health.

Just over half of the fluid in your body exists inside your cells. This intracellular fluid is slightly alkaline and has a pH of about 7.[2] The majority of the fluids that exist outside your cells, including your blood, are even more alkaline at a pH of about 7.4. Overall therefore, for total health, the body needs to be maintaining an alkaline pH. If, however, over time, the amount of acid in the body exceeds the body's capacity to neutralise and remove it, the body will automatically resort to other measures in an attempt to maintain an alkaline pH. This includes dumping acid in certain body tissues (fat is a favourite) and drawing on minerals, such as magnesium, potassium and calcium from other locations – this includes bones, soft tissues and body fluids. Each of these minerals (in most people) will shift the body towards alkalinity. So what specific circumstances would lead to an acid strain within the body?

The causes of body acidification

Diet

The mismatch between our genetically inherited nutritional requirements and the food that passes our mouths is the single most important factor contributing to body acidification.[3] Genetically, we are still hard-wired to exist on the predominantly plant-based hunter–gatherer diet. The switch 10,000 years ago, to a predominantly grain-based diet heralded the movement from a diet that alkalised the body, to one that had an overall acidifying effect on the body. As time has passed and the intake of grains and animal products has continued to rise, and consumption of plant-based products fallen, this acidic load has become worse.

The effect that a particular food has on the acid–alkaline balance of the body is not so much to do with whether a food or drink is intrinsically alkaline or acidic, but whether after being metabolised (broken down) by the body it leaves a net positive acidic load (in which case it acidifies the body) or a net negative acid load (in which case it alkalises the body).[4] Although this is an oversimplification, as a general rule of thumb, foods that contain the minerals of sulphur, phosphorus, chlorine and iodine are acid-forming, and foods that contain sodium, potassium, calcium, magnesium and iron are alkaline-forming. In practical terms this means that fruits and vegetables are alkalising grains, and meat, fish, seafood, nuts, milk, dairy and eggs are acidifying. The overall ratio of acidifying to alkalising foods will ultimately determine the effect of food on your body. In the Western world this ratio is about 80 per cent to

20 per cent. For total health this ratio needs to be reversed to nearer 20 per cent to 80 per cent.

Age

The net acid load of the modern Western diet and its acidifying effects on the human body are exacerbated as we get older.[5] This is mainly due to an age-related decline in kidney function. The ability of kidneys to retain bicarbonates (which alkalise) and excrete acids (which is acidified) gets progressively more impaired, leading to a worsening of the body acidification with age. This might in part explain why degenerative diseases, which are thought to be related to over-acidification, occur in the elderly population.

Stress

Chronic stress and worry activates the sympathetic nervous system and stimulates the release of cortisol from adrenal glands and glucagons from the pancreas. Both increase the metabolic rate of the body's cells, leading to increased production of carbon dioxide and other waste products.

Pre-existing disease

Virtually any disease, acute and chronic, can contribute to the acidification of the body.

Toxins

Yeasts and fungi, such as candida, are known to produce toxins, such as acetylaldehyde, uric acid, alcohols and lactic acid.[6] These have an acidifying effect on the body, as do heavy metals, such as mercury and cadmium, and pesticides, which interfere with the normal cellular metabolism.

Detoxification systems

The body's cells are producing acid waste all the time as part of the normal metabolic process. That doesn't normally pose a problem for the body as long as its organs of detoxification are working optimally; this includes, primarily, the lungs, liver and kidneys, but also the intestines, lymphatics and the skin. Any problem with these, such as constipation (intestines), inactivity (lymphatics and skin), or shallow breathing (lungs) can contribute to acidification of the body.

Others

Smoking, excessive exercise,[7] alcohol, drugs of abuse, medications and some supplements can contribute to acidification.

Body acidification and disease

Although the amount of published research on the relationship between low-grade acidity and disease is limited, the following have been suggested:

Inflammation

Acids are known to cause irritation and inflammation of the cellular tissues and membranes. Some practitioners believe that acid waste accumulations are responsible for the inflammation and pain associated with arthritis, interstitial cystitis, colitis and neuritis, for example. One study investigated the relationship between the pH of joint fluid in patients with rheumatoid arthritis and the severity of joint inflammation. The researchers found that the more acidic the fluid the greater the amount of inflammation in the joints.[8]

Electrical charge

William Philpott, a pioneer within the field of biomagnetics, states that fatty acids, which are normally negatively charged on the outside, become positively charged in response to a more acidic environment. This makes them stick to the negatively charged blood vessel wall (opposites attract) and this contributes to atheroma and heart disease.[9]

Enzyme inactivation

Enzymes are critical to health and life; they catalyse the millions of chemical reactions that go on in the body every second and are responsible for creating proteins – the building blocks of the body. They are, however, extremely pH sensitive. When pH falls outside the optimum range, their function is compromised, leading to a reduction in health. One example is the cells power stations – the mitochondria. The production of energy (ATP) is considerably reduced in response to changes in oxygen, pH and the presence of toxins. This can lead to symptoms such as fatigue and reduced exercise tolerance.[10]

Storage of acid in tissues

When the threshold of the body's ability to buffer acid is exceeded, it becomes stored in the extracellular matrix – the space that surrounds the cells. A classic example of this would be gout, a condition in which acidic wastes – called uric crystals – are deposited in the joint of the big toe.[11]

Depletion of minerals

One of the minerals used to buffer acid is calcium. If the body is in a constant state of acidic stress and mineral supplies of calcium are low, then this can lead to permanent loss of calcium from the bones, and to the eventual development of osteoporosis. One study reported in the American Journal of Clinical Nutrition, for example, found an association between the consumption of cola and osteoporosis in women. The more cola that was consumed on a regular basis the lower the bone mineral density in the hips of women. One of the theories put forward is that the phosphoric acid content in the cola (which is also found in dairy and grains) acidifies the blood and that causes calcium to be mobilised from the bones in an attempt to maintain pH balance.[12]

Growth of micro-organisms

In his book *The pH Miracle*, Robert Young talks about how the overacidification of the blood and body tissues encourages the proliferation of organisms called microzyma. It is his belief, and one shared by some other scientists, that viruses, bacteria and fungus are not discrete, separate organisms, but the same organisms – microzyma – at different stages of development. The factor that controls which stage they are in is the pH of the environment within which they find themselves – hence the importance of bringing the body into pH balance. As the body gets more acidic, these microzyma transform from viruses to bacteria and eventually into yeasts, fungi and mould. They do this in order to survive the acid environment within which they find themselves. Yeasts and fungi feed on the sugar in our diet and use this to create waste products, which, in turn, further add to the acidic load, and the vicious cycle continues, unless broken. By alkalising the body, Dr Robert Young has shown that fungi and yeasts revert back to their original and less harmful viral and bacterial forms.[13]

Is your body acidic?

It's actually difficult to know for certain whether parts of your body's tissues are acidic or not. I'm not convinced of the accuracy of the saliva and urine tests that some companies recommend, although they might help you to monitor your treatment programme. And, of course, it's not practical or realistic to measure the acidity of your tissues directly. However, having said that, it is my own clinical experience – and that of other integrated medical practitioners – that the majority of people with chronic health challenges do benefit from a pH-balancing programme. The goals of such a programme are to:

1. Reduce the acidic load on the body.

2. Increase the alkaline reserves of the body (the ability of your body to adjust to and compensate for changes in body pH) by providing alkaline minerals.

3. Restore the body's tissues and fluids to their optimum pH range. In most cases this means slightly alkaline.

How to pH balance your body

If you suspect that your body might be in need of pH balancing, try the following recommendations. (If you have a serious condition such as cancer, I would strongly encourage you to work with an integrated medical doctor.)

Step 1 • Switch to an alkaline diet

Earlier on I talked about how the effect of a particular food on the body's pH depends, not on whether it is alkaline or not, but on whether it has an acidifying or alkalising effect after it has been metabolised by the body. For example, lemon juice is acidic, but has an alkalising effect on the body. As a general rule of thumb, to pH-balance your body you should try to eat a diet that consists of about two-thirds by volume of alkaline-forming foods and the rest acid-forming. For most people, that means eating more vegetables and fewer grains. The division of foods into acid- and alkaline-forming foods are based on the work of Dr Thomas Kremer.

Acid-forming foods

Grains (oat flakes, buckwheat whole grain, rye, spelt, wheat, bran, millet, rice – particularly brown rice – and corn), meat (particularly liver, rabbit and canned corn beef), eggs, cheese (especially parmesan, emmental, processed, cheddar and hard cheeses), milk and yoghurt (only mildly acidic), nuts (walnuts, pecans, sweet almonds, cashews, pistachios, Brazil nuts and peanuts), seeds, lentils, peas, tofu, chick peas (only slightly acid forming), and cola.

Alkaline-forming foods

This includes all vegetables (spinach, swiss chard and beet greens are the most alkaline-forming), beans (especially white, pinto, lima, mung, and kidney), fruits (figs, plums, prunes, raisins and avocados are the most alkaline-forming), the grains (buckwheat flour and quinoa), green beans, the nuts (hazelnuts, fiberts and macadamias), whey, garlic, celery, basil, chives, parsley, ginger, curry powder, black pepper, apple vinegar, and honey.

One caveat, though, is to remember that these food choices are based primarily on the effect on pH. However, as we saw in Barrier 1, nutrient content and individual metabolic requirements can mean that one person's health will thrive on incorporating meat and dairy into their diet, whereas this will have the opposite effect on another person. My advice to you is to use the above recommendations in conjunction with the healthy-eating recommendations in Barrier 1.

Step 2 • Take alkalising supplements

It's difficult to make a one-size-fits-all recommendation when it comes to supplements, as certain minerals (for example, calcium), can have different effects depending on the metabolism of the person who is taking it. In one person it might have an alkalising effect, in another an acidifying effect. And just to complicate things further, the *type* of calcium will have different effects; for example, calcium hydroxide and carbonate will usually alkalise the blood; calcium lactate will acidify it. You can see how complicated it can get! However, from experience I have found that the following products will help the majority of people who take them.

- **Alkaline salts**, containing magnesium, potassium and calcium carbonate, are an effective way to support the body's own buffering system. Studies examining the effect of long-term supplementation with potassium bicarbonate in post-menopausal women found that it was able to significantly reduce the rate of age-related bone loss and increase levels of growth hormone.[15] (See Resources, page 420, for recommended products.)

- **Greens powders** containing alkalising chlorophyll, such as wheatgrass and barley grass added to your bottle of water is a great way of keeping your body alkaline throughout the day (see Resources, page 420, for recommended products).

- **Liquid chlorophyll** is a good alkaliser (see Resources, page 420, for recommended products).

Step 3 • Hydrate your body

One of the most common health recommendations you will come across is to drink your six to eight glasses of water a day. Whereas there is no scientific evidence to base this on, what I have seen consistently with my own patients is that those who drink at least 2 litres (3½ pints), or even 3 litres (5¼ pints) of water a day feel great for doing so. Of course, quality of water is also important – Barrier 4 makes some suggestions on this. Overall my advice is this: if your energy levels are high and your health is great, continue what you are doing, if they aren't, increase the amount of water you drink and monitor how you feel. You might be pleasantly surprised.

Step 4 • Move your body

Moderate amounts of exercise are alkalising to the body, whereas excessive amounts of exercise are acidic due to the release of lactic acid. As a general rule of thumb feeling worse after exercise tends to mean that your acid load is greater than your body's ability to remove it. If this applies to you, cut back on the exercise a little, give yourself two weeks on your pH-balancing programme and then try exercising again – you should feel better now.

Step 5 • Manage your stress and relax your body

Learning how to breathe deeply, meditate, and calm the body and mind are all effective strategies for alkalising the body. This works because these all stimulate the parasympathetic nervous system – the part of the nervous system that governs repair and relaxation. See instant stress release in my The Mind–Body Toolbox (page 368) for more detail.

Step 6 • Cleanse your body

The presence of heavy metals and other toxins in the body can interfere with the metabolism of the body's cells and contribute to the creation of acids. Constipation allows more toxins to be reabsorbed into the body, and infections can add to the toxic load by generating toxins – all of these need to be addressed. See Barrier 4 on Toxicity for advice.

Step 7 • Treat any underlying imbalances

The presence of any imbalance, whether it is nutritional, environmental, hormonal or emotional, can contribute to acidity. For example, chronic tension held within the body can result in mico-spasms within different muscles. The resulting reduction in blood flow leads to acidification of the local tissues. You can change your diet and take your alkalising supplements, but not addressing the underlying tension will hold you back from experiencing the highest level of improvement possible. If you are unsure which imbalances are affecting your body or you are unsure how to go about treating them, my advice would be to work alongside an integrated medical doctor or nutritional therapist. They can help you prioritise the changes and support you in your return to total health.

Now that you have reached the end of this chapter, my advice is to reread it one more time. While doing so highlight those sentences (using a highlighter pen) that you feel are important to you. Once you've done this write down at least five steps or actions that you are going to take, and spend a moment visualising yourself implementing them. Once you have completed this, move on to your next barrier.

MIND–BODY ESSENTIALS

- Body acidification (the low-grade acidifying of our body's fluids) can be a significant barrier to total health.

- Fatigue, skin problems, hair loss, osteoporosis, obesity, migraines and arthritis are just a few of the signs that your body might be acidic.

- The most effective way to alkalise your body is to eat a diet that consists mainly of plant-based alkalising foods and to limit your intake of acidifying foods such as grains and animal products. There are exceptions to this rule, which is why it is very useful to know your metabolic type (see Barrier 1).

- Recommended mind–body tools to accompany this chapter are: instant stress release (page 368), sleep (page 384), meditation (page 376), conscious breathing (page 314) and relaxation (page 380).

- For recommended reading see Resources, page 425.

Digestive health imbalance

Simon had been suffering from stomach problems and abdominal bloating for the last 15 years of his life. He had seen countless doctors, had a flexible camera inserted top and bottom, and tried just about every gut health supplement on the market. He was eating a healthy diet, drinking vegetable juices twice daily and taking high-potency multivitamin–mineral supplements and essential fatty acids. What's more he exercised regularly and had read everything he could lay his hands on when it came to gut health. On paper he was the model of holistic living, but, despite this, something was still wrong. In fact as the weeks and months went by he felt things were getting worse, not better. He came to me to see if I could work out what was going wrong.

Usually when I get a complex case such as this, my first thoughts are to look for the obvious thing that might have been overlooked. With a little more questioning, two things became apparent. Despite eating a healthy diet and taking some good-quality supplements, his digestive tract was not absorbing nutrients properly. Further investigations confirmed this, and I started him on a programme similar to the one I am about to share with you, to rectify this problem. The real breakthrough, however, came when I helped him to understand that his high levels of stress were contributing to his stomach problems. I will go into a little more detail in a moment, but in a nutshell I told him that the gut has its own brain, a centre of intelligence that is very much tuned into, and an active part of, our emotional guidance system. Prolonged periods of stress, such as he was experiencing, not only causes the bowel to release inflammation-causing chemicals into the body, but it can also cause deterioration in the gut immune system. This can make the body very unwell, and predispose that person to many of the gut imbalances covered in this chapter. You can take all of the supplements you want (which he had done), but unless you also deal with any underlying emotional issues, the gut will rarely heal fully. Simon was committed to his own health, and as a result of that he also addressed two other barriers – unmet emotional needs and psychological stress – in addition to following the advice in this chapter. Within three months, his bowels were working normally and all bloating and diarrhoea had gone.

I have come across a number of patients whose gut problems, including food allergies, were primarily related to psychological causes, and even emotional trauma. These are not to be missed; otherwise gut problems can go on for years and cause unnecessary upset and suffering. If you do have a longstanding gut problem please do bear this in mind. Ask yourself whether stress or emotions could be playing a part in your symptoms. You could even go one step further and use the symptom dialogue mind–body tool (page 391) to have a dialogue with your gut. Remember: your gut is a source of intelligence, that's proven, and because of that it can, and, more accurately, does, constantly speak to you. Our challenge is to listen!

Digestion and health

In every year that goes by more evidence emerges linking digestive health imbalances with disease. Cancer, arthritis, heart disease, weight problems, fatigue, autism, headaches, backaches, bad breath, foul body odour, bloating, abdominal gas, haemorrhoids, constipation, diarrhoea, depression, mood swings, irritability, skin problems, sciatic pain, insomnia, hypertension, frequent colds, allergies, asthma, prostate trouble, hypoglycaemia and menstrual problems are just some of the conditions linked to poor digestive health.[1] Furthermore, it's not just the gut that gets affected by the health of the digestive system. Digestive problems can:

- **Reduce absorption of nutrients** because of a build-up of sticky mucus plaques, inflammation of the cells lining the gut wall, and existing nutritional deficiencies, which prevent enzymes from working properly.[2]

- **Result in undigested food particles entering the bloodstream,** which in turn leads to an activation of the immune system and the release of chemicals causing inflammation.[3]

- **Cause a build-up of fermenting and decomposing food.** This provides a breeding ground for disease-causing bacteria, parasites and yeast, and drip-feeds numerous toxins into the bloodstream.

- **Place a considerable amount of stress on other organs of detoxification** such as the liver, lymphatic system, kidneys and skin.[4]

Before we get into improving the health of your gut, I want to give you a quick lesson in anatomy.

The digestive system

The digestive tract consists of over 8.2m (27ft) of tubing stretching from the mouth to anus. In partnership with various glands and organs, such as the liver, pancreas, gall bladder and salivary glands, it acts as the body's gatekeeper. It also meticulously prepares, digests and absorbs nutrients, hosts a significant proportion of your immune system and provides a home to an army of friendly bacteria that manufacture vitamins. It also boosts immunity, aiding recovery from infections, and repairing and promoting the health of the digestive tract, and it helps to reduce the severity of inflammatory conditions.

The gut brain

There is much more to your guts than waste, digestion and nutrient absorption – the gut has a mind of its own![5] The gut brain lives in the tissue lining of the oesophagus, stomach, and small and large intestines. It consists of a complex network of over 100 million nerves and produces considerable quantities of neurotransmitters and neuropeptides (the chemicals that communicate mood). In fact, the gut brain is so advanced that it can actually think independently of the brain, store memories and influence the way the emotional brain functions. This explains the gut feelings we can get. Every time we encounter a new situation, the gut brain, like the emotional brain, scans it to see if it is in any way a potential threat. By comparing it to the memory of past experiences it will let you know its conclusion through gut feelings. Comfort in the area of the solar plexus (just above your belly button) says 'no problems here'. Discomfort, however, says 'potential threat, ignore at your peril'. But here's the interesting part: unlike the emotional brain, the gut brain isn't censored by the rational, thinking part of the brain. This means that under certain circumstances gut feelings are a more reliable indicator and assessment of a situation than our own brain. Maybe you can recall the consequences of a time when you ignored your gut feeling?

Bearing this in mind, when it comes to restoring gut health, a comprehensive programme must look at the way we manage our emotions and deal with stress, as each of these can influence and be influenced by the health of the gut; for example:

- The presence of candida and parasites can contribute to irritability and depression, as can food allergies. Conversely, moderate amounts of stress have been shown to inhibit the production of stomach acid. This leaves the body more vulnerable to infection and interferes with nutrient absorption.[6]

- People with generalised anxiety disorder are much more likely to experience ulceration of the stomach and duodenum. This occurs in a dose-dependent way; that is, the greater the anxiety the greater the chance of having an ulcer.[7]

- Some researchers have found that fear inhibits the movement and activity of the upper part of the gastrointestinal tract, while stimulating the tail end of the colon – anyone who has had diarrhoea when anxious and fearful can associate with this. Anger, however, is associated with contractions of both the upper and lower part of the bowel and an increase in the secretion of stomach acid – this might explain the association between anger and ulceration.[8]

- Other clinicians have found a link between the suppression of emotions and irritable bowel syndrome.[9]

As you go through this chapter bear in mind the intimate relationship between your emotional world and your gut health. Ask yourself questions. For example, 'How much is my irritability contributing to my irritable bowel syndrome?', 'Is it possible that stagnation in my life is contributing to the stagnation in my bowels [constipation]?' 'Is my oversensitivity a factor in my food allergies?' There are, of course, no right or wrong answers, but what I do know from experience is that if there are emotional components to your digestive health imbalance and they are acknowledged, then healing takes place much quicker and deeper.

How to improve your digestive health

There are eight gut imbalances, which individually and collectively can have a significant impact on your digestive health, and therefore total health. Each of these may or may not be an issue for you right now, so I have provided you with questionnaires for each. The higher your score the greater the likelihood that it is an issue for you. If, after going through this chapter, three or more of these eight factors apply to you, it might be an idea to seek the help of a practitioner experienced in integrated approaches to digestive health, otherwise it might get a little confusing.

The eight gut imbalances are:

1. Low stomach-acid levels

2. Low digestive-enzyme levels

3. Leaky-gut syndrome

4. Dysbiosis (when there is an imbalance between the good and bad bacteria in the gut)

5. Food allergies and intolerances

6. Candida

7. Parasites

8. Incompatible food combinations

In addition to these eight, I would encourage you to read the following chapters as well, because of their absolute importance to gut health: unmet physical needs (particularly exercise and healthy eating) (page 350 and Barrier 1), relaxation (page 380), conscious breathing (page 314), meditation (page 376) and emotional mismanagement (Barrier 13). Specific recommendations for gut-related disease, such as IBS and colitis, are provided in the quick reference chart, Option 2: Health Condition Guide on pages 33–43.

1. Low stomach-acid levels

Your stomach produces an impressive 3 litres (5¼ pints) of acidic fluid each day. This stomach acid has a lot of important roles, including the digestion of protein, defending your body against infection and helping the absorption of nutrients, such as calcium, vitamin B_{12} and iron. Whereas it is true that some people produce too much stomach acid, the majority of people with stomach imbalances, especially those over the age of 60, produce too little. Low stomach-acid levels are considered to be an important contributor to indigestion, and many other conditions including arthritis, asthma, chronic autoimmune disease, coeliac disease, diabetes, eczema, gall-bladder disease, hives, osteoporosis, pernicious anaemia, psoriasis, rheumatoid arthritis, rosacea, Sjögren's syndrome, thyroid imbalance, Crohn's disease, acne, hives, allergies, autism, depression, constipation, diarrhoea, inflammatory bowel disease, skin problems such as eczema and psoriasis, and irritable bowel syndrome.[10] It's important to know about!

How to assess your stomach-acid levels

Try the stomach-acid test

One easy, but admittedly not very accurate, way to test for a deficiency is the stomach-acid test. Next time you get indigestion, add a teaspoon of lemon juice to some warm water and sip on it. If this helps, it suggests that you are deficient in stomach acid and would therefore benefit from betaine hydrochloride (stomach-acid replacement) supplementation. Don't do this test if you have suspected stomach ulcers.

Arrange a Heidelberg capsule test

The Heidelberg test determines your ability to secrete hydrochloric acid. To do this you swallow an instrument the size of a large capsule, which has a string attached to it for retrieval. The instrument then transmits information about the pH of the digestive tract and how it changes when you drink a bicarbonate solution. This test has to be arranged through your doctor.

Take the low-stomach-acid questionnaire

The following symptoms are associated with having insufficient or low amounts of stomach acid:

QUESTIONNAIRE: low stomach acid

For each question score 0 for no; 1 for occasionally; 3 for yes, then total up the section.

Do you:

1. Get indigestion? ☐
2. Have a coated tongue? ☐

▶

3. Experience burping, bloating, gas and/or burning immediately after meals? ☐

4. Have an itchy rectum? ☐

5. Have undigested food in your stools? ☐

6. Feel nauseous after taking supplements? ☐

7. Have dilated blood vessels on your cheeks or nose? ☐

8. Have excessive amounts of wind? ☐

9. Have iron-deficiency anaemia? ☐

10. Have weak or cracked nails? ☐

11. Have constipation or diarrhoea? ☐

12. Experience a sense of fullness immediately after eating? ☐

13. Are you aged 50 or more? ☐

Total score ☐

A score of 7 or more suggests that low stomach-acid levels might be contributing to your symptoms.

How to treat low stomach acid

If the stomach-acid test, capsule test, and/or questionnaire indicate that you might have low stomach-acid levels, you should consider following the steps below.

Step 1 • Treat the underlying cause/contributors

There are several factors to consider and each one should be evaluated and addressed, preferably with the help of a nutritional therapist or an integrated medical doctor. They include:

- **Helicobacter pylori** This common bacteria is known to decrease the stomach's production of protective mucus and increase pH in the stomach, both of which can contribute to chronic indigestion, gastritis and ulceration.

- **Excess alcohol** Either eliminate alcohol altogether or limit to one or two drinks a week.

- **Non-steroidal anti-inflammatory drugs (NSAIDs)/steroids** Reduce or stop if possible (discuss with your doctor before doing so).

- **Food allergies/intolerances** See solution 5, page 107.

- **Diet high in processed foods** and low in whole foods. See Barrier 1.

- **High intake of animal protein** Limit your intake of red meat to once or twice a week.

- **Chronic stress** See Barrier 9.

- **Environmental chemicals and pollutants** See Barrier 4.

- **Zinc deficiency** The production of stomach acid is reliant on zinc, a deficiency of which can lead to low stomach-acid levels. Supplement with 30mg of zinc picolinate a day.

Step 2 • Take betaine hydrochloride

Betaine hydrochloride, from beetroot, is essentially stomach acid, and is one of the most immediate ways to resolve the symptoms associated with low stomach acid. Start by taking one capsule with your main meal. If this doesn't aggravate your symptoms, at every subsequent main meal take one more capsule. Continue to increase the dose until you reach either five tablets or you experience warmth in your stomach. Warmth indicates that the dose is slightly too high, and that you need to reduce the dose by one tablet. This is the dose that you should now be taking for large main meals. For smaller meals take less.

If you start following the advice above, your own stomach-acid production will kick in, you will notice the warm feeling again, and you should continue to reduce the dose to zero. This might take a couple of weeks. If you have, or suspect that you might have, ulcers or your symptoms get worse in any way, do not do this test.

2. Low digestive-enzyme levels

In conjunction with stomach acid the body produces a variety of digestive enzymes to help break down large complex food molecules into smaller, absorbable particles. The types of digestive enzymes produced depends on how far down the digestive tract food is. For example, the salivary glands produce ptyalin to break down carbohydrate, the stomach produces pepsin to break down protein, and the pancreas (the main digestive enzyme-secreting gland) produces a variety of enzymes to break down fat, protein and carbohydrate. Food allergies and nutrient deficiency-related diseases are strongly related to low levels of digestive enzymes.[11]

How to assess your digestive-enzyme levels

Take the digestive-enzyme questionnaire

The following symptoms are associated with having an insufficient or low amount of digestive enzymes:

QUESTIONNAIRE: digestive enzymes

For each question score 0 for no; 1 for occasionally; 3 for yes, then total up the section.

Do you:

1. Get abdominal bloating or swelling?

▶

2. Experience abdominal discomfort or pain? ☐

3. Get indigestion? ☐

4. Experience wind after meals? ☐

5. Have undigested food in your stools? ☐

6. Have any skin problems? ☐

Total score ☐

A score of 5 or more suggests that low digestive-enzyme levels might be contributing to your symptoms.

How to treat low levels of digestive enzymes

Step 1 • Treat the underlying cause/contributors

There are several factors to consider and each one should be evaluated and addressed, preferably with the help of a nutritional therapist or an integrated medical doctor. They include:

- **Overeating** Over a period of time this can put too much strain on the body. Reduce your portion size.

- **Excessive amounts of cooked foods** Increase your intake of enzyme-rich raw vegetables and fruits.

- **Failing to chew properly** Chewing helps to break food down into smaller pieces, it stimulates the release of amylase enzyme from the salivary glands, plus it activates the enzymes that are present in your food. Get into the routine of chewing your food at least ten times before swallowing.

- **Vitamin and mineral deficiency** Enzymes require adequate levels of various vitamins and minerals. Take a multivitamin–mineral. See Barrier 1.

Step 2 • Take a digestive-enzyme supplement

Digestive-enzyme supplements can cause an almost immediate improvement in symptoms. Most enzyme formulas contain amylase, lipase and protease, and possibly others such as glutenase (to break down gluten), lactase (to break down lactose) and amylo-glucosidase (to digest wind-causing compounds in certain vegetables). If you are not a vegetarian, the best enzyme supplement to take is one that contains pancreatin, an enzyme supplement derived from the pancreas of cow or pig. It might not sound appealing, but it works exceptionally well. If you are vegetarian, stick to a plant-based enzyme formula, such as Nutri's Similase. Digestive-enzyme supplements are best taken just before food and probably for no longer than a period of four to eight weeks. If you have food allergies, you might need to take them for longer.

3. Leaky-gut syndrome

The lining of your gut is a semi-permeable membrane across which it selectively uptakes properly digested fats, proteins and carbohydrates. However, in leaky-gut syndrome, the spaces in between the cells that line the intestines become irritated, inflamed, and, as the name suggests, leaky. These normally tight junctions allow larger molecules, such as bacteria, toxins and partially digested food to pass through into the blood; the body reacts to them as foreign invaders, and the immune system becomes activated, leading to widespread inflammation and a worsening of other digestive problems, such as irritable bowel syndrome. The following conditions are associated with leaky-gut syndrome: any autoimmune disease, Crohn's disease, acne, hives, allergies, autism, depression, constipation, diarrhoea, inflammatory bowel disease, skin problems such as eczema and psoriasis, rheumatoid arthritis and irritable bowel syndrome.[12]

How to assess leaky-gut syndrome

Arrange a gut permeability test

This is not essential, as so many people have leaky gut, and would therefore be better off using the money they would pay for the test to spend on supplements instead. However, if you do want to get tested you can request your nutritional therapist to arrange a gut permeability test. This involves drinking a solution containing small and large molecules and then collecting your urine for a 24-hour period. If the integrity of the gut wall is intact it should contain only the small molecules.

Take the leaky-gut questionnaire

The following symptoms are associated with having a leaky gut:

QUESTIONNAIRE: leaky gut

For each question score 0 for no; 1 for occasionally; 3 for yes, then total up the section.

Do you:

1. Have any food allergies or intolerances?

2. Drink alcohol on more than three days a week?

3. Have you taken NSAIDS or steroids for more than a week?

4. Experience any digestive problems such as wind, indigestion, bloating or irregular bowels?

5. Experience mood swings, anxiety, fuzzy or foggy thinking and/or poor memory?

6. Have recurrent infections?

►

7. Experience tiredness, fatigue and/or muscle aches and joint pains? ☐

8. Have any skin problems? ☐

Total score ☐

A score of 5 or more suggests that leaky gut syndrome might be contributing to your symptoms.

How to treat leaky-gut syndrome

Step 1 • Treat the underlying cause/contributors

There are a lot of factors to consider and each one should be evaluated and addressed, preferably with the help of a nutritional therapist or an integrated medical doctor. They include:

- **Impaired gut immunity** IgA is a specific type of antibody made in the gut in response to the presence of potential invaders. IgA levels can be boosted with the use of the supplement n-acetyl glucosamine and a probiotic (see the section on dysbiosis, page 103).

- **Intestinal infections** Yeast, candida and parasites. See Barrier 7.

- **Excess alcohol** Either eliminate alcohol altogether or limit to one or two drinks a week.

- **NSAIDS/steroids** Reduce or stop if possible (discuss with your doctor before doing so).

- **Food allergies/intolerances** See gut imbalance 5 for solutions.

- **Dysbiosis** See gut imbalance 4 for solutions.

- **Lack of stomach acid and/or digestive enzymes** See gut imbalance 1 and 2 for solutions.

- **Diet high in processed foods** and low in natural whole foods. See Barrier 1.

- **Chronic stress** This depletes IgA levels, plus affects stomach-acid and digestive-enzyme levels. See Barrier 9.

- **Environmental chemicals and pollutants** See Barrier 4.

- **Nutritional deficiencies** See Barrier 1.

Step 2 • Repair the damage

The following supplements are recommended to help repair and regenerate the lining of the digestive system:

- **Glutamine** is the primary fuel and source of nourishment for the lining of the digestive system. Take 1–5g one to three times a day.

- **Butyric acid** feeds the cells of the intestinal lining and is essential in maintaining the integrity of the gastrointestinal wall. Take 1,200mg a day.

- **Zinc** is required to help maintain the natural defences of the intestinal mucosal barrier and for tissue repair. Take 30mg a day.

- **Probiotics** such as acidophilus and bifidobacteria will also help to maintain a high level of gut health (see dysbiosis below for more information).

4. Dysbiosis

Our guts are teeming with microscopic bacteria – over a hundred trillion to be precise. When our immune system is strong and gut function intact, we live in harmony with these bacteria. We provide food, water and shelter and they in turn repay us by helping to develop and mature the immune system, manufacturing vitamins, keeping disease-promoting bacteria in check, aiding recovery from infections, repairing and promoting the health of the digestive tract and helping to reduce the severity of inflammatory conditions. When things are balanced and calm all is well. However, if our immune system weakens, because of stress or toxicity, or our gut function deteriorates because of mineral, stomach-acid and/ or digestive-enzyme deficiencies or we expose ourselves to steroids,

NSAIDS or antibiotics, the situation reverses. Disease-promoting bacteria, such as E.coli and Klebsiella, and other microbes such as candida and parasites take hold and start to produce toxins, which interfere with the normal functioning of the digestive tract. This state of imbalance is called dysbiosis and is believed to be an underlying factor in many diseases, including rheumatoid arthritis, irritable bowel syndrome, ankylosing spondylitis and inflammatory bowel disease.[13]

How to assess if you have dysbiosis

Arrange a comprehensive digestive stool analysis test (CDSA)

Like the test for leaky gut syndrome this one is not essential, but if you do want to go ahead with it I'd recommend doing it under the supervision of a nutritional therapist. You provide a sample of your stool and the CDSA test will tell you how well you are digesting and absorbing your food, whether you have blood in your stool, which bacteria and yeasts are in there and how your intestinal immune function is doing. It will also identify which antibiotic and antifungal preparations (whether herbal or drug) that micro-organism is sensitive to.

Take the dysbiosis questionnaire

The following symptoms are associated with having dysbiosis:

QUESTIONNAIRE: dysbiosis

For each question score 0 for no; 1 for occasionally; 3 for yes, then total up the section.

Do you:

1. Have any food allergies or intolerances?

▶

2. Have constipation or diarrhoea? ☐

3. Experience indigestion? ☐

4. Experience any digestive problems such as
wind, indigestion, bloating, or irregular bowels? ☐

5. Have or suspect that you have candida and/or
parasites? ☐

6. Feel tired and fatigued? ☐

7. Consider yourself to be stressed? ☐

8. Have bad breath? ☐

Total score ☐

A score of 5 or more suggests that dysbiosis might be contributing to your symptoms.

How to treat dysbiosis

Step 1 • Treat the underlying cause

The main causes to identify and treat are:

- **Lack of health-promoting bacteria** Take a probiotic supplement (see page 106).

- **Lack of stomach acid or digestive enzymes** leads to undigested food fermenting in the gut. See gut imbalance 1 and 2 for solutions.

- **Environmental chemicals and pollutants** See Barrier 4.

- **Constipation** Increase your fluid intake, add linseeds to your diet and take aloe vera.

- **Candida and parasites** See Barrier 7.

- **Diet high in animal protein and sugar** See Barrier 1.

- **Psychological stress** See Barrier 9.

- **Antibiotics** kill good and bad gut bacteria, therefore use only when necessary and take a probiotic for six months afterwards.

Step 2 • Repopulate your bowel with probiotics

Probiotics (meaning 'for life') refers to over 400 strains of bacteria that naturally reside in our intestines and collectively help to encourage a healthy digestive balance. They manufacture vitamins, boost immunity, aid recovery from infections, repair and promote the health of the digestive tract and help to reduce the severity of inflammatory conditions. Fermented products, such as live yogurt, miso and sauerkraut, and probiotic supplements, are highly effective in restoring balance and harmony to the digestive tract. The most important probiotic strains are lactobacillus acidophilus and bifidobacterium bifidum.

Some of their many benefits include inhibiting the growth of harmful bacteria, promoting healthy digestion and nutrient absorption, easing the symptoms of irritable bowel syndrome, enhancing immune function, and increasing the body's resistance to infection. Probiotic bacteria also produce substances called bacteriocins, or antibiotic-like substances, which are powerful enough to neutralise Escherichia coli bacteria, some strains of which are linked to diarrhoea and various infections. Probiotics need to be taken for at least six months in order to repopulate the bowels effectively.

Step 3 • Supply your bowel with prebiotics

The good intestinal bacteria such as lactobacillus and bifidobacteria feed on short-chain carbohydrates called fructo-oligosaccharides (FOS). FOS has been shown to help ease constipation and inhibit the attachment of disease-promoting bacteria and parasites to the bowel wall. The recommended dose is 1g a day. Foods high in FOS include bananas, onions and asparagus.

5. Food allergies and intolerances

Food allergies and intolerances are thought to affect 40 per cent of the general population, and an even higher percentage of people who have digestive problems.[14] However, these figures are hotly disputed, with nutritional therapists tending to believe that food allergies and intolerances are very common, and dieticians believing the contrary.

What are food allergies and intolerances?

Allergies generally fall into five different types. Of those, types 1 and 3 are involved in creating the symptoms associated with food allergies. A food allergy refers to an immune-system response to one or more proteins within a specific food. The classic true allergy is type 1, or immediate-onset, allergy. In this case a food substance such as peanut or prawn triggers an immediate release of histamine and other inflammatory chemicals from a group of antibodies called IgE. These give rise to symptoms including an itchy red rash, shortness of breath, and wheezing and swelling of the lips, mouth and throat, as well as stomach cramps, vomiting and diarrhoea. The reactions can be severe and life threatening.

More commonly, and possibly accounting for 80 per cent of food allergies, are type 3, or delayed-onset, allergies. These are also referred to as intolerances. Involving another type of antibody called IgG, the symptoms, which include facial puffiness, tiredness, intestinal cramps, bloating and food cravings, occur anywhere between two hours and two days after ingestion. Over 100 different diseases ranging from depression and fatigue to inflammatory bowel disease and eczema have been linked to IgG food allergies.

Why do food allergies and intolerances come about?

Different people will have different reasons why they suffer from food allergies. Some allergies will be related to the presence of candida and parasites, others to medications, alcohol and processed foods or alcohol, and others to stress, toxicity and lack of stomach acid or digestive enzyme. I had two particularly interesting patients whose allergies had their origins in traumatic events. In both cases they had unconsciously associated food that coincidentally was present in the room when the trauma happened. Every time they subsequently ingested that food, the emotion of the trauma triggered an allergic response. By using one of the emotional releasing techniques I talk about later on, both were able to completely heal themselves of their allergies. However this is rare – in the case of IgG-type related food allergies, it is believed that the majority come about because of undigested food particles finding there way into the bloodstream via a leaky gut. The immune system mounts an offensive, and this leads to many of the allergy symptoms mentioned previously.

The most common food allergies and intolerances

You can be allergic to almost anything, but the most common allergies are to cow's milk and cheese, wheat, gluten (found in oats, wheat, rye and barley), corn, beef, yeast, eggs, garlic, nuts, kiwi fruit and soya.

How to assess if you have food allergies / intolerances

Because food allergies are complex processes there is no one test that can give you a definitive answer as to whether your health and body are being affected by food allergies. My advice is to start by filling in the questionnaire below, and if that is positive then you can move on to blood testing. Some practitioners recommend the elimination diet as an alternative to blood testing. In this diet you remove all suspected foods from your diet for 14 days, and then reintroduce them every third day while watching out for reactions. Whereas there is no doubt that this approach can work, the considerable majority of people find it too laborious and difficult to use.

QUESTIONNAIRE: food allergies/intolerances

For each question score 0 for no; 1 for occasionally; 3 for yes, then total up the section.

Do you:

1. Suffer from eczema or itchy rashes? ☐

2. Experience excess mucus or catarrh formation in the throat, nose or sinuses? ☐

3. Have cravings for certain foods such as chocolate, cheese or doughy foods? ☐

4. Experience irritable bowel syndrome? ☐

5. Suffer from migraines or regular headaches? ☐

6. Have recurrent, unexplained symptoms? ☐

7. Have fluid retention? ☐

8. Have dark circles under your eyes and/or facial puffiness? ☐

9. Feel lethargic soon after eating? ☐

10. Did you have problems such as colic, glue ear, ear infections, eczema or asthma as a child? ☐

Total score ☐

A score of 8 or more suggests that you might have a food intolerance. You should either consult with a nutritional therapist or consider purchasing one of the two following blood tests.

IgG Elisa blood test

As the name suggests this blood test measures levels of IgG antibodies to various different foods. This is helpful to know because about 80 per cent of food allergies are mediated by IgG. See Resources, page 418, for testing laboratories. All they need from you is a small sample of blood, which you can collect yourself in the comfort of your own home. They will then analyse it and tell you which foods you are reacting to. Once you have your results back, you should avoid the allergy-provoking foods for at least three months, after which most can be reintroduced on a rotation basis.

Food Allergen Cellular Test (FACT)

This test measures levels of the inflammatory chemicals released from white blood cells when exposed to various food allergens. The nice thing with this test is that it will pick up IgG and IgA immune responses and other non-immune responses. This makes it the allergy test of choice. The only downside, apart from cost, is that you will need to have blood taken from you in order to have the test done. For more information contact the Individual Wellbeing Diagnostic Laboratories (see Resources, page 418).

What next?

Once you know which foods you are allergic to, the usual recommendation would be to avoid them strictly for at least three months and then, with the exception of wheat and cow's dairy, you can reintroduce them into your diet, but taking care not to eat a food group (for example, wheat) more frequently than every fourth day. While there's no doubt this process helps, the total-health approach goes one step further by addressing the underlying causes and contributors.

How to treat your food allergies or intolerances

Step 1 • Treat the underlying cause

The main causes to identify and treat are:

- **Leaky-gut syndrome** See gut imbalance 3 for solutions.

- **Lack of stomach acid or digestive enzymes** See gut imbalance 1 and 2 for solutions.

- **Environmental chemicals and pollutants** See Barrier 4.

- **Candida and parasites** See gut imbalances 6 and 7 for solutions.

- **Psychological stress** See Barrier 9.

- **Dysbiosis** See gut imbalance 4 for solutions.

Step 2 • Keep to a healthy diet

Slowing down while eating, chewing well, eating smaller portions and sitting down to eat while relaxed, all help to reduce stress on your digestive tract, as does limiting alcohol, caffeine and processed foods. Eating regular meals, increasing your intake of whole grains, fruit and vegetables (as long as you are not allergic to them) will all help, as does drinking a minimum of 1–2 litres (1¾–3½ pints) of filtered water a day. For more information on healthy eating see Barrier 1.

Step 3 • Choose healthy alternatives

Here are some alternatives to the main food allergens:

- **Instead of cow's dairy produce**, try goat's milk, sheep's milk, organic whole soya milk, almond milk, rice milk, quinoa milk.

- **Instead of wheat**, try rye, barley, oatcakes, quinoa, buckwheat, millet.

- **To avoid gluten**, try rice, quinoa, buckwheat, millet, corn, potato flour, sago, tapioca.

If you have an intolerance, for example to lactose, you might find that you can drink one glass of milk a day, however more than one glass might trigger symptoms. The key is to learn what your threshold is and to not go over it.

The following cookbooks have some good meal suggestions:

- *Healthy Gluten-free Eating: The Ultimate Wheat-free Recipe Book* by Darina Allen

- *The Everything Gluten-free Cookbook: 300 Appetizing Recipes Tailored to Your Needs!* by Rick Marx and Nancy T. Maar

Step 4 • Reduce inflammation in your body

One of the ways food-allergy symptoms come about is through the release of inflammation-promoting chemicals called prostaglandins. A diet high in saturated fat, trans-fatty acids and omega-6 fats all increase the likelihood of this happening, while a diet rich in omega-3 fatty acids reduces it by promoting the secretion of anti-inflammatory chemicals. Taking omega-3-rich sources such as fish oil, and/or using organic flax seed oil or organic essential-balance oil will be enough to reduce inflammation. If you are suffering from an inflammatory related condition such as arthritis, joint pain, eczema or asthma, try adding DLPA Complex from Higher Nature. It contains three natural and effective anti-inflammatory and pain-killing supplements: bromelain, astaxanthin and the amino acid DLPA.

Step 5 • If you are experiencing symptoms of food intolerance

Try an Alka-Seltzer or a glass of water with one teaspoon of alkaline salts. Both can help reduce some of the symptoms. Type 1 (true allergies) are life threatening and require adrenaline and medical support.

6 and 7. Candida and parasite infections

These are covered separately in Barrier 7.

8. Incompatible food combinations

Dr Hay's food combining theory is one of the most hotly debated approaches in the field of nutrition. Some people regard it as scientifically unfounded, others swear by it. In my own clinical practice I rarely refer to it, however, I know people who have followed the principles and experienced a considerable improvement in their symptoms. For this reason I am going to include it, and I will leave you to come to your own conclusions.

The basic premise of food combining is that the three different food groups – proteins, fats and carbohydrates – all require different conditions for digestion. Protein, for example, requires the highly acidic environment of the stomach, whereas carbohydrates require the alkaline environment of the mouth and small intestine. What Dr Hay observed, and many others confirmed subsequently, is that protein-rich foods such as meat, eaten at the same time as carbohydrate-rich foods such as potato, put a considerable strain on the digestive system, because of their completely contrasting requirements for digestion. When we are young this combination rarely causes a problem; however, as we age and the efficiency of our digestive system decreases, this combination can lead to digestive imbalance and incomplete digestion of food. The latter is, as we have now learnt, a significant contributor to food allergies. Based on this observation and numerous others, a set of food-combining rules have been formulated. My own advice is to try these out if you do suffer from digestive upset, and see how you get on. The key elements in Dr Hay's original theory, expounded in the 1930s, was to eat 'alkaline-forming foods', eat fruit on its own, avoid refined and heavily processed foods, and don't mix protein-rich and carbohydrate-rich foods. The rules don't need to be followed strictly unless you suffer from moderate to severe digestive problems. They are as follows.

1. Eat fermenting fruits (such as strawberries, peaches, plums, melons and mangoes) and acidic fruits (such as oranges, pineapple and grapefruit) in between meals, as a snack. Fruits that don't ferment readily, such as apples, bananas and pears can be mixed with complex carbohydrate-rich foods such as oats.

2. Eat melons alone as they don't combine well with any other food.

3. Eat one protein-type per meal, for example avoid eating meat with cheese or fish.

4. Eat protein-rich foods such as meat, fish, cheese and eggs either by themselves or with non-starchy vegetables, such as asparagus, green beans, green peas, broccoli, peppers, Brussels sprouts, cabbage,

celery, cucumber, aubergine, spinach, mushrooms, carrots and cauliflower.

5. Eat mainly alkaline-forming foods such as fruits and vegetables.

Now that you have reached the end of this chapter, my advice is to re-read it one more time. While doing so highlight those sentences (using a highlighter pen) that you feel are important to you. Once you've done this write down at least five steps or actions that you are going to take, and spend a moment visualising yourself implementing them. Once you have completed this, move on to your next barrier.

MIND–BODY ESSENTIALS

- To benefit from the foods we eat and the supplements we take we need to be able to absorb them effectively.

- Numerous research studies have linked problems of the digestive system to serious health problems both of the body and mind. The health and function of the gut is intimately linked to our emotional state. Stress, psychological trauma and emotional upset can all influence the gut. Indeed, these can sometimes be the underlying cause of gut problems. Addressing these issues is an important part of recovering good gut health.

- Eating a nutrient-dense, wholefood diet, minimising the use of processed foods, caffeine, alcohol, antibiotics and NSAIDS, and managing your stress, are the foundations of good digestive health.

- Recommended mind–body tools to accompany this chapter: emotional freedom technique (page 332), focusing (page 356), creative visualisation (page 319), symptom dialogue (page 391), meditation (page 376), conscious breathing (page 314) and relaxation (page 380).

- For recommended reading see Resources, page 426.

Toxicity

Sarah described herself as being 'allergic to the world'. She had seen six different doctors over a ten-year period as she desperately struggled to understand and find a treatment for her hypersensitivity to chemicals. Just one whiff of perfume would leave her eyes streaming, her heart pounding and her head thumping. Her mood would turn dark almost instantly. In fact, this was so bad she described herself as being 'a bit of a Jekyll and Hyde'. She felt like a completely different person, just because of some chemical in her environment. So what was going on?

Sarah was suffering from multiple chemical sensitivity (MCS), a condition in which an already toxic body struggles to cope with chemicals in the environment. If we pour water into a container that is already full, the water naturally spills out. Well, this is what happens in someone with MCS. Their body's ability to detoxify and cope with toxins is so stretched that the slightest exposure to chemicals – such as perfumes, cosmetics, petrol, food additives and cleaning agents – overloads their bodies and spills out as these incapacitating symptoms. It is not uncommon to find that people with MCS seek refuge in a near-sterile environment. It really is a debilitating and isolating disease.

Of course, this is an extreme example, but it does bring into sharp focus the influence that our environment can have on our health and quality of life. Toxins can also have a very powerful effect on our mood. This is important to bear in mind. I have had at least six patients with depression that was mainly related to mercury toxicity, and at least 30 others whose energy levels and general mood were negatively affected by toxins in their diet and environment. If you have identified toxicity as one of your barriers and are experiencing problems with your mood, memory or ability to concentrate, I would strongly encourage you to follow the recommendations that I make. My belief, which is shared by some other open-minded practitioners, is that toxicity represents one of the greatest and most significant health challenges, not only to ourselves but also to future generations.

Our toxic world

The air we breathe, the food we eat, the water we drink, the cosmetics we use, the products we clean with, the clothes we wear, and the places in which we live and work drip-feed toxins into our bodies, but because their effects on our health can be delayed for years or be extremely subtle, hardly anyone knows it's happening. Although it is absolutely imperative that we eat more nutritious food, exercise more and take care of our emotional needs, to my mind all of us need to wake up to the slow poisoning that is going on, especially in those that are most vulnerable – our children.

What is toxicity?

When I use the word 'toxicity' I am mainly referring to chemicals that originate from our environment that interfere with the healthy functioning of the body. Most of this chapter is dedicated to these. However, in the broadest and most holistic sense, toxicity can also come about from:

- **Heavy metals** from amalgam fillings, vaccines, antiperspirants, cigarette smoke, paint, copper and lead pipes, and food packaging.

- **Household chemicals** from household cleaners, air fresheners, disinfectants, drain cleaner, furniture polish, wax, paints, personal-care products such as bleaches, dyes, scents and hairsprays.

- **Building materials and products** Adhesives, carpeting, upholstery, manufactured wood products, photocopy machines, pesticides and cleaning agents may emit volatile organic compounds (VOCs), including formaldehyde.

- **Medications** The side effects from medicines and prescribed drugs.

- **Environmental toxins** Pollution from the air we breathe, the food we eat (pesticides, colourings, additives) and the water we drink.

- **Electromagnetic toxins** from PCs, lighting, televisions, freezers, Wi-Fi, pylons and microwaves.

- **Industrial toxins** from the outputs of large industrial plants.

- **Bacteria, fungus moulds, yeasts and parasites** from our food and water supply and body acidification.

- **Intestinal toxins** from gut dysbiosis.

- **Internally generated toxins** from the body's own metabolic processes; the amount produced increases considerably in the presence of nutritional deficiencies.

As you can see, this is a massive subject, so I'm going to keep focused mainly on the influence of toxic chemicals on the body, as the evidence is most abundant here.

How much of a problem is toxicity?

Over a 70-year period between 1930 and 2000, global production of man-made chemicals increased from 1 million to 400 million tons each year.[1] Little is known about the toxicity of most of these chemicals. An estimated 70,000 synthetic chemicals are in everyday use. Most chemicals have never been assessed for their effect on health or the environment. [2]

There is evidence linking chemical toxicity to a wide range of conditions, including autism, attention deficit hyperactivity disorder, chronic fatigue syndrome, multiple chemical sensitivities, multiple sclerosis, memory loss, childhood cancers, premature puberty, low sperm counts, testicular cancer, breast cancer, undescended testicles, multiple myeloma, non-Hodgkin's lymphoma, infertility, birth defects, asthma and learning disabilities.[3]

A report published in 1996 by the environmental think-tank World Resources Institute, found a considerable amount of evidence to suggest that pesticides are suppressing the immune responses to bacteria, viruses, parasites and tumours, making millions of people significantly more vulnerable to disease.[4] Additionally, the World Health Organization (1992) reports that roughly three million pesticide poisonings occur annually and result in 220,000 deaths worldwide.[5]

A report based on tests of ten samples of umbilical cord blood found an average of 287 contaminants in the blood, including mercury, fire retardants, pesticides and the Teflon chemical PFOA. Of the 287 chemicals detected, 180 cause cancer in humans or animals, 217 are toxic to the brain and nervous system, and 208 cause birth defects or abnormal development in animal tests. The dangers of pre- or post-natal exposure to this complex mixture of carcinogens, developmental toxins and neurotoxins have never been studied.[6]

Another study led by Mount Sinai School of Medicine in New York, in collaboration with the Environmental Working Group and Commonweal, found an average of 91 industrial compounds, pollutants and other chemicals in the blood and urine of nine volunteers, with a total of 167 chemicals found in the group. Of the 167 chemicals found, 76 cause cancer in humans or animals, 94 are toxic to the brain and nervous system, and 79 cause birth defects or abnormal development.[7]

How the body deals with toxins

Our body is designed to detoxify toxins, and, given the extraordinary amounts of natural and man-made toxins we expose ourselves to every day, it does a pretty excellent job. At the heart of the body's detoxification system, is the liver. It filters bacteria and immune complexes out of the blood and either converts toxins into water-soluble products that can be removed via the kidneys or enzymatically breaks them down into parts that no longer pose a threat to the well-being of the body. Other important contributors to the detox process include the intestines, which remove toxins from the bowel, kidneys, which remove water-soluble toxins, and skin, which removes fat-soluble toxins.

How toxins cause disease

Whether a toxin or combination of toxins causes problems within your body depends on a lot of different things, including the toxicity of the toxin, the amount, and the presence and combination of other toxins. In addition to these, factors relating to your own body play a very big role. They include:

Impaired detoxification

The ability of any given toxin to cause health problems is closely related to the efficiency and effectiveness of the body detoxification systems, particularly the liver. For example one Italian study tested the liver detoxification enzyme activity of a group of chemical plant workers among whom there was an excessively high rate of bladder cancer.[8] The researchers found a direct correlation between those that developed bladder cancer and those with a less efficient detoxification system. So, despite the workers being exposed to pretty much the same levels of chemicals, it was those with impaired liver detoxification who went on to develop cancer.

Nutritional imbalances

Nutritional deficiencies predispose an individual to disease in the presence of certain toxins.[9] For example:

- **Magnesium** deficiency increases the toxicity of some drugs.

- **Selenium** can protect the body against the toxic effects of mercury.

- **Calcium** can protect the body against the toxic effects of aluminium and lead.

- **Vitamin C** can protect the body against the toxic effects of cadmium, lead and arsenic.

- **Zinc** can protect the body against the toxic effects of lead and cadmium.

- **Antioxidants** can help reduce the inflammation and damage caused by the release of toxins in the body.

Epigenetic inheritance

Chemicals in the bodies of your parents, grandparents and even great-grandparents might be affecting your health now, through a phenomenon called epigenetic inheritance.[10] Epigenetic inheritance refers to the passing down of biological information from one generation to the next that is not encoded in the DNA but attached to the DNA. These epigenetic changes influence the way DNA works. For example, one study found that environmental toxins can reprogramme the activity of animals' genes in a way that can be passed down at least four generations.[11] A group of pregnant rats were exposed to a combination of pesticides and insecticides – two synthetic chemicals that are known to interfere with the normal functioning of reproductive hormones. The male rats that were born had low sperm counts and fertility, but despite this were still able to mate with females. Their male offspring also had low sperm counts, and the cycle continued, with more than 90 per cent of each male offspring in subsequent generations being affected. One of the interesting findings from this experiment was the fact that a low sperm count didn't come about from an alteration to the sequence of the DNA (which is what happens with most genetically inheritable conditions), but from an alteration in the chemicals attached to DNA – it is this that changes the way genes work. The researchers proposed that this epigenetic inheritance might be one of the mechanisms that are responsible for the considerable increase in diseases such as breast and prostate cancer and infertility.

Genetic inheritance

Our genes play a big part in determining how effectively our bodies respond to toxins, in fact so much so that the rate at which toxins are inactivated by the liver might vary by as much as fivefold, and that's among healthy individuals.[12] This goes some way to explain why two people might be exposed to a similar load of toxins but be affected very differently. Fortunately, just because someone has a inherited tendency to, say, slow detoxification, it doesn't mean that they are stuck with it; adequate nutritional supplementation and lifestyle change, as we are about to find out, can correct it to a degree.

What is the solution?

Whereas it isn't possible to completely avoid all toxins (and neither for most people is it necessary), you can make some simple adjustments to your lifestyle and environment that will considerably reduce the degree to which you are affected. In addition to this we can all support our body's attempts to get rid of toxins and restore balance. The approach I use with my patients is very straightforward and I have provided an outline of it here. It involves two steps that are used alongside one another. If you are, however, experiencing severe symptoms, or you are unsure as what is causing your health challenge I would encourage you to seek the help of an integrated medical doctor specialising in environmental medicine or a nutritional therapist.

Step 1 • Reduce your toxin load

Clean up your diet

Hydrogenated and trans-fatty acids, aspartame, artificial colours, flavourings and preservatives can be a source of stress on the body. Most non-organic foods are contaminated with pesticides, and most tap water with chemicals, hormones and residues of various medications, so wherever possible go for organic food and filtered water. (See Barrier 1 for more information.)

Remove allergens

In the digestive health imbalance section (Barrier 3) we explored how food allergies and intolerances can be a significant source of stress to the body, with the most common being to dairy, wheat, soya, corn and eggs. If you suspect that you might have a food allergy, my advice would be to arrange for an IgG or FACT blood test and then exclude those foods that test positive for at least three months.

Balance your gut

Intestinal dysbiosis – an imbalance between the health-promoting and disease-promoting bacteria in your gut – encourages candida, parasites and other microbes to produce toxins, many of which are linked to certain diseases. (See Barriers 3 and 7 (pages 89 and 180) for more information.)

Reduce your exposure to air pollution

Air pollution can be a serious contributor to ill health, particularly if you are susceptible (for example, if you are elderly or you have a chronic disease), and/or you live next to a busy road, or in the city, or near to a power plant or chemical factory. Air pollution is composed of many environmental factors, which include carbon monoxide, nitrates, sulphur dioxide, ozone, lead, second-hand tobacco smoke and particulate matter. Particulate matter (also known as particle pollution) is composed of solid and liquid particles within the air, and is a significant contributor to inflammation, heart disease and even death rates. The Environmental Protection Agency (EPA) has declared that 'tens of thousands of people die each year from breathing tiny particles in the environment'.[13] A report released by the Health Effects Institute and published in *Science* magazine shows that death rates in the 90 largest US cities rose by 0.5 per cent with only a tiny increase in particles less than 10 micrometers in diameter.[14] If you are at risk or concerned about air pollution – here's my advice:

- **Avoid smoky environments** Research has established that exposure to the second-hand smoke of just one cigarette per day accelerates the progression of atherosclerosis – one of the main contributors to heart disease.[15]

- **Open your windows** Some research suggests indoor pollution is much more of a problem than outdoor pollution. Keeping your windows open helps air to circulate.

- **Purchase a couple of plants that are known to purify the air** They include English ivy, philodendrons, potted chrysanthemums, spider plants, aloe vera and Chinese evergreen.

- **Avoid artificial air fresheners**, use natural essential oils or toxic-free products instead.

- **A negative air ioniser device** generates millions of negatively charged particles, which may help to improve quality of sleep, reduce severity of migraines and allergies, and ease asthma symptoms (see Resources, page 424).

Reduce your exposure to electro-pollution

One of the unseen threats to our health is that posed by electro-magnetic pollution. Our bodies are being bombarded with EMFs (electromagnetic frequencies) and ELFs (extremely low frequencies) from numerous different sources, such as computers, telephones, mobile phones, power lines, cellphone relays, transformers, radios, radio transmitters, televisions and microwave ovens. Whereas there is to my knowledge no absolute proof that these cause specific diseases, there is emerging evidence that they are a source of strain on the body, and mobile phones, for example, when used frequently and for long periods of time, can modify and damage certain structures in the brain.[16] There is at present very little evidence available to guide us on what a safe level of exposure consists of and even less evidence on the long-term effects of electro-pollution. So, until we know more, the advice I give to my patients is to play safe by making some simple adjustments:

- Start by limiting your use of your mobile phone. Use a land line phone whenever possible, avoid placing your mobile on your belt or top pocket, turn it off when not required and keep it away from the side of your bed when sleeping at night-time.

- Stay a minimum of 46cm (18in) away from televisions and computer screens. Turn them off when not in use.

- Buy a cactus plant, *Cereus peruvianus*, which naturally restores an electromagnetically disturbed environment back to near normality.

- Move all electric clocks, clock radios, and telephone answering machines at least 1.2m (4ft) away from the head of the bed.

- Avoid using electric blankets, microwaves and blow hairdryers. Don't let your children play near power lines, transformers, radar domes or microwave towers.

- There is some preliminary evidence to suggest that devices such as Qlink can help to strengthen the body's own electromagnetic fields and help protect normal brain function in users of mobile phones (see Resources, page 424).

Swap your household cleaning products

One of the most common causes of poisoning in the UK is the ingestion or exposure to household cleaning products. Most household products are toxic – the skull and crossbones on the packaging gives it away! The majority have not been tested for combined or accumulated effects nor for their effects on unborn children. In a nutshell most standard household cleaning products are a potential hazard and source of chemical toxins. There are a lot of safer non-toxic alternatives that can be used instead (see Resources, page 424). If you do use conventional cleaning products make sure that they are stored in their original containers out of reach of children. Always follow the directions on the labels.

Go chlorine-free

Chlorine has been added to the water supply for a hundred years to kill bacteria. There's no doubt it works, but at what cost? There is an increasing amount of evidence linking chlorine and its by-products such as trihalomethanes (TTHMs) and haloacetic acids to health problems. These include increased risk of bladder and rectal cancer, and heart disease.[17] Using a water filter will remove chlorine, but it's important to remember to change the filter every so often! However, it's not just the water that we drink that we have to watch, we also take chlorine into our bodies from the inhalation of steam and via absorption through the skin when we shower. If you do shower regularly and want to reduce your exposure to chlorine you could consider purchasing a shower filter from Healthy House (see Resources, page 424).

Go fluoride-free

Fluoride is a known toxin, which has been added to the water supply (for about 10 per cent of the UK population) and toothpastes in order to help prevent tooth decay. Whereas fluoride in toothpastes can help reduce decay, there is accumulating evidence that fluoride in water does not prevent tooth decay, and in certain vulnerable groups, such as the elderly, children, people with deficiencies of magnesium and calcium, and people with heart or kidney disease, it can cause significant health problems. These include: increased risk of osteoporosis, dental fluorosis (damage to the enamel of the teeth), infertility, reduced IQ, increased risk of hip fractures and increased risk of osteosarcoma (bone cancer) in boys.[18] You can check whether your water supply is fluoridated by asking your water supplier. If it is, my advice would be to invest in a reverse osmosis water system – a system that removes fluoride as well as heavy metals, chlorine and other chemicals (see Resources, page 424). Please note that most conventional water filters do not remove fluoride. Other ways to reduce your intake of fluoride is to switch to fluoride-free toothpastes (the Aloe Dent and Kingfisher range are both good) and to limit your intake of processed cereals and fruit juices, some of which can have high fluoride levels.

Use non-toxic personal care products

Deodorants, tampons, moisturisers, lipstick, hair dye, nail polish, perfumes, shower gels are made from chemicals, many of which are known carcinogens, allergens and hormone disruptors.[19] Of particular concern is the evidence linking tampons with toxic shock syndrome, a potentially fatal infection of the blood caused by the toxin TSST-1 (see Resources, page 424).[20] Fortunately, there are an increasing number of companies specialising in non-toxic personal care products (see Resources, page 424).

Reduce your exposure to mercury

Amalgam fillings, which contain 50 per cent mercury by weight, and fish laden with mercury are thought to be responsible for the increase in mercury-related health problems seen by practitioners such as myself. Mercury toxicity has been linked to depression, autism, lupus, memory problems, behavioural problems, birth defects, kidney disease, immune suppression, Alzheimer's, chronic fatigue syndrome, infertility and allergies.[21] Another study found high blood levels of mercury in patients with Alzheimer's disease when compared with non-AD patients.[22]

If you have mercury fillings, and experience any long-term health problems, I would encourage you to consider having your analgam fillings removed. However, this should only be carried out by a dentist who follows the guidelines set out by the British Society for Mercury-Free Dentistry. If you go to www.mercuryfreedentistry.org.uk they have a list of such dentists. The reason this is important is because mercury can be released during the removal process and this can make the toxicity problem worse.[23] When offered a choice of replacement fillings, choose composite 'white' filling instead or, even better, fillings that are completely free from metals. You should also be on an appropriate detox programme at the same time (see Step 2).

All fish and seafood contain mercury; however, only those with the highest levels need to be avoided – these include swordfish, shark, king mackerel and tilefish. These are probably not on your regular menu anyway, but tuna might be. Tuna is also high in mercury, and the UK Food Standards Agency recommends that all women who are planning to become pregnant, or who are pregnant or breastfeeding, limit their intake of tuna to one fresh tuna steak or two medium-size cans per week.[24]

Another significant source of mercury used to be found in thimerosal, a common constituent of vaccines. If you choose to have your children vaccinated, always ask for information on the contents of the vaccine before proceeding.

Reduce your exposure to cadmium

Cadmium is a mineral whose levels are starting to increase within the general population due to contamination of our food and water supply. It's also found in cigarette smoke, and the air we breathe as an industrial pollutant. Excess cadmium levels, particularly when combined with low zinc levels, have been associated with depressed immune function, high blood pressure, bone and joint aches and pains, and kidney stones.[25] You can reduce your exposure to cadmium by minimising smoking and exposure to cigarette smoke, limiting your consumption of refined foods, shellfish, coffee, tea and soft water.

Reduce your exposure to lead

Lead is the most common toxic mineral, and believed to negatively impact the health of 20 per cent of men and 10 per cent of women. While lead pollution is less than what it used to be, mainly due to the introduction of lead-free petrol and the reduction of lead in paint, it still remains a considerable problem. Our intake of lead today comes from a variety of sources, including lead contamination of foods grown near industrial plants or roads, water from lead pipes, cosmetics, pesticides and the solder in tin cans. Chronic lead toxicity has been associated with hyperactivity and learning disorders in children, and general symptoms such as fatigue, muscle weakness, headaches, depression, memory loss and insomnia.[26] Symptoms are worse when combined with a deficiency of calcium, zinc and iron. You can reduce your exposure to lead by having your water tested (if you think you might have lead pipes), limiting your intake of foods from tin cans, not storing foods in pottery (because some glazes contain lead), and limiting your exposure to areas of high air pollution.

Avoid geopathic stress

Geopathic stress is a term used to describe a disruption or distortion in the Earth's natural electromagnetic field. Some researchers claim that this field is essential to our health, but when disturbed – due to natural geological faults, underground flowing water, mineral deposits, noxious sites and man-made excavations and construction – it becomes a strain on our immune system. Geopathic stress is increasingly being recognised as a contributory factor in serious chronic illness such as cancer, inflammatory arthritis, chronic fatigue syndrome and neuro-degenerative disease.[27] Its presence is apparently suggested by two or more of the following: an illness resistant to the appropriate healthcare treatment, an illness that improves when away from home for a prolonged period of time, an illness that starts or deteriorates shortly after moving house, a problem with mould in the house, growths of lichen and moss on the roofs, lawn and walls of the house, your cat prefers a particular spot on your bed or favourite seat (cats are attracted to geopathically stressed areas, dogs are repelled) and/or the presence of underground streams. Geopathic stress can be formally diagnosed with use of a geo-magnetometer or through dowsing.

Step 2 • Detox your body

This step really depends on which toxins are causing the problem. For example, if the toxic load is mainly due to yeasts, parasites or intestinal toxins, then treating them as outlined in Barrier 7 is the solution. However, as a rule of thumb, a general detoxification would involve:

- Healthy eating (Barrier 1)

- Alkalising your body (Barrier 2)

- Exercise (see page 350)

In addition to the above you could consider supporting your detoxification systems with supplements that are designed to improve the functioning of the liver and intestines. I would normally recommend taking these for a minimum of three months.

Liver

- **The herb milk thistle** is the most well-researched supplement for protecting the liver and supporting the production of new liver cells. Take 120mg of silymarin three times a day.

- **Artichoke and dandelion** both help to promote the flow and production of bile from the liver. Bile helps removes toxins from the liver. They work particularly well when combined with milk thistle.

Recommended products: Kiki Liver Rescue (contains all three), Higher Nature's Milk Thistle and Artichoke, or Health Direction Livatone Plus.

Intestines

- A lactobacillus probiotic will help to repopulate the bowels and support healthy bowel movements.

- Psyllium husk is a soluble fibre that is great for binding to toxins in the gut and helping them to be removed. In addition it also helps with constipation and diarrhoea, and can lower raised LDL cholesterol.

- Organic aloe vera is rich in amino acids, enzymes, vitamins and minerals and is my number-one favourite choice for people with digestive imbalance. It helps to cleanse the bowel and is good for constipation and removing bowel residues.

- If candida or parasites are a problem, look at Barrier 7.

Recommended products: Optima Maxicol (contains psyllium and probiotics), Higher Nature's organic aloe vera and Solgar psyllium seed husks powder.

Vitamin/mineral/antioxidant/EFA support

Our bodies need optimum levels of vitamins, minerals, antioxidants and essential fatty acids for many reasons, including: protecting our cells from the damaging free radicals that are created by toxins; enabling our detoxification systems to work effectively; and to repair damage. My advice is to start a high-potency supplement formula that provides your body with all of the vitamins, minerals and antioxidants and to take supplementary essential fatty acids (see Barrier 1 for further suggestions). If you are removing mercury from your body, make sure you take at least 200mcg of selenium a day and the amino-acid glutathione – this will help remove it.

Removal of heavy metals

If your body is experiencing heavy metal toxicity, or you think it is, my advice would be to work alongside an integrated medical doctor who has experience in heavy metal detoxification. Failing that, you could consider using a supplement called NDF (see Resources, page 424). To read more about it visit the website www.healthydetox.org.

NDF contains a combination of chlorella, coriander and non-dairy PolyFlor probiotics, all of which, individually and in combination, bind to toxic metals and help them to be removed from the body. The supplement comes with a full set of instructions, which will guide you through the dosages. If you are undergoing removal of amalgam fillings I would start this about seven days beforehand.

Now that you have reached the end of this chapter, my advice is to reread it one more time. While doing so highlight those sentences (using a highlighter pen) that you feel are important to you. Once you've done this write down at least five steps or actions that you are going to take, and spend a moment visualising yourself implementing them. Once you have completed this, move on to your next barrier.

MIND–BODY ESSENTIALS

- Toxicity from chemicals in your environment and within your body poses one of the greatest threats to your total health.

- All of us without exception have a cocktail of chemicals within our bodies. While it was once thought that the levels of these chemicals were too low to have a significant impact on our health, we now know that this is not true.

- If you have heavy metal toxicity or are going to have your mercury amalgam fillings removed, work with a healthcare professional.

- Recommended mind–body tools to accompany this chapter: exercise (page 350) and creative visualisation (page 319).

- For recommended reading see Resources, page 426.

Chronic inflammation

Gloria was an angry and stressed woman – her words not mine! She had experienced some strange and bizarre symptoms for a period of six months and was fed up because no one could put a finger on what was happening. She had joint aches and pains that came and went; eczema that flared up for a couple of days then disappeared. And all of her tests had come back negative, apart from one called CRP. This test indicated that her body was inflamed, although what was causing the inflammation was a mystery. From my perspective as an integrated medical doctor, I was concerned about Gloria because I know that chronic inflammation puts her at high risk for future health problems. Some researchers are now suggesting that chronic inflammation is a significant contributor to more than a 100 different diseases, including cancer, heart disease and Alzheimer's disease.[1] Unless the underlying cause of Gloria's inflammation was identified and treated, the chances are that she would develop one of these diseases. Her vague symptoms were a wake-up call, an invitation to prevent a more serious problem from developing.

Gloria's 'inflammatory' personality, combined with high levels of stress and a passion for cakes, biscuits and alcohol had created a significant level of inflammation within her body. My job was to create an integrated and anti-inflammatory programme that would address all of these issues. The programme I used to do this is the same one I am about to share with you. Before I do that, however, I want to remind you that our physical body can reflect our emotional state back to us. Gloria was a classic example of this. She was literally bubbling with stress and anger, and not surprisingly this was spilling over into her body as inflammation. At least there was congruence between mind and body! She had no problems with understanding how her emotions were contributing to the inflammation, and fortunately she agreed to do the mind-based work as well. She identified stress, unmet emotional needs, denying reality and psychological stress as her other barriers. Her commitment was great, and within six months she was symptom-free and feeling like a new woman. The moral of the story here is to ask yourself if your inflammatory body is a symptom of an inflammatory mind and/or lifestyle. For many people it won't be, but for many others, the answer is yes.

What is inflammation?

Inflammation is the immune system's first line of defence in your body's war against infection and injury. For example, if you accidentally cut yourself, or part of your body becomes infected, the damaged cells release chemicals into the surrounding area. A couple of things then happen. The local blood vessels dilate and become more permeable – this leads to the characteristic redness, heat and swelling of inflammation. The white cells – the cavalry and first line of defence of the immune system – get activated and start secreting a potent mix of inflammatory chemicals, designed to kill off any bugs that might be present. They also act as a waste-disposal system by digesting and removing the damaged cells. In the meantime, the healthy cells that surround this battlefield switch on their protective sprinkler system, by releasing anti-inflammatory chemicals and proteolytic enzymes to break down the digestive enzymes being secreted by the white cells. Once the damaged cells are removed and the sprinkler system has accomplished its job, repair and regeneration of the area commences. In a well-nourished, healthy individual the inflammation settles, optimum function is restored and we get on with our life. That's how it should be.

The challenge for the majority of the adult population is that their bodies provide a fertile ground in which inflammation continues to persist. Diets high in refined oils, processed foods and sugar, and low in fish, fruits and vegetables, along with obesity, lack of sleep and stress, are just some of the factors that tip the balance in favour of inflammation. Rather than the inflammatory process being switched on and off as when required, in these people chronic inflammation bubbles on in the background; like molten lava it seeps slowly through the body damaging everything it comes into contact with – including DNA, blood vessels, and even the cells that comprise the brain. And it is this damage that is now believed to be the mediator of so many different types of diseases, which collectively belong to the so-called inflammation syndrome.

How does inflammation cause disease?

Once chronic inflammation is established it starts to wreak havoc throughout the body. For example, until recently it was believed that atherosclerosis (deposits of cholesterol in artery walls resulting from elevated cholesterol levels in the blood) was the root cause of heart disease. Now the consensus among cardiologists is that inflammation of the lining of arteries is more likely to be the cause.[2] Furthermore, the deposits of cholesterol might actually be the body's attempt to patch up the defects caused by inflammation. An article published in the journal *Oncology* commented on the evidence to support the conclusion that chronic inflammation can predispose an individual to cancer, by damaging the cells' DNA and repair mechanisms, preventing cellular destruction and stimulating the formation of blood vessels – a process known as angiogenesis. The longer the inflammation persists, the higher the risk of associated carcinogenesis.[3] Another debilitating condition, Alzheimer's disease, which is the most common form of dementia, is known to result from an inflammatory process that destroys brain cells. This leads to the characteristic deterioration in brain function and memory.[4]

Assessing your levels of inflammation

Working out whether you have chronic inflammation in your body is not as straightforward as you might have thought. Chronic inflammation doesn't have the redness, swelling, pain and tenderness that are symptomatic of acute inflammation. Also, in many people, chronic inflammation actually doesn't cause any obvious symptoms. To help you work out whether you need to address inflammation in your body, therefore, I've suggested four different ways in which you can assess your levels of inflammation:

1 Do you have an inflammatory related disease?

This is an obvious one, if you have one or more of the following then you have inflammation: anaemia, allergies, arthritis, asthma, Alzheimer's disease, autoimmune disease, cancer, colitis, depression, diabetes, fibromyalgia, heart disease, kidney failure, lupus, prostatitis, psoriasis, sinusitis or stroke.

However, this list is far from complete, so if you know you have a condition related to inflammation that is not mentioned here, that will count as well.

2 Fill in the inflammation questionnaire

The questionnaire on page 24 has been designed to identify whether inflammation might be a factor that is influencing your health. If you haven't already filled it in, I would encourage you to do so now.

3 Get your doctor to measure your hs-CRP levels

High-sensitivity C-reactive protein (hs-CRP) is a blood protein that both promotes and reflects the level of inflammation in the body. Several studies have shown that plasma CRP concentrations are increased many years in advance of first coronary and cerebrovascular events in healthy and high-risk individuals.[5] Data from the Physicians' Health Study, a clinical trial involving 18,000 apparently healthy physicians, found that elevated levels of CRP were associated with a threefold increase in the risk of heart attack.[6] Another study – the Harvard Women's Health Study – found CRP to be a more accurate predictor of heart problems than cholesterol levels in predicting coronary problems.[7] Women in the group with the highest CRP levels were more than four times as likely to have died from coronary disease, or suffer a non-fatal heart attack or stroke. This group was also more likely to have required a cardiac procedure such as angioplasty or bypass surgery than women in the group with the lowest levels. This test is becoming more popular and widely available and is often taken at the same time as a cholesterol test. The results need to be interpreted according to your particular circumstances, but generally hs-CRP levels are as follows:

Less than 1.0 mg/L = low risk for cardiovascular disease

Between 1.0 and 2.9 mg/L = intermediate risk for cardiovascular disease

Greater than 3.0 mg/L = high risk for cardiovascular disease

4 Measure your AA/EPA ratio

Your blood AA/EPA ratio is a good marker of silent inflammation (undetected low-grade inflammation). AA (arachidonic acid) is a potent pro-inflammatory chemical derived from omega-6 essential fatty acids, and EPA is one of the active anti-inflammatory components of omega-3 essential fatty acids. One hundred years ago the ratio of omega-6 to omega-3 in the human diet was roughly equal; however, excessive consumption of processed foods and refined oils, and a much reduced consumption of fish and vegetables, has led to a dramatic change in this ratio – for the average Westerner it is near to 20:1. This is believed to be a major factor in the current epidemic of inflammatory diseases.

The AA/EPA test is best organised through your nutritional therapist or an integrated medical doctor. It is also a useful way of monitoring how your treatment programme is going.

- An AA/EPA ratio of 1.5 is considered to be ideal, since this is the ratio found in the Japanese population, which has one of the greatest longevity and the lowest incidences of cardiovascular disease.

- The average AA/EPA of someone on a Western diet is approximately 10.

- For patients with inflammatory conditions and neurological disorders, the AA/EPA ratio can be in excess of 20.

How to treat chronic inflammation

If you have scored greater than 10 on the inflammation questionnaire (page 24), or are known to have an inflammatory condition, or have a AA/EPA ratio of more than 1.5 or an hs-CRP level of greater than 1.0, try the following to reduce inflammation within your body safely and effectively:

Step 1 • Improve your omega-3 to omega-6 ratio

Restoring the balance of omega-6 to omega-3 to a ratio of roughly 2:1, is one of the most effective ways to treat chronic inflammation and help the body recover from inflammation-based diseases. Here's how:

- Increase your intake of omega-3 fatty-acid rich foods such as oily fish (salmon, herring, sardines and mackerel), flaxseed, walnuts, Brazil nuts, green leafy vegetables, grass-fed meat and omega-3 enriched eggs. See Barrier 1 for more advice on healthy eating.

- Decrease your intake of omega-6 rich products such as refined vegetable oils (corn, soy, safflower and sunflower), processed foods and grain-fed meat.

- Supplement your diet with fish oil at a dose of between 3,000mg and 10,000mg a day depending on the severity of inflammation. Because contamination of fish oils with toxins such as PCBs, dioxins and mercury is such a problem, you should buy a brand that is mercury-free and has negligible levels of toxins. Recommended brands include Higher Nature, Nutri, Solgar and Biocare.

- Increase your intake of anti-inflammatory foods such as nuts, seeds, beans, fruits and vegetables.

Step 2 • Stabilise your blood-sugar levels

The effect of consuming refined carbohydrates, sweets and sugary drinks is to inflammation as petrol is to fire: it makes it a lot worse! High levels of sugar in the blood stimulate the release of insulin from the pancreas gland, which in turn increases the production of the pro-inflammatory hormone PGE2. Controlling and maintaining a relatively stable blood sugar and insulin level is therefore an important part of reducing inflammation. Here are some ways to achieve that:

- **Reduce your consumption of refined carbohydrates**, this includes sugar, confectionery, cakes, biscuits, pastries, fruit juice and fizzy drinks.

- **Eat some protein** with snacks and your main meals, as this will help to stabilise your blood-sugar levels. For example, eat a handful of walnuts with a piece of fruit, hummus with oatcakes, and some oily fish with a jacket potato and steamed vegetables.

- **The mineral chromium polynicotinate** at a dose of 200mcg to 400mcg a day can help to stabilise blood-sugar levels. Foods that contain chromium include: black pepper, broccoli, dried beans and whole grains.

Step 3 • Increase your antioxidant intake

Antioxidants are substances that neutralise free radicals, which are highly reactive chemicals that damage the body's cells and promote inflammation. The body naturally generates trillions of these free radicals each day, but in the presence of natural antioxidants such as vitamins C, A and E, and beta carotene, they rarely cause a problem. However, if the level of antioxidants is insufficient to keep in check the amount of free-radical activity, inflammation and cellular damage soon follows. Here are some suggestions for increasing your intake of antioxidants:

- Decrease the amount of free-radical activity by limiting your exposure to pollution, avoiding smoking and passive smoking, environmental toxins and pesticides and avoiding eating chargrilled, processed and fried foods.

- Increase your intake of antioxidant-rich foods, such as kidney beans, pinto beans, avocados, olives, blueberries, prunes, blackberries, strawberries, kiwi fruit, pecan nuts, kale, spinach, Brussels sprouts, broccoli, red pepper and onions.

- Green, white and rooibos tea are all antioxidant-rich drinks. Make sure that you use boiled water that has been allowed to cool slightly, as boiling water destroys the antioxidants. Aim for at least three cups a day.

- Herbs such as oregano, turmeric, garlic, ginger and holy basil are potent sources of antioxidants. Researchers with the US Department of Agriculture found that on a per-gram fresh-weight basis, oregano and other herbs ranked even higher in antioxidant activity than fruits and vegetables. Oregano has 42 times more antioxidant activity than apples, 30 times more than potatoes, 12 times more than oranges and 4 times more than blueberries![8]

- Take a broad-spectrum antioxidant supplement that contains some of the following: vitamin C, vitamin E, beta carotene, mixed carotenes, selenium, zinc, bioflavonoids, cysteine and methionine (sulphur-containing amino acids), CoQ10, grapeseed extract, glutathione, alpha lipoic acid, astaxanthin, Acetyl-L-Carnitine. See Barrier 1 for more information.

Step 4 • Take anti-inflammatory supplements

Before you reach for the ibuprofen, you should be aware of the ever-increasing amounts of research linking non-steroidal anti-inflammatories (NSAIDs) to serious side effects, including accelerated joint damage, gastrointestinal bleeding and increased risk of heart disease when taken at high dosages for prolonged periods of time. Fortunately, there are plenty of alternative, safer options, such as:

- **Bromelain** (standardised to 2,000mcu) at a dose of 200mg three times daily on an empty stomach. It is good for acute joint pain, sinusitis, post-surgery, sports injuries, cellulite and thrombophlebitis.

- **Astaxanthin** at a dose of 1–2mg twice daily. It is good for rheumatoid arthritis, carpel tunnel syndrome, repetitive strain injury, post-exercise soreness.

- **Vitamin C**, at a dose of 1–3g daily in divided dosages. It is good for minor injuries, muscle soreness, reflex sympathetic dystrophy and as a general anti-inflammatory.

- **Flavanoids**, such as grapeseed extract, pycogenol and quercetin at a daily dose of 200mg to 400mg three times a day. Because they are synergistic with vitamin C they are ideally taken in combination. Quercetin is good for prostatitis and interstitial cystitis.

- **Vitamin E** (mixed tocopherols), at a dose of 400IU per day. It is good for menstrual pain and as a general anti-inflammatory.

- **GLA** (gamma-linolenic acid), at a dose of 400mg–1g per day. It is good for people with eczema, rheumatoid arthritis, asthma, allergies and ulcerative colitis. Because GLA is synergistic with EPA they should ideally be taken together.

- **EPA** (eicosa-pentaenoic acid) at a dose of 1,000–2,000mg per day. It is good for arthritis, Alzheimer's disease, depression, menstrual pain, kidney stones, colitis, and as a general anti-inflammatory.

- **MSM**, at a dose of 1–3g daily. It is particularly good for osteoarthritis.

- **Devil's claw** (standardised to contain 3 per cent iridoid glycosides) at a dose of 750mg three times daily. It is good for back pain, arthritis, joint pain and gout.

- Other anti-inflammatories include: turmeric, white willow bark, nettle leaf extract and boswellia.

The supplement DLPA Complex from Higher Nature contains astaxanthin, bromelain and the amino-acid painkiller DLPA. Together they provide a very effective natural anti-inflammatory. I often use this with omega-3 fish oils in my patients with chronic inflammation.

Step 5 • Treat the underlying contributors and causes of inflammation

This list is by no means comprehensive, but it gives you an idea of the possible reasons behind your chronic inflammation. Because there are so many possibilities, it is probably best to work with a health practitioner, who can exclude or identify which are relevant to you.

- **Infection** Severe infections or microbes that are able to survive the onslaught of the immune system will perpetuate the immune inflammatory response. See Barrier 7 for more information.

- **Animal protein**, such as meat, eggs, cheese and dairy, are rich in arachidonic acid, a chemical that accelerates the production of pro-inflammatory prostaglandins.

- **Trans-fatty acids**, as found in doughnuts, margarine, biscuits, crackers, fried food and many processed foods, interfere with the enzyme delta-6-desaturase which is needed for the production of anti-inflammatory prostaglandins.

- **Sugar** Raised blood-sugar levels, either because of high consumption (usually due to fizzy drinks and confectionery) and/or diabetes and insulin resistance, are known to raise levels of the pro-inflammatory chemicals IL-6 and CRP.

- **Vegetable oils and many processed foods** are rich in omega-6 essential fatty acids, which in a body relatively deficient in omega-3 essential fatty acids generate significant quantities of pro-inflammatory compounds.

- **Leaky-gut syndrome** The cells lining the gut wall are usually tightly bound together; however, in leaky-gut syndrome, they become loose and 'leaky', allowing undigested food particles to squeeze between them and into the bloodstream. The body's immune system launches a defence and in the process sparks an inflammatory response.

- **Allergies** of any kind – food, hayfever, dust mite, and so on – provide a constant source of irritation and stress to the body's immune system.

- **Stress** Chronic and severe acute stress floods the body with pro-inflammatory chemicals.

- **Stomach-acid/digestive-enzyme deficiency** can result in nutrient deficiencies and undigested food particles (which can contribute to food allergies).

- **Constipation** results in a build-up of toxins in the large intestine, which then get absorbed into the bloodstream.

- **Food additives,** which includes flavourings, preservatives and stabilisers, can all exacerbate inflammation. Top culprits are tartrazine, sulfites, monosodium glutamate (MSG), salicylates and aspartame.

- **Environmental toxins** Chemical toxins and irritants can accumulate in various parts of the body and become a potent source of irritation.

- **Chronic disease** Any chronic disease can be a source of strain on the body and its resources, and predispose it to inflammation.

- **Genetic inheritance** There are a number of inherited conditions that predispose an individual to inflammation. One of the most common is atopic eczema. Sufferers have a defect in the enzyme delta-6-desaturase, a key enzyme involved in the production of anti-inflammatory prostaglandins.

- **Nutrient deficiencies** Following on from the example above, nutrient deficiencies can also prevent enzymes from working properly. For example, low levels of zinc and magnesium slow down the rate at which the delta-6-desaturase enzyme works.

- **Obesity** A waist size of greater than 86cm (34in) in women and 102cm (40in) in men is indicative of abdominal obesity and a greatly increased risk of chronic inflammation. Fat cells, particularly those around the tummy, make large amounts of pro-inflammatory chemicals, including IL-6 and CRP.

- **Exercise** Excessive amounts of exercise have been shown to considerably increase inflammation. (See Exercise, page 350, for more information.)

- **Sleep deprivation** Even just a modest amount of sleep deprivation has been shown to adversely affect hormone and cytokine levels.

Now that you have reached the end of this chapter, my advice is to re-read it one more time. While doing so highlight those sentences (using a highlighter pen) that you feel are important to you. Once you've done this write down at least five steps or actions that you are going to take, and spend a moment visualising yourself implementing them. Once you have completed this, move on to your next barrier.

MIND–BODY ESSENTIALS

- Chronic inflammation is a significant contributor to many diseases, including cancer, heart disease and Alzheimer's disease.

- A diet high in fruits, vegetables, oily fish and olive oil, and low in refined carbohydrates and oils such as sunflower, soy and corn, is the foundation for reducing inflammation.

- Fish oils, evening primrose oil and a broad-spectrum antioxidant supplement are the foundations of a good anti-inflammatory supplement programme.

- Recommended mind–body tools to accompany this chapter: sleep (page 384), creative visualisation (page 319), instant stress release (page 368), meditation (page 376), conscious breathing (page 314) and relaxation (page 380).

- For recommended reading see Resources, page 426.

Hormonal imbalances

Sophie felt exhausted. She struggled to get out of bed in the mornings, her whole body felt heavy and she felt depressed, which she assured me was very unusual for her. Her spark had gone and she didn't know what to do about it. Her GP had tested her for a low-functioning thyroid, but the blood test didn't reveal any problems. She was fed up with being this way and had come to me for some help.

Despite her 'normal' blood test, Sophie was displaying all the common signs and symptoms of a thyroid and adrenal problem. Both of these glands, as we will discover in a minute, play an essential role in generating energy and helping us cope with stress. Sophie's hormones had become out of balance following years of eating a poor diet and failing to get enough sleep – on average six hours a night. Plus, she was stressed out. Her husband had left her two years ago, her 24-year-old son was still living with her, and she was in a job that she didn't enjoy. The combination of stress and failing to take care of her physical and emotional needs had upset the delicate balance of her hormones and this resulted in her symptoms. I started Sophie on an integrated programme to tackle the underlying problems, as well as the hormonal imbalances. She had a shaky start, mainly because she kept forgetting to take her supplements, but after some gentle coaxing from me, and pressure from her son, she eventually stuck to the programme. It wasn't an overnight change, but within seven months, her energy was back, her mood was lifted and her hormones had returned to their healthy levels and rhythms.

If, like Sophie, you've identified hormones as one of your barriers, then help is at hand. About one in five of my patients have a significant hormonal imbalance, and I've found over the years that correcting them using an integrated approach is an essential part of achieving total health. One of the keys to successful hormonal balancing is to consider what emotional or lifestyle imbalances could be contributing to the hormonal imbalances. Your mood is intimately linked with your hormones, with stress being one of the most potent sources of upset to hormonal balance. What is stressing you at the moment? What is interrupting the flow of life for you at the moment? What are you resisting in your life? Bear these in mind as you move through this chapter.

Let's start by taking a look at some background information on hormones.

What are hormones?

Hormones are molecules of information that are produced by one part of the body (a gland) and circulated to another part to tell it something. As extraordinary as it might sound, the movements and quantities of these millions of information molecules are co-ordinated. When in harmony – that is, the hormone-producing glands are speaking and hearing properly – the body is mobilised towards good health, to total health. When the opposite happens, ill health and disease set in.

One of the greatest challenges facing anyone who is committed to total health is the challenge of balancing their hormones. Hormonal flow is exquisitely sensitive to upset and interference. Processed diets, stress, nutritional deficiency, medications, inactivity, toxins, moods and infections all affect hormonal balance. To this I would also add falling out of sync with our environment. We are all aware of nature's natural rhythms – the four seasons, night and day, and so on – well, our own bodies have their natural rhythms that take their cue internally from genes, and externally from our environment.[1] For example, the light of morning triggers the body's production of various hormones, such as cortisol, and the neurotransmitters serotonin – these lift mood, increase energy and get you ready for the day ahead. However, when this relationship is interfered with; for example, by working night shifts or getting to bed late, and getting out of bed late, the natural ebb and flow of hormones gets interrupted. This strain sets the seeds of disease and illness.

Hormonal imbalance problems

The list of problems related to hormonal imbalances is pretty much endless. It includes general conditions such as fatigue, hair loss, inflammation, irritability and loss of libido, to more specific diseases such as fibroids, endometriosis, hormone-related cancers, PMT, polycystic ovaries, and breast and prostate disease, decreasing sperm count, depression, insomnia, anxiety and addictions.[2] Most authorities would agree that all of these are on the increase and that hormone-related problems are a major cause of ill health and concern.

How to overcome hormonal imbalance

This is a big subject and one that I can't cover comprehensively in one chapter. I have decided to concentrate on the hormonal imbalances that I most commonly encounter in my own clinic. Having said this, because of the complexity of hormones, and because hormonal imbalances tend to be symptoms of other imbalances, I would strongly encourage you to work alongside an integrated medical doctor or nutritional therapist. The hormonal imbalances covered are those of adrenal and thyroid glands, insulin and sex hormones.

Adrenal and thyroid glands

They say great things come in small packages, well, there are no finer examples of that than your adrenal and thyroid glands. As part of the body's elaborate and complex endocrine system, these two hormone-producing organs influence virtually every aspect of your well-being. Mood, energy levels, weight and libido, are all intimately connected to the health of your thyroid and adrenal-gland function and your body's ability to utilise the hormones that they produce. When they work optimally and in harmony your health flourishes. However, when they enter a state of imbalance, usually because of chronic stress, inflammation and/or nutritional imbalances, deterioration in health soon follows. Indeed many practitioners working within the field of nutritional and integrated medicine will tell you that adrenal and thyroid problems are endemic. Fortunately, the majority, if diagnosed correctly, will respond to taking some supplements and making a few simple lifestyle changes.

Adrenal imbalance

What are the adrenals?

The adrenals are two small pyramid-shaped glands sitting on top of your kidneys. Despite their small size, they are vitally important to your health and well-being: they help your body respond to stress, maintain the body's energy, regulate the immune system, and keep your blood sugar, fluid levels and blood pressure within a healthy range. The interior part of the adrenal glands – the adrenal medulla – produces the hormones adrenaline and noradrenaline: the so called fight-or-flight hormones. These help your body respond effectively to acute stress. The exterior part of the adrenal gland – the adrenal cortex – is concerned with helping your body adapt to chronic stress. It manufactures over 30 different steroids, including cortisol, DHEA and cortisone, and helps control the body's use of fats, proteins and carbohydrates, regulate insulin levels, reduce inflammation and influence immune-system function.

What is adrenal fatigue?

Healthy adrenal glands secrete very precise amounts of steroid hormones. However, too much physical, emotional, environmental and/or psychological stress can cause an imbalance in the function of the adrenals, and result in adrenal fatigue or insufficiency, a condition arising when the adrenal glands are no longer coping with the demands placed upon it. This gives the classic symptoms of adrenal fatigue: low energy, tiredness, insomnia, irritability, cravings, anxiety and difficulty concentrating. Typically, many people with adrenal fatigue get into a habit of relying on stimulants such as caffeine, sugar or sodas to keep them going, and then alcohol or marijuana to wind themselves down at the end of the day. As time goes on it becomes harder and harder to get going and to relax and so greater amounts of stimulants and relaxants are required, and the stress–adrenal fatigue cycle continues.

What causes adrenal fatigue?

Essentially anything that causes prolonged physical, emotional and/ or psychological stress can cause adrenal fatigue. This includes:

- Work pressure

- Relationship difficulties

- Chronic repressed emotions

- Emotional trauma

- Chronic illness, infection, surgery, inflammation, pain

- Grief, loss, financial difficulties

- Depression and anxiety

- Allergies and intolerances

- Toxicity

- Lack of quality sleep

How to assess your adrenal health

Take an adrenal stress index (ASI) saliva test

One of the easiest ways to check adrenal-gland function is to measure the level of DHEA and cortisol in a saliva sample taken at four different times during the day. The levels and ratios of each are then measured and compared with what would be expected in a healthy person. (For more information about this test see Resources, page 423.)

Blood-pressure test

If you have an automated blood-pressure device at home, try this test. Lie down and keep still and relaxed for about five minutes. Take your blood pressure and record the result. Keeping the blood-pressure cuff on, stand up and take your blood pressure immediately. The top number (the systolic blood pressure) would usually increase or remain constant. A decrease in its value can be an indicator of adrenal fatigue. Repeat twice to confirm your results.

Take the adrenal-fatigue questionnaire

QUESTIONNAIRE: adrenal fatigue

For each question score 0 for no; 1 for occasionally; 3 for yes, then total up the section.

Do you:

1. Feel tired for no obvious reason? ☐

2. Experience light-headedness on standing? ☐

3. Feel more awake at night? ☐

4. Crave salty food, sugar or liquorice? ☐

▶

5. Feel stressed, restless, overwhelmed and/or exhausted? ☐

6. Have a reduced libido? ☐

7. Tremble when under stress? ☐

8. Find it hard to lose weight? ☐

9. Have dark circles under your eyes or are your eyes sensitive to bright lights? ☐

10. Spend the whole day rushing from one thing to another? ☐

11. Suffer from interrupted sleep or insomnia? ☐

12. Experience anxiety, irritability, nervousness, phobias or panic attacks? ☐

13. Get absentminded or feel that your short-term memory lets you down? ☐

14. Keep yourself going on sugar, caffeine and/or nicotine? ☐

Total score ☐

A score of 10 or more suggests that you are experiencing some adrenal fatigue. My advice would be to confirm this with the ASI saliva test.

How to revive your adrenal glands

If the saliva test, blood-pressure measurements and/or questionnaire indicate that you have adrenal fatigue, follow the eight steps described below. Also bear in mind that recovering from adrenal fatigue is not going to happen overnight; depending on your health and degree of adrenal fatigue it can take anywhere from between three months to two years – it requires a real commitment.

Step 1 • *Identify and resolve your main sources of stress*

Facing reality (Barrier 12) and taking action to deal with the underlying causes of your stress (Barrier 9) are the keys to stopping further adrenal fatigue. In addition to this you should also:

- Go through the list of 'causes' of adrenal fatigue, and identify which are relevant to you. If you are unsure, seek the help of an experienced healthcare practitioner.

- Next, identify the first step to addressing that cause; for example, phoning to make an appointment with your doctor; sitting down with your boss to talk about problems at work; talking to the Citizen's Advice Bureau.

- Now visualise yourself doing this first step and take action within 48 hours. Enlist a friend or family member to support you.

- If you can't take action to change the cause of stress, try accepting this fact fully. Stress arises when we resist reality. For more information on this read the book *Loving What Is* by Bryon Katie.

Step 2 • *Sleep well*

Sleep is a wonderful healer and rejuvenator. If you get less than eight hours of sleep a night or you have problems getting to sleep or staying asleep, consider taking valerian, or 50–100mg of 5-HTP (but don't take it with antidepressant medications). The sleep mind–body tool has further suggestions.

Step 3 • *Switch to healthy foods*

Providing your body with high-quality nourishment, and maintaining a stable blood-sugar level is an essential part of helping your adrenal glands to recover. Turn to Barrier 1 for more suggestions. In a nutshell, this means:

- Cutting back on refined carbohydrates, such as sugary snacks and white bread.

- Eating small amounts of meat, dairy and potatoes.

- Making fresh fruit, vegetables, whole grains, oily fish and olive oil the bulk of your diet.

- Avoiding foods to which you are intolerant – wheat and cow's dairy produce are the top culprits (see Barrier 3).

Step 4 • Avoid stimulants

Sugar, caffeine, nicotine, chocolate, alcohol and refined foods are significant contributors to adrenal fatigue. Do whatever you can to reduce your consumption of these, at least until you feel much better. If you think you are addicted to any of these, take a look at Barrier 10.

Step 5 • Take adrenal support supplements

The adrenal gland, like all of the body's organs, requires optimum amounts of vitamins, minerals and essential fatty acids to stay healthy. As a general rule of thumb you should consider supplementing with a 50mg B vitamin complex, an additional 500mg of vitamin B_5, 1,000–3,000mg of vitamin C with bioflavanoids, and 1,000–3,000mg of omega-3 fish oil. To these I would add one of the following.

- **Rhodiola and Ashwagandha** This is my preferred adrenal-support formula, as it contains two adaptogenic herbs, the first, rhodiola, also called arctic root, and the second, ashwagandha, Indian ginseng. Adaptogenic means it helps the body to restore balance, fight fatigue and boost energy levels.

- **Ginseng** is another adaptogen that has been used for thousands of years in traditional Chinese medicine as a tonic to help the body reach its full potential for health. There are a few different types of ginseng, but the ones most useful for helping recharge the adrenals are Siberian and American ginseng. The supplement B-Vital from Higher Nature contains these with all of the B vitamins as well as vitamin C.

- **L-theanine** is nature's alternative to valium and a very effective supplement for calming the bodymind. Take 200mg once or twice a day.

If your saliva test confirms your DHEA levels are low, you could consider the following. Please note, however, that this should only be done under the supervision of a doctor, and DHEA levels need to be monitored at least every six weeks:

- **DHEA** is the most abundant steroid hormone in the body. In addition to being a precursor to the sex hormones (testosterone, oestrogen and progesterone), it also has been found to stimulate immune function, decrease cholesterol levels, increase insulin sensitivity and help the body recover from stress.[3] In addition to being very good at supporting adrenal gland function, it can be a particularly effective treatment for someone with an autoimmune disease, such as systemic lupus erythematosus (SLE). The recommended dosage is between 10mg and 25mg twice a day. (**Note** DHEA should not be taken if you have a hormonally related disease, such as breast, uterine or prostate cancer or endometriosis.)

The need for these supplements should be reviewed every three months – ideally with the help of a nutritional therapist or an integrated medical doctor.

Step 6 • *Exercise gently*

Exercise is a great stress reliever. During exercise, levels of stress hormones decrease, DHEA levels increase and anxiety/depressive states are lifted. It is important, however, to not over-exercise, as this can stress your adrenal glands further. Yoga, walking and swimming are ideal. See the Mind–Body Toolbox chapter on exercise (page 350) for further suggestions.

Step 7 • *Make time to relax*

Building some form of relaxation into your daily routine is an important part of helping your bodymind to relax and recharge itself. Think of something you could realistically do most days to help you unwind – meditation, massage, a hot bath, reading and going for a walk are all simple, but effective ideas. See the relaxation mind–body tool for further suggestions (page 380).

Step 8 • Address other imbalances

Adrenal imbalance rarely occurs in isolation. You should also check for other metabolic imbalances such as thyroid imbalance and oestrogen imbalance. It's also important to treat chronic sources of stress to the body as well, such as allergies (see Barrier 3), and candida and parasites (Barrier 7). Making sure these are identified and treated effectively will help the adrenal gland recover much quicker.

Thyroid imbalance

An estimated 5 per cent of the population suffer from hypo-thyroidism (an under-functioning of the thyroid gland), and the majority don't know about it.[4] Women are at the greatest risk, developing thyroid problems seven times more often than men, with the risk increasing with age and for those with a family history of thyroid problems. If left untreated, thyroid imbalances can leave people at risk of heart disease, infertility and osteoporosis.[5]

What is the thyroid gland?

Your thyroid is a butterfly-shaped gland that straddles your wind-pipe, with one lobe either side. The cells that make up the thyroid gland combine the mineral iodine with the amino-acid l-tyrosine to create two hormones: thyroxine (T4) and the biologically more active triiodothyronine (T3). The '3' and the '4' refer to the number of iodine molecules in each thyroid hormone molecule. Once released by the thyroid gland these hormones travel throughout the body, and regulate the enzymes involved in controlling the rate at which energy is produced. In general, the higher the level of thyroid hormones, the greater the amount of energy and heat produced. This in turn affects heart rate, blood pressure, growth, appetite, mood, mental sharpness, body temperature and even libido. There's hardly any physiological process that isn't affected by thyroid hormones.

What is hypothyroidism?

An underactive thyroid, or hypothyroidism, occurs when the thyroid gland fails to make sufficient thyroid hormone to meet the body's demands. When your thyroid is not working properly or the thyroid hormones aren't able to exert their effects on the body's cells – usually because of a mineral deficiency – many bodily functions start slowing down. This gives the classic hypothyroid symptoms of low energy, low temperature, extreme tiredness, intolerance to cold weather, mental drowsiness, weight gain, depression, low libido, thinning hair and constipation. The most common cause of hypothyroidism is autoimmune thyroiditis, a condition in which the body's own immune system starts attacking the thyroid gland. The symptoms are much the same as classical hypothyroidism except that weight and/or body temperature tends not to be a problem, and anxiety and allergies are more of a problem. Autoimmune thyroiditis, which is also called Hashimoto's disease, can also result in the thyroid gland swelling to two to three times its normal size.

What causes thyroid imbalances

There are many different factors that can affect thyroid function, they include:

- Auto immune disease (Hashimoto's disease)

- Selenium, iodine or zinc deficiency

- Adrenal fatigue, usually because of excessive cortisol levels (due to stress)

- Chronic inflammation

- Pregnancy

- Fluoridated water

- Soya products – these are known to suppress thyroid function

- External radiation to the head and neck area

- Medications such as lithium and amiodarone

- Radioactive iodine treatment for hyperthyroidism

- Surgical removal of the thyroid due to cancer or nodules

- Mercury amalgam fillings

- Compromised liver and/or kidney function

- Glandular fever

- Pesticides, heavy-metal toxicity, smoking and other environmental chemicals

- Prolonged illness

- Starvation or fasting

- Allergies

How to assess your thyroid health

Take a blood test

In theory, measuring blood for indicators of thyroid function should be an easy and accurate way to assess your thyroid function. The markers measured usually include TSH (thyroid stimulating hormone), T4 (thyroid hormone), T3 (active thyroid hormone) and anti-microsomal and anti-thyroglobulin antibody test (to check for an autoimmune cause). However, many integrated medical doctors, myself included, have come across many patients with 'normal' thyroid test results, despite scoring positively on the questionnaire and temperature test. So what's going on? Some of these patients will have mineral deficiencies that are preventing the thyroid hormones from working effectively, so supplementing these through diet and supplements is necessary. Others need to have their free T3 and free T4 tested, as these indicate the actual amounts of thyroid hormones that are available to exert their influence on the cells of the body. T3 and T4 are bound to proteins and are therefore not available to the body's cells. Free T3 levels of less than 260 pg/ml, free T4 levels of less than 0.7 and/or TSH levels above 2.0 in the presence of the signs and symptoms of thyroid imbalance are strongly suggestive of hypothyroidism. (To arrange a total thyroid screen test see Resources, page 422.)

Barnes Test

Devised by an American doctor called Broda Barnes, the Barnes Test is based on the theory that in the absence of an infection the body's temperature is mainly determined by the level of thyroid hormones, with low thyroid function being reflected in a low body temperature.[6] The procedure involves measuring your underarm temperature with a mercury thermometer immediately upon waking up in the morning for three consecutive mornings. Leave the thermometer in place for ten minutes. Men and post-menopausal women can take their temperature on any day, as long as they don't have an infection. Because pre-menopausal women's temperatures tend to fluctuate with the hormonal cycle, Dr Barnes suggests that the most accurate time to assess temperature is on the second, third or fourth day of the period.

Normal body temperature in the morning is between 36.6°C and 36.8°C (97.8°F and 98.2°F). A temperature of 36.4°C (97.4°F) or less, in combination with some of the hypothyroid symptoms, is suggestive of a low functioning thyroid.

This test is useful in that it provides a measure of the effect of thyroid hormones on the body. These functional tests are, in the main, much more useful than measuring levels of a particular hormone alone.

Take the thyroid-imbalance questionnaire

QUESTIONNAIRE: thyroid imbalance

For each question score 0 for no; 1 for occasionally; 3 for yes, then total up the section.

Do you:

1. Get easily chilled (especially hands and feet)?

▶

2. Gain weight easily despite eating little or find it hard to lose excess weight? ☐

3. Find it hard to get up in the morning? ☐

4. Experience low energy levels? ☐

5. Have a family history of thyroid problems? ☐

6. Experience a sore throat, or nasal congestion? ☐

7. Suffer from constipation, gas, bloating, or indigestion? ☐

8. Have dry skin or hair? ☐

9. Suffer from depression and/or irritability? ☐

10. Sleep a lot? ☐

11. Experience fogginess of thinking, poor memory or concentration? ☐

12. Have muscle aches and/or joint pains? ☐

Total score ☐

A score of 10 or more suggests that you are experiencing some degree of hypothyroidism. My advice would be to double check and confirm this, using the Barnes test.

How to revive your thyroid gland

If your blood tests, temperature test and/or questionnaire indicate that you have hypothyroidism, I would strongly encourage you to seek help from a nutritional therapist or integrated medical doctor. Failing that, follow the eight steps described below. Also bear in mind that, like recovering from adrenal fatigue, your treatment programme might require you to take supplements and/or medications for years, or even the rest of your life. Here are the main steps to reviving your thyroid gland:

Step 1 • Avoid thyroid-suppressing foods

Goitrogens are substances found in foods that interfere with the function of the thyroid gland. These foods include soya, walnuts, peanuts, almonds, millet, pine nuts, cabbage, mustard and apples, and foods from the brassica family such as cabbage, turnips and radishes. Your intake of these foods should be limited. However, when these are cooked, the compounds that cause thyroid imbalance are inactivated. Turn to Barrier 1 for more healthy-eating suggestions.

Step 2 • Eat thyroid-supporting foods

Thyrotrophs are foods that help stimulate thyroid hormone production and the conversion of T4 to T3. These should be eaten regularly, and include egg yolk, seaweeds (kelp and dulse), mushrooms, garlic, seafood and wheatgerm. Coconut oil is also thyroid stimulating and should be used to cook with.

Step 3 • Take thyroid-support supplements

If you have classical hypothyroidism (low temperature, low energy, low mood and high weight), you want to consider taking the following supplements to boost and support thyroid activity. They should include:

- **A multivitamin–mineral** See Barrier 1. Supplementing with minerals and vitamins such as selenium, iron, zinc, copper and the B vitamins helps to ensure that your thyroid hormones are achieving their maximal effect within the body.

- **An omega-3 essential fatty acid supplement**, such as flaxseed or fish oil, increases the body's sensitivity to thyroid hormones and decreases inflammation – which in turn might contribute to the autoimmune attack on the thyroid gland.

- **L-tyrosine** is the energising amino acid. It provides the thyroid with the food to make its hormones, plus it gets converted into the neurotransmitters dopamine, adrenaline and noradrenaline. Take 500–1,000mg L-tyrosine three times daily away from food (before breakfast, mid-morning and mid-afternoon). If you find it too stimulating (for example, you feel agitated), you can drop the mid-afternoon dose.

- **Kelp** is a potent source of iodine and is useful if a deficiency of iodine is suspected. Take one to two capsules a day. Do not take if you have Hashimoto's thyroiditis, as it will aggravate it.

If you have autoimmune thyroiditis, the treatment must be conventional. Synthetic T4 (synthroid) +/- synthetic T3 (usually called Cytomel) is the best treatment and this must be done under the supervision of a doctor. Some doctors will, however, not treat this if the TSH, T4 and T3 are normal.

When taking the above treatments, it is important to monitor your progress by repeating the temperature test every week for the first six weeks, blood tests every three months as well as monitoring your symptoms and how you feel.

Step 4 • Exercise

Regular aerobic exercise, such as a 30-minute brisk walk three times each week, helps to increase the secretion of thyroid hormones, and increase the body's sensitivity to those thyroid hormones. I have had patients report that regular yoga is also helpful. See the exercise mind–body tool (page 350) for further suggestions.

Step 5 • Address other imbalances

Thyroid imbalance is usually accompanied by other metabolic imbalances such as adrenal imbalance and oestrogen imbalance. It's also important to treat chronic sources of stress to the body as well, such as allergies (Barrier 3) and candida and parasites (Barrier 7). Low-functioning thyroid is also a relatively common cause of raised LDL cholesterol. Making sure these are identified and resolved will help the thyroid gland recover much quicker.

The relationship between thyroid and adrenal function

Because thyroid and adrenal function is intimately linked, you tend to find that when one is imbalanced, the other attempts to compensate. For example, if the adrenals go into overdrive because of chronic stress, the thyroid will attempt to restore some balance, by reducing thyroid hormone secretion and turning down the rate of metabolism (the rate at which energy is produced). Conversely, if the thyroid fails, the adrenals have to work even harder to keep the rate of metabolism up. Hence, the importance of testing the function of both, and treating both if required.

MIND–BODY ESSENTIALS

- An under-functioning thyroid and adrenal gland is a common problem, and should be considered if you experience any of the following: fatigue, weight gain, insomnia, depression and/or anxiety.

- Supplements for a low-functioning adrenal gland can include a multivitamin and mineral, vitamin C, vitamin B complex, Siberian ginseng, rhodiola and DHEA (under medical supervision).

- Supplements for a low-functioning thyroid gland can include a multivitamin and mineral, L-tyrosine and kelp.

- Recommended mind–body tools to accompany this section: creative visualisation (page 319), Bach Flower Remedies (page 298), meditation (page 376), conscious breathing (page 314) and relaxation (page 380).

- For recommended reading see Resources, pages 426–7.

Female hormonal imbalances

Up until two years ago Elaine described herself as the life and soul of the party. Her health was good and her mood generally buoyant. But then things started to deteriorate, her husband noticed it first. She started to become impatient and irritable about the smallest of things. She became depressed, experienced profuse sweating at night and, according to her (but said with a smile), her desire for sex took a dive – something was most definitely wrong!

Elaine was of course going through the peri-menopause, a period of considerable hormonal and emotional change just prior to the cessation of her body's ability to ovulate. Like millions of women before her, Elaine was now faced with a challenge that required her to make some adjustments to her lifestyle, ones that would not only placate her symptoms but would also help her sail through into the next phase of her life – the menopause.

The total-health approach

My role, when any women who comes to me asking for help with a hormone-related problem, is to understand the root of the problem, explain clearly what's going on and then suggest which changes and which supplements can help. This is what I did with Elaine and I'd like to do with you now.

The first thing is to realise that to deal effectively with female hormonal problems, such as PMS, menopause, fibroids or endometriosis, we are required to look beyond the hormones as well. Nutrient levels, stress, smoking, irregular sleep cycles, and disease, as well as toxins, relationships and levels of happiness are intricately tied up with hormonal flow. All of these things need to be explored. The second thing, and this is really important, you should never treat hormonal problems without knowing exactly which hormones are imbalanced. For example, I recently had two patients wanting help to treat their peri-menopausal symptoms. These included hot flushes, tiredness and depression. So, from their history, it would be easy to think that they have the same problem, but their hormone testing revealed very different underlying imbalances. They both had a high oestrogen to progesterone ratio, but one was due to high levels of oestrogen and the other due to low levels of progesterone. For the first woman the focus of her treatment plan, therefore, was on reducing her oestrogen levels, and for the second woman, on increasing her progesterone levels. The treatment programme I used with them is similar to the one I am going to share with you in a moment.

So to start us off I'm going to talk generally about the two main female hormones oestrogen and progesterone, explore the phenomena of oestrogen dominance, and then provide some general guidance on restoring hormonal balance. For advice on how to resolve specific female health issues, such as fibroids, or PMS, I'd recommend you take a look at Option 2: Health Condition Guide on pages 33–43, once you've finished reading this section.

Oestrogen and progesterone

I'm going to discuss the two main female hormones, oestrogen and progesterone together because their relationship holds the key to understanding female hormonal health and imbalances.

- **Oestrogen** actually consists of three hormones: oestradiol (E2), the main oestrogen made by women's ovaries before menopause; oestrone (E1), a weaker oestrogen produced both in the ovaries and in fat tissue from other hormones, and the main oestrogen found in women after menopause; and oestriol (E3), the weakest of the three main forms of oestrogen, made in the body from other oestrogens. When your oestrogen levels are optimum, here's what you can expect: improved skin tone, better mood, mental clarity, sex drive, good digestion, vaginal lubrication and a reduced rate of bone loss.

- **Progesterone** works in harmony with oestrogen, but also against it. For example, progesterone protects against the cancer-promoting effects of oestrogen on the endometrium, and the inhibition of thyroid hormone activity. In addition to preparing the uterus for egg implantation and maintaining pregnancy, optimum levels of progesterone are associated with helping to build and maintain bone, regulating fluid balance, supporting thyroid function, increasing energy and sex drive, promoting appetite, and protecting against breast cancer and osteoporosis.

During a normal 28-day menstrual cycle, oestrogen and progesterone, and the hormones that control their release, LH and FSH, co-ordinate the maturation and release of an egg, with the preparation of the uterus wall lining. Oestrogen dominates in the first half of the cycle, with levels peaking at ovulation, and falling thereafter. Progesterone levels start rising just prior to ovulation and continue rising to a peak. If there is no pregnancy, progesterone levels drop, you have a period and the whole cycle begins again.

So, getting the balance right between the two is therefore an important part of fulfilling your total health potential.

What are the signs of oestrogen/progesterone imbalance?

The higher the ratio of oestrogen to progesterone, the higher the risk of health problems such as headaches, migraines, anxiety, cloudy thinking, food cravings, irregular bleeding, breast tenderness, weight gain, water retention and depression.

What causes oestrogen/progesterone imbalance?

Causes of too little progesterone	Causes of too much oestrogen
Chronic stress	Herbs such as black cohosh and damiana
Under-active pituitary gland	Xeno-oestrogens, particularly pesticides
Under-active thyroid gland	Foods contaminated with growth hormone
Ovarian problems	Constipation, liver problems HRT, birth control pills

How to assess if you have a sex-hormone imbalance

The only accurate way to test your hormone levels is to get a blood or saliva test conducted by a reputable laboratory. You can, however, use the questionnaire below to help you decide whether further testing is necessary.

QUESTIONNAIRE: sex-hormone imbalance (for women)

For each question score 0 for no; 1 for occasionally; 3 for yes, then total up the section.

Do you:

1. Experience premenstrual mood swings? ☐

▶

2. Use or have you used, birth control pills or hormone medication? ☐

3. Experience irregular, lengthy or uncomfortable periods? ☐

4. Have a history of miscarriage or infertility? ☐

5. Have painful or lumpy breasts? ☐

6. Experience cyclical headaches or migraines? ☐

7. Gain weight easily or find it hard to lose weight? ☐

8. Experience peri-or post-menopausal discomfort (such as hot flushes, weight gain, sweats or insomnia)? ☐

9. Have acne, excessive facial hair and/or are known to have PCOS (polycystic ovarian syndrome)? ☐

Total score ☐

A score of 6 or more indicates that you should consider hormone saliva testing.

Hormone saliva test

Saliva tests are one of the most effective ways of diagnosing whether you have an existing oestrogen/progesterone imbalance (as is a blood test). In addition to progesterone and oestrogen, it is also helpful to know your levels of testosterone (I discuss this later), the adrenal hormones DHEA and cortisol, and melatonin – all of these influence female hormones. Contact Individual Wellbeing Diagnostic Laboratories (see Resources, page 422) and they will send out the kit; you provide a saliva sample and return it to them. The test I recommend is the comprehensive female hormone panel.

How to treat your oestrogen/progesterone imbalance

If your test results show that you have an oestrogen/progesterone imbalance, then I would strongly encourage you to seek help from a nutritional therapist or integrated medical doctor who has experience in female hormonal imbalances.

Step 1 • Treat the underlying imbalances

To ensure long-term well-being, you need to be addressing:

- **Nutritional deficiencies** These include deficiencies in minerals such as magnesium, B vitamins, vitamin E, vitamin C and essential fatty acids.

- **Candida overgrowth** This can be a significant contributor, especially if you have a history of taking antibiotics and/or the oestrogen contraceptive pill. See Barrier 7 for more information.

- **Digestive health problems** Low stomach acid, enzyme deficiency and leaky gut syndrome are all contributors. See Barrier 3 for more information.

- **Toxins** We are exposed to thousands of toxins each day via the food we eat, water we drink, air we breathe and products we use. Some of these, especially those found in certain plastics, are known to interfere with hormonal balance and the body's biochemistry. See Barrier 4 for more information.

- **Alcohol** Women who drink more than 12 units of alcohol a week are known to have higher oestrogen but lower progesterone levels than those who drink less. Moderate consumption of alcohol has been linked to decreased fertility.

- **Processed diets and stimulants** See Barrier 1 for more information.

- **Stress** Prolonged periods of stress interfere with hormonal balance. Cortisol, the main stress hormone, for example, is known to compete with progesterone and reduce its activity within the body. See Barrier 9 for more information.

Step 2 • Reduce your exposure to xeno-oestrogens

Xeno-oestrogens are chemicals found in our environment that are known to interfere with hormonal balance, impair immune function and increase the risk of cancer.[7] Because their shape is similar to our body's own natural supply of oestrogen, they can stimulate those receptors and lead to problems.

- **Go organic** Pesticides are the single greatest source of xeno-oestrogens.

- **Stay clear of fatty food** such as full-fat cream/dairy and fatty meat, as xeno-oestrogens are concentrated here. If you eat meat, leave the skin and drain off the fat.

- **Growth hormones** given to animals are another source of xeno-oestrogens. Steer clear of drinking non-organic milk and eating non-organic meat.

- **Drink pure water** that is known to be free from hormone-disrupting chemicals. Plastic bottles leach these chemicals into them. If you do drink from them make sure that the bottle has not been left out in the sun or heated.

- **Limit your use of plastic clingfilm** wherever possible, use glass storage jars instead of plastic and never microwave food in a plastic bowl.

Step 3 • Eat the right kinds of food

- **If your oestrogen levels are too low**, the following foods can help to raise oestrogen levels naturally: apples, plums, cherries, coconut, tomatoes, potatoes, olives, yams, carrots and brown rice.

- **If your oestrogen levels are too high**, fermented soya foods such as tempeh and miso can help to normalise excessive amounts of oestrogen. They contain substances called genisteins, a type of phyto-oestrogen that blocks oestrogen from binding on to their receptors. Other phyto-oestrogens include apples, flaxseed, nuts, celery, whole grains and alfalfa.

By following the healthy eating programme in Barrier 1, you can stabilise blood-sugar fluctuations, as these can trigger symptoms such as hot flushes, fatigue and irritability.

Step 4 • Exercise regularly

A regular moderate-intensity exercise programme that incorporates weight bearing and works against gravity (such as jogging and dancing) and resistance training (such as weights) can help to reduce hot flushes and prevent the bones from thinning. See the exercise mind–body tool (page 350) for further suggestions.

Step 5 • Take supplements to balance your hormones

In addition to taking the foundation nutritional supplements mentioned in Barrier 1, you should also consider the following. If you are in any doubt as to what is best for you, seek the help of a nutritional therapist or doctor specialising in women's hormone imbalances.

- **Natural progesterone** This cream has been widely popularised by the late Dr John Lee, a medical doctor who spent the majority of his life pioneering natural approaches to managing female hormone-related conditions, such as PCOS (polycystic ovarian syndrome), the menopause, PMS and fibrocystic breast disease.[8] One study found that 83 per cent of women using progesterone experienced a significant improvement in their menopausal symptoms, compared to 19 per cent on placebo.[9] Progesterone cream should be used under the supervision of an integrated medical doctor and its effects should always be monitored through the use of saliva testing. For more information see Resources, page 423.

- **Vitex agnus castus** is one of the most widely recommended herbs for women with hormonal imbalances. It acts on the hypothalamus and pituitary glands by increasing luteinizing hormone (LH) production and mildly inhibiting the release of follicle stimulating hormone (FSH). The result is a shift in the ratio of oestrogen to progesterone, in favour of progesterone. It is therefore most commonly used with women who have symptoms relating to progesterone deficiency – this can include women with premenstrual syndrome, abnormal menstrual cycles, polycystic ovary syndrome, and peri-menopausal and menopausal symptoms.[10] The usual dose is 4mg a day of a standardised extract containing 6 per cent of adnusides.

- **Black cohosh** is commonly used to treat the symptoms of the menopause, such as hot flushes, sleep disturbances and sweating. It is also known to raise levels of the happy-mood neurotransmitter serotonin, so it is helpful particularly if symptoms are accompanied by a depressed mood. How black cohosh works is unclear.[11] The usual dose is 20–40mg a day, containing 1 or 2mg of 27-deoxyactein. It should not be used if you have any pre-existing liver problems.

- **Dong quai**, also known as Chinese angelica, and the female ginseng have been used for thousands of years in traditional Chinese medicine. Despite its popular use in treating symptoms relating to the menopause, to date there has been conflicting evidence concerning its effectiveness.[12] This might be because it is designed to be used in conjunction with other herbs such as agnus castus or chamomile. (**Note** Dong quai can thin the blood so it shouldn't be taken if you are on warfarin.) The recommended dose is 600mg a day.

Testosterone imbalances in men

This section is mainly focused on testosterone levels as they relate to men. Whereas testosterone levels do have a significant role to play in the health of women, I do not advocate attempting to treat testosterone imbalances in women without professional advice and supervision. My own experience with helping men with testosterone imbalances, however, is that as long as the levels are being monitored the following advice can be used safely and effectively.

Testosterone, a hormone produced by the adrenal glands and testis in men, can have a significant effect on the way that you feel and on the health and growth of the body. For example, testosterone influences sex drive, calcium deposition in the bones, muscle growth, strength, stamina, red cell production and even cholesterol levels.[13] From the age of 30 onwards, levels of biologically active (free) testosterone starts dropping at a rate of between 1 and 2 per cent per year, until the age of 70. By the time a man reaches 80, he has a 1 in 2 chance of having a testosterone level low enough to be causing health problems.

In men, low testosterone levels lead to a lowering of libido, motivation and energy, depression, deteriorating memory, excess weight around the middle, impotence, infertility, high cholesterol, soft erections and loss of muscle mass. With the obvious exception of the soft erections, the effects on women are similar.

In women high testosterone levels can be a feature of a genetically inherited condition called polycystic ovarian syndrome. This gives rise to the classic signs of excessive hair growth, acne, weight gain and failure to ovulate.

What causes testosterone imbalance?

As we age, levels of testosterone do naturally fall, but there are specific factors that are known to accelerate this decline. These factors include:

- Stress

- Thyroid and adrenal imbalances

- Smoking

- Nutritional deficiencies

- Lack of dietary fibre

- Environmental toxins

- The hormone oestrogen

- Andropause – the male menopause

How to assess if you have low testosterone

The only accurate way to test your testosterone levels is to get a blood or saliva test conducted by a reputable laboratory.

QUESTIONNAIRE: low testosterone (for men)

For each question score 0 for no; 1 for occasionally; 3 for yes, then total up the section.

Are you:

1. Over the age of 50?

2. Losing weight unintentionally?

3. Losing muscle mass?

4. Experiencing a lower sex drive?

5. Experiencing softer erections?

6. Experiencing increasing fatigue and deteriorating stamina?

7. Experiencing enlargement of your breasts?

8. Experiencing any prostate problems, such as difficulty urinating, or poor urine stream?

9. Having any memory lapses or periods of forgetfulness?

Total score

If you score 8 or more, this suggests you should consider a saliva test or seeing a nutritional therapist or integrated medical doctor for advice.

Testosterone saliva test

Saliva tests for testosterone are one of the most effective ways of diagnosing whether you have an existing testosterone imbalance (as is a blood test). Contact Individual Wellbeing Diagnostic Laboratories (see Resources, page 423) and they will send out the kit; you provide a saliva sample and return it to them.

How to treat your low testosterone

If your test results show that you have low levels of testosterone, then I would strongly encourage you to seek help from a nutritional therapist or integrated medical doctor who has experience in male hormonal imbalances.

Step 1 • Treat the underlying cause

The main causes to identify and treat are:

- **Psychological stress** See Barrier 9

- **Environmental chemicals and pollutants** See Barrier 4

- **Smoking** See Barrier 10

- **Adrenal/thyroid imbalances** See the first part of this chapter

Step 2 • Avoid foods that lower testosterone or increase oestrogen

Avoid:

- **Excessive consumption of alcohol** (more than 21 units per week).

- **Saturated fatty foods**, such as red meat and full-fat dairy, cow's milk, sugar and refined carbohydrates such as biscuits, cakes, pastries and white bread can all interfere with testosterone levels – these should be avoided/limited.

- **Go organic** Pesticides can have oestrogen-like effects in the body – oestrogen has been associated with prostate enlargement and prostate cancer.

- **Oats can help to raise free testosterone**, and vegetables containing a chemical called indole-3-carbinole, such as broccoli, kale and Brussels sprouts, can help to prevent the negative effects of oestrogen.[14]

- **Drink nettle tea** Researchers have found that testosterone can bind to a type of protein called sex hormone binding globulin (SHBG). If it does, it no longer becomes available to have biological effects within the body. Nettle root has been found to bind to SHBG thus making more free testosterone available in the body.[15]

- **Being overweight** can reduce testosterone levels, so try combining the healthy eating programme (Barrier 1) with exercise (page 350) to help you lose fat and gain muscle mass.

Step 3 • Exercise regularly

Moderate-intensity exercise, five times a week for at least 30 minutes each time has been shown to boost levels of free testosterone in men of all age groups. See the exercise mind–body tool for further suggestions. It's important to include weight training in addition to cardiovascular work.

Step 4 • Take supplements to raise testosterone

There are a couple of options available to you, but whichever option you choose it is important you monitor your testosterone levels at least every three months. It is possible to raise testosterone too high – this would lead to symptoms such as hair loss, acne, oily skin and hair, weight gain and irritability. Do not use any of these if you have or suspect you might have prostate cancer. And remember to check regularly your testosterone levels and PSA (a blood marker that can indicate prostate cancer).

- **Zinc** 50mg helps to stop the conversion of testosterone into oestrogen, as well as helping to raise testosterone levels and boost sperm count. In one study 37 infertile men with decreased testosterone levels and associated low sperm counts were given 60mg of zinc daily for 50 days. In 22 of these patients, testosterone levels significantly increased and mean sperm count rose from 8 million to 20 million.[16]

- **Testosterone replacement therapy** is available on prescription or privately, and is available as patches, gel, capsules, oral lozenges, injections and implants. It's crucially important that you don't use any synthetic testosterone product – this includes methyltestosterone – as these have been associated with increased risk of cancer and liver problems.

- **The herb saw palmetto** has been used to treat benign prostatic enlargement; it works by inhibiting the enzyme that converts the testosterone into dehydrotestosterone, a hormone that stimulates prostate cell growth. It also blocks oestrogens and should be used alongside testosterone replacement therapy.[17]

MIND–BODY ESSENTIALS

- Sex hormone imbalances are common among the Western population. Nutritional deficiencies, chronic stress, alcohol, smoking and particularly environmental toxins are known to interfere with the precise regulation and co-ordination of hormonal flow.

- As a general rule of thumb hormonal imbalances will improve with a wholefood, natural diet, regular moderate exercise, cessation of smoking and moderation of alcohol, stress management and nutritional supplementation.

- Of the specific treatments available for correcting hormonal imbalances in women, natural progesterone, agnus castus and black cohosh are the most promising.

- Of the treatments available for testosterone imbalance in men, zinc, testosterone replacement therapy and saw palmetto are the most promising.

- Recommended mind–body tools to accompany this sectioin: creative visualisation (page 319), Bach Flower Remedies (page 298), meditation (page 376), conscious breathing (page 314) and relaxation (page 380).

- For recommended reading see Resources, pages 426–7.

Insulin imbalance – metabolic syndrome

I recently gave a public lecture in which I talked about a condition called metabolic syndrome. Despite the fact that it affects 25 per cent of the British population and is a big risk factor for heart disease, stroke, high blood pressure, polycystic ovary syndrome, Alzheimer's disease and type II diabetes, only two people in an audience of 100 had heard about it[18] – and 50 per cent of the audience were doctors and nurses! It was a stark reminder to me how essential health knowledge can take a long time to filter through to the people who need to hear about it.

What is metabolic syndrome?

Metabolic syndrome (or syndrome X as it is also known), is not a disease but a collection of metabolic imbalances, and a by-product of obesity, chronic inflammation and stress. The most common features of metabolic syndrome, and the tell-tale signs that show you might be affected by it, are:

- Excess body fat around the middle.

- High levels of fats in the blood that are known to be associated with disease.

- Reduced levels of the 'good' fat high-density lipoprotein (HDL) cholesterol.

- Raised blood pressure.

- Blood that has an increased tendency to clot.

At the heart of metabolic syndrome is insulin resistance.

Insulin resistance

Insulin is a hormone produced by specialised cells in the pancreas, in response to raised blood sugar. One of insulin's main jobs is to drive glucose plus other nutrients into the cells of the body, especially muscle cells. Insulin resistance is said to be occurring when those same cells lose their sensitivity to insulin. As to why this happens is still unclear, but the research shows that a combination of genetic factors, obesity, inactivity, high cortisol levels due to stress and a diet high in sugar and refined foods are all significant players. Of these, obesity is considered to be the most significant. Whereas most people tend to think of the rolls of fat that they carry around their waist as inert – that is, it just sits there and does nothing – the truth is quite the opposite. Researchers have found that fat is a living tissue that is constantly exchanging and influencing the rest of the body through hormones called adipokines.[19] In addition to regulating the appetite and metabolic rate, adipokines also influence inflammation. This is important to know because the fatter you are, the greater the number of hormones produced and the higher the level of inflammation within the body. This is a problem, because it is this chronic low-grade inflammation (that I talked about in Barrier 5) that makes the body more resistant to the effects of insulin.[20]

As your cells become resistant to insulin, blood-sugar levels increase, and the pancreas is forced to produce more insulin to compensate, leaving you with a hormonal imbalance. The higher insulin levels result in more glucose being stored as fat, plus it prevents cells from breaking down fat. This double whammy makes it very hard to lose weight – in fact if you really struggle to lose weight, this might be the reason why!

The result: your waistline gets bigger, levels of good (HDL) cholesterol levels go down, inflammation levels rise, blood pressure goes up (due to retained sodium and constricting blood vessels), and the blood becomes thicker. Before you know it metabolic syndrome has crept up on you and you are a walking time bomb for more serious disease.

Do you have metabolic syndrome?

Because metabolic syndrome can progress to killers such as diabetes, heart disease and cancer, diagnosing it early and treating it fully offers you a great escape – an opportunity to prevent the inevitable deterioration in health. Here are two other ways to diagnose it.

Blood test

The definitive test for metabolic syndrome is a comprehensive insulin resistance blood test. Your healthcare provider might be able to provide this for you; alternatively you can arrange the test via Individual Wellbeing Diagnostic Laboratories (see Resources, page 422). The test involves you fasting for eight hours then having a sample of blood taken from you. The lab will then measure the levels of various markers. Whereas guidelines differ slightly as to what results constitute metabolic syndrome, one set of criteria indicate that a diagnosis can be made if you have three or more of the following:[21]

- Your waist measures more than 102cm (40in) if you are a man, or more than 86cm (34in) if you are a woman.

- The level of fats called triglycerides in your blood is 1.7 mmol/L before breakfast.

- Your level of good (HDL) cholesterol is less than 1 mmol/L if you are a man, or less than 1.3 mmol/L if you are a woman.

- The level of glucose in your blood is more than 6 mmol/L before breakfast.

- Your blood pressure is 130/85 or higher.

Metabolic-syndrome questionnaire

Another less accurate way to assess the possibility of you having metabolic syndrome is to fill in the following questionnaire.

QUESTIONNAIRE: metabolic syndrome

For each question score 0 for no; 1 for occasionally; 3 for yes, then total up the section.

Do you:

1. Struggle with your weight despite watching what you eat?

▶

2. Experience forgetfulness, poor memory or mental confusion, particularly after eating? ☐

3. Store most of your body fat around your middle? ☐

4. Crave sugary or starchy foods? ☐

5. Have a waist size of more than 102cm (40in) if you are a man, or 86cm (34in) if you are a women? (score 6) ☐

6. Experience drowsiness or a drop in energy or mood after meals? ☐

7. Regularly feel tired despite having a good night's sleep? ☐

8. Have high blood pressure or high cholesterol? ☐

9. Have a history of early heart disease or diabetes in your family? ☐

Total score ☐

If your blood test comes back positive and/or you scored 6 or more on the questionnaire then I would recommend that you follow my metabolic-syndrome programme.

How to treat metabolic syndrome

Step 1 • Treat the underlying cause

The main causes to identify and treat are:

- **Obesity** See Barrier 1. In my experience most people who are obese will benefit from reducing their carbohydrate intake (and exercising).

- **Chronic inflammation** This is really important to address; see Barrier 5.

- **Physical inactivity** See mind–body tool 7.

- **Psychological stress** See Barrier 9.

- **Sex/adrenal/thyroid imbalances** See the first part of this chapter.

Step 2 • Take supplements

When used in combination with a metabolic-type diet, exercise and an inflammation-reducing programme, supplements can really help your body to recover from metabolic syndrome. Here are the ones that I use most often use with my own patients:

- **Chromium** is essential to insulin and helps to drive blood glucose into the body's cells. A number of studies have found that supplementation of chromium can improve insulin sensitivity, cholesterol levels and blood-sugar levels.[22] Depending on the severity of the metabolic syndrome I usually recommend 400–1,000mcg of chromium polynicotinate a day.

- **The active components of fish oil**, EPA and DHA, are known to help burn fat and improve the efficiency with which the body uses glucose. When used in high enough dosages fish oil can also help reduce the low-grade inflammation that is often seen in people with metabolic syndrome.[23] The usual dose is 3,000mg a day.

- **The antioxidant alpha-lipoic acid** can improve insulin resistance and increase glucose uptake into muscle cells. The dose is 100mg per day.[24]

- **Coenzyme Q10**, 30mg daily may help to improve the function of insulin-producing cells in the pancreas, as well as lower blood pressure and raise HDL cholesterol levels.[25]

- **L-glutamine** If cravings are a problem for you, try taking 1,000mg of the amino acid L-glutamine three times a day. It's great for reducing cravings and helps to keep the blood sugars stable.[26]

Now that you have reached the end of this chapter, my advice is to re-read it one more time. While doing so highlight those sentences (using a highlighter pen) that you feel are important to you. Once you've done this write down at least five steps or actions that you are going to take, and spend a moment visualising yourself implementing them. Once you have completed this, move on to your next barrier.

MIND–BODY ESSENTIALS

- Metabolic syndrome is a major risk factor for heart disease, cancer, diabetes and many other disease conditions.

- The number-one risk factor for developing metabolic syndrome appears to be the combination of obesity and chronic low-grade inflammation.

- Successful reversal of the metabolic syndrome involves combining fat loss through a personalised nutrition and exercise programme, plus the addition of supplements that will increase insulin sensitivity and reduce inflammation.

- Recommended mind–body tools to accompany this section: exercise (page 350), emotional freedom technique (page 332), and instant stress release (page 368).

- For recommended reading see Resources, pages 426–7.

Candida and parasites

Patrick, a 45-year-old self-employed man, had experienced tiredness, fuzzy thinking and abdominal bloating for over three years. Although his GP was very supportive and understanding, all tests turned up negative and he was told that it was probably all down to the stress that he had been experiencing for quite some time. He was advised to take some time off and to see if that helped, which he did – but it didn't. Fortunately Patrick had seen an article that I had written for a self-help group called the National Candida Society, and because of what he read he contacted me. The symptoms he was experiencing fitted almost exactly the symptoms of a common yeast infection called candida, that I was writing about. The tests I arranged confirmed the diagnosis, and three months after starting the programme all of his symptoms without exception had resolved, and he was back at work. What's more the experience had made him re-evaluate his life and his priorities, and as a result he decided to take a part-time nutritional course, to learn more about how nutrition can help people achieve total health.

Patrick's candida infection, like most illnesses, was really a signpost to other deeper imbalances – in his case failing to take care of his body and emotional needs. When he addressed those with my support and guidance, and dealt with the candida using nutritional and psychological approaches, his body responded very quickly and positively.

In this chapter I am going to share with you the same integrated treatment programmes that I use with my patients for two factors that can contribute to ill health— candida and parasites.

Candida infection

Candida is yeast that quietly resides in our intestines. As long as the body remains in a healthy state, it rarely causes problems. However, in some people, usually those who have been exposed to prolonged treatment with antibiotics and steroids, or who have experienced prolonged periods of stress, it can overgrow and transform into a more pathogenic fungus form. In its fungal form it develops long rootlike structures called rhizoids, which invade the local gut wall. In addition to this these pathogenic or disease-causing forms produce various toxins that can damage the lining of the gut and cause a wide range of debilitating and distressing symptoms, such as abdominal bloating, food allergies, fuzzy thinking, thrush, depression, hormone imbalances and fatigue.[1]

How do we get candida?

Factors that predispose a person to candida include a history of anti-biotic usage (antibiotics kill off healthy bacteria, but candida remain due to their natural resistance), steroids, the contraceptive pill, poor diet, compromised immune function, psychological stress and impaired thyroid function/adrenal function.[2]

How to assess if you have candida

There are a couple of ways in which you can work whether candida is contributing to your symptoms or not. The first and easiest is to complete the candida questionnaire.

QUESTIONNAIRE: candida

For each question score 0 for no; 1 for occasionally; 3 for yes, then total up the section.

1. Do you suffer from yeast infections, such as thrush? ☐

2. Do you suffer from rashes on your body? ☐

3. Do you experience foggy-headedness? ☐

4. Do you have bloating or abdominal distension? ☐

5. Have you previously or do you use birth control pills or hormone medication? ☐

6. Do you have uncomfortable periods – cramps, lengthy, heavy bleeding, tender breasts? ☐

7. Have you used antibiotics extensively (at any time in your life)? ☐

8. Have you used steroids or birth control pills for more than one year? ☐

9. Do you have chronic fungus on nails, skin or suffer from athlete's foot? ☐

10. In the past have you had recurring sinus or ear infections? ☐

11. Do you suffer from chronic fatigue? ☐

12. Are your stools of an unusual colour, shape or consistency? ☐

Total score ☐

If you score more than 8 I would suggest you arrange to have a saliva test.

Saliva test

An IgA antibody saliva test is probably the most effective way of diagnosing whether you have an existing candida problem. If you contact

Individual Wellbeing Diagnostic Laboratories (see Resources, page 423) they will send out the kit; you provide a saliva sample and return it to them. Although they also offer a blood test, most of my patients find this test better because it doesn't involve taking blood.

How to treat candida

Once the diagnosis of candida has been made, the priority is to remove the candida while treating and resolving the underlying conditions that allowed it to grow in the first place.

Step 1 • Treat the underlying cause

The main causes to identify and treat are:

- **Dysbiosis** See Barrier 3.

- **Leaky-gut syndrome** See Barrier 3.

- **Lack of stomach acid** or digestive enzymes See Barrier 3.

- **Environmental chemicals and pollutants** See Barrier 4.

- **Parasites** (these can co-exist). See later on in this chapter.

- **Psychological stress** See Barrier 9.

Having treated over 100 patients with candida, a common feature among virtually all of them is a history of excessive amounts of mental and physical activity, and a failure to meet there own emotional needs. Over time this stress compromises the gut's immune system, and leads to behaviours that promote candida growth such as excess consumption of carbohydrates and sugars. If this resonates with you I would encourage you also to read Barrier 8, unmet emotional needs.

Step 2 • Start an anti-candida diet

As long as you are tackling the underlying causes of candida overgrowth and taking anti-candida supplements you shouldn't have to be on this restrictive diet for more than six weeks. I have many patients coming to me after two to three years of being on an anti-candida diet, and because the underlying issues weren't being addressed, they have become intolerant to virtually every type of food they have eaten! Avoid the following foods completely for the first six weeks of the programme:

- Sugar, including fruit juices, fruits, honey, maple syrup, corn syrup, chocolate and sucrose.

- Yeast-containing foods, such as dried fruit, peanut butter, chocolate, cakes, wheat, cow's dairy produce, mushrooms, mouldy cheese, tomato ketchup and no alcohol for the first six weeks (if you are feeling much better after that try the occasional gin or vodka in moderation).

- Foods to which you are allergic or intolerant – see Barrier 3.

For some recommended cookbooks, see Resources, page 427.

Step 2 • Take an anti-candida formula

The following need to be used for at least four to six months and need to be done in conjunction with dietary change and while addressing the underlying causes:

- **Oxygenated magnesium products.** I've used these with patients for over six years, and I've yet to find anything more effective. When oxygenated magnesium peroxide reaches the intestines it releases oxygen, which kills the candida. My advice is to start slowly with it (one or two capsules first thing in the morning) then increase by one capsule every third day, up to a maximum of five a day. If you develop diarrhoea or the symptoms get markedly worse, reduce your dose by one. After four months I gradually tailor the dose down eventually to zero (this only works if the underlying imbalances are dealt with). After two weeks, I would recommend you taking a combination of a lactobacillus sporogenes probiotic to repopulate the bowels, organic aloe vera juice to cleanse and provide nutrients for the bowel, and a glutamine supplement to repair the leaky gut. (See Resources, page 420 for suppliers.)

- **Threelac** This is the alternative to oxygenated magnesium, I've personally never used it, but some practitioners find it to be very useful. It contains a unique combination of lactic acid-producing bacterial strains of probiotics. The recommended dosage is one sachet per day for ten days, moving to two sachets per day for the next two months.

- **Candigest plus** consists of seven enzymes, which are designed to digest the protective wall of the candida, break down the carbohydrates on which it feeds and digest the interior of the candida cell. It can be used very effectively in combination with any of the supplements above. I tend to use it with magnesium peroxide.

Step 3 • Support your body's cleansing process

As the candida starts to die, you might start to experience deterioration in your symptoms. This period usually last for up to seven days or so. To support your body while going through this try the following:

- Drink 2–3 litres (3½–5 ¼ pints) of water a day.

- Take the herb milk thistle to support liver function and aloe vera to help the gut.

- Drink an alkaline salt solution, such as Higher Nature's Alkaclear, just before going to bed. This can ease the symptoms and you could actually continue taking this throughout the entire six-month programme outlined in Step 2.

Step 4 • Switch to coconut oil

The medium-chain saturated fatty acids in organic virgin coconut oil are an effective treatment against candida. You can eat it straight from the spoon if you like – it doesn't taste that bad. Take a tablespoon three times a day for the first week, and then reduce to two tablespoons a day for a further three weeks.

Step 5 • Troubleshooting

In about 10 per cent of people with candida, significant improvements don't happen for a variety of reasons. More often than not it's because they have mercury toxicity and/or parasites. If you think this might apply to you my advice would be to seek some professional help from a nutritional therapist or integrated medical doctor.

Parasite infections

A parasite infection is a commonly overlooked cause of health problems, including irritable bowel syndrome, abdominal bloating, diarrhoea, abdominal pain, foul-smelling stools, allergies, fatigue and indigestion.[3] If you have any history of international travel then this is definitely one that you should take a look at. An estimated 40 per cent of the world's population are thought to be infected by one or more different parasites. The most common parasites are: [4]

- *Blastocystis hominis* Great Smokies laboratory in the USA, who specialise in parasite detection, found this parasite in about 20 per cent of samples they received. It tends to cause problems only when someone's immune system has been weakened. Symptoms include fatigue, anorexia, weight loss, flatulence, irritable bowel syndrome and chronic fatigue.

- *Dientamoeba fragilis* causes diarrhoea and abdominal discomfort.

- *Giardia lamblia* A study in the *Journal of Nutritional Medicine* showed that 27 per cent of patients studied with chronic fatigue had *Giardia* infection. In addition to fatigue it can also cause diarrhoea and anorexia.

The most common way of acquiring parasites is by ingesting parasite eggs through food, fruits and vegetables grown on contaminated soils, drinking or walking through contaminated water, from household pets, sex with infected partners, eating raw or undercooked meat or fish, poor food preparation and sanitation.

How to assess if you have parasites

One of the biggest challenges faced by a health practitioner is finding an accurate way to assess whether their patients have parasites or not.

The stool test described on page 188 is one of the classic tests. However, it can provide false results; that is, give a negative test when parasites are present. It just depends on whether that particular stool sample contained parasites or not, and on the accuracy of the test. As a general rule of thumb I will use the following questionnaire with my patients, and if they score highly then I will either commence treatment straight away or arrange a stool test and then start treatment.

QUESTIONNAIRE: parasites

For each question score 0 for no; 1 for occasionally; 3 for yes, then total up the section.

Do you:

1. Experience restless sleep? ☐

2. Have any skin problems, such as rashes or itches? ☐

3. Grind your teeth when asleep? ☐

4. Have cravings for certain foods such as chocolate, cheese or doughy foods? ☐

5. Feel tired most of the time? ☐

6. Experience bloating or excess wind? ☐

7. Have anaemia? ☐

8. Experience muscle aches or pains? ☐

9. Suffer from migraines or regular headaches? ☐

10. Experience constipation or diarrhoea? ☐

11. Travel abroad? ☐

12. Have any food allergies? ☐

13. Have recurrent, unexplained symptoms? ☐

▶

14. Have anal or rectal itching? ☐

15. Get a fever for no obvious reason? ☐

16. Have dark circles under your eyes? ☐

17. Have foul-smelling stools? ☐

Total score ☐

A score of 20 or more may suggest parasites. You should consider further testing.

Comprehensive parasitology

This stool test reports all bacterial flora (beneficial, imbalanced and pathogenic), yeasts, and intestinal parasites (worms, eggs, lava and protozoa), and may be used to monitor treatment for bacterial, yeast or parasitic infections. You will be sent a container to place the sample in, and then you post it back to the laboratory. For more information contact Individual Wellbeing Diagnostic Laboratories (see Resources, page 420).

How to treat your parasites

Once the diagnosis of parasites has been made, the choice of treatment will really depend on which parasites you have. As for many of the other imbalances that I've discussed so far, it's important not only to kill the parasites but also to treat and resolve the underlying conditions that allowed them to grow in the first place.

Step 1 • Treat the underlying cause

The main causes to identify and treat are:

- **Dysbiosis** See Barrier 3

- **Leaky-gut syndrome** See Barrier 3

- **Lack of stomach acid or digestive enzymes** See Barrier 3

- **Environmental chemicals and pollutants** See Barrier 4

- **Candida** (these often coexist) See the beginning of this chapter

- **Psychological stress** See Barrier 9

Step 2 • Take an anti-parasite formula

Patience is part and parcel of treating parasites – the most effective anti-parasite programmes need to be followed for at least three months. The two that I recommend (from which you should choose one) are:

- **Biotics Research ADP** Contains an extract of the herb oregano. The dosage is three times a day just before meals for one week, then three tablets, three times a day just before meals for four weeks. After 14 days on ADP, add in Biotics probiotic Biodophilus-FOS and Colon Plus Capsules. The latter contains psyllium, flaxseed, apple pectin, lactobacillus acidophilus, bromelain and other nutrients known to help normalise bowel flora and function.

- **Nutri's wormwood and black walnut** contains a number of known and effective anti-parasite herbs including wormwood, fennel, fenugreek, garlic and black walnut leaves. Follow the instructions that come with it. After two weeks start Nutri's psyllium and apple pectin to cleanse the bowels, Nutri's Enterogenic Concentrate, to repopulate the bowels with probiotics, and Nutri's permeability factors to repair any leaky gut caused by the parasites.

Step 3 • Cut down on sugars

Sugar is one of parasites' favourite foods, so for the duration of the parasite programme you should exclude all obvious sources of sugar, including fruit juice and chocolate. A piece of fruit such as an apple or pear once or twice a day is fine. Better still, follow the healthy-eating plan in Barrier 1.

Step 4 • Prevent re-infection

Once the parasites have been successfully treated (you should know because you will feel significantly better), you should consider precautions to prevent a further parasite infection. Here are a some tips:

- When travelling, take a lactobacillus probiotic supplement and an anti-parasite formula, such as Higher Nature's Paraclens, to prevent infection.

- Drink clean, pure water.

- Avoid raw or under-cooked beef, chicken, pork and fish.

- Avoid fruit and vegetables that are not properly washed. Don't eat the skin of fruits. In countries where drinking the tap water is not recommended do not eat salads or raw vegetables.

- Wash your hands after handling pets or working outdoors.

- Never let your pets lick your face or your plates.

- Worm your pets regularly.

Now that you have reached the end of this chapter, my advice is to re-read it one more time. While doing so highlight those sentences (using a highlighter pen) that you feel are important to you. Once you've done this write down at least five steps or actions that you are going to take, and spend a moment visualising yourself implementing them. Once you have completed this, move on to your next barrier.

MIND–BODY ESSENTIALS

- Health problems that don't resolve with treatment, or ongoing digestive imbalances, particularly bloating, should arouse suspicion that candida and/or parasites might be present.

- Switching to a low-sugar, low-yeast, low-processed, high-wholefood diet is an important part in helping your body to recover.

- Of the many supplements available to treat candida and parasites I have found oxygenated magnesium (for candida), oregano, wormwood and black walnut (for parasites) in combination with a probiotics formula to be the most effective.

- Recommended mind–body tools to accompany this chapter: creative visualisation (page 319), Bach Flower Remedies (page 298), meditation (page 376), conscious breathing (page 314) and relaxation (page 380).

- For recommended reading see Resources, page 427.

Unmet emotional needs

Mike had a long history of clinical depression stretching back some 22 years. Like many people with depression he had taken antidepressants, found some benefit, but relapsed a couple of months after stopping them.

This cycle of on–off depression is very common in my experience and a very clear indicator that the underlying reason for the depression hasn't yet been addressed. My job as an integrated medical doctor is to work out what the underlying cause is. In Mike's case it was fairly straightforward.

I classify the underlying causes of depression into two camps: biological and psychological. The biological can include things like nutrient deficiencies, allergies, hormonal imbalances, medications and toxic influences. Someone with a biological depression tends to have quite severe depressive symptoms, is generally unresponsive to talk therapy approaches and is less likely to experience a remission. Mike's questionnaire results and history suggested that he did not have a biological depression. His underlying cause was psychological, and, more specifically, unmet emotional needs. The long-term solution to resolving Mike's depression was to start getting his emotional needs met.

What are emotional needs?

I came across the idea of emotional needs after having read about the Human Givens psychotherapy approach to mental health.[1] At the heart of the Human Givens approach is the idea that we experience distress when we are not meeting our innate emotional needs. There are many of these emotional needs, all of which are connected to our survival and evolution. I've described the main ones below:

- **The need for security** This includes the security of living in a safe environment and neighbourhood, and the safety of knowing that you are physically and emotionally safe in the presence of the people that surround you. This includes people at home and your place of work.

- **The need for intimacy** The desire to experience emotional, sexual and psychological closeness or intimacy is one of our most powerful drives, and yet frequently the one that gets ignored, denied or repressed. Intimacy (literally meaning 'into-me-see'), arises when two individuals drop their persona and defences and allow themselves to be present with one another.

- **The need for positive attention** You just have to watch a child, to witness how powerful this need is. Children need attention, and will do everything in their power to get the attention of their parent, either through behaving themselves and performing well or, if that fails, through misbehaving. Either way, they need attention and so do we as adults. However, to thrive as human beings we also need to allow ourselves to receive positive attention as well.

- **The need to feel socially connected** We are intrinsically social creatures and need to feel that we are part of something beyond our immediate family group. Having a wider social network (friends) and enjoying the company of people with similar or common interests is a key need if we are to create total health. Having a network of friends and participating in groups or community-related projects are well known to protect against depression.

- **The need for control** A person who feels that they have some degree of control in respect of their life situation (work, finances and relationships) is able to withstand stress and life's challenges much more effectively than someone who has little or no control. For example, people with little or no control at work experience higher levels of stress and anxiety than those with more control.

- **The need for status** In any given social situation we each need to feel that we have our place and purpose, a sense that we are being recognised and respected for who we are. This needs to include our place within the home and at work.

- **The need to feel competent** Self-esteem (the estimation of ourselves) is intimately tied up with feeling competent and having a sense of accomplishment in what we do. This can apply in many aspects of our life, including relationships, lovemaking, work, recreation and sports.

- **The need for positive meaning and purpose** This is the big one! Our minds are constantly trying to attach meaning to what we do and what we experience. When something has meaning, it takes on importance and adds depth and flavour to our life – for better or for worse. Something that holds a positive meaning for you – for example, a vision to make a success of your business – enables you to look beyond and find solutions to problems and challenges that would otherwise be blockages to your development and success. Tied in with meaning is purpose: the feeling of determination and drive that comes from having a vision and belief in what you are doing.

That's one half of the equation. The second half is that to help us meet these needs nature endowed us with specific resources:

- The ability to develop, learn and acquire new knowledge and insight.

- The ability to build rapport, empathise and connect with others.

- Imagination, which enables us to solve problems, plan our futures, instruct the subconscious mind and alter memories that might be adversely affecting us.

- A conscious, rational mind that can analyse, make plans and control our emotions.

- The ability to 'know': understand the world unconsciously through metaphorical pattern matching.

- An observing self: a part of us that can step back from, and observe, our emotions and thoughts.

- Dreaming is nature's way of discharging stress. Expectations that aroused the autonomic nervous system during the day and were not discharged are metaphorically completed in dream stories during REM sleep, leaving us refreshed and ready for the new day.

Using these resources to meet your emotional needs in a healthy and balanced way is one of the most important keys to fulfilling your total health potential. A failure to meet our emotional needs leads to emotional and psychological distress, whether we are aware of it or not. If left unresolved, this accumulated distress often deteriorates into anxiety, addictions, depression and, in the predisposed, psychosis. The key to mental health, therefore, is to identify which emotional needs need to be met.

Identifying unmet emotional needs

If you've identified this as one of your barriers, then your first step is to make an assessment of the degree to which your emotional needs are being met right now, by filling in the emotional needs questionnaire below. Read through each question slowly and spend a few moments thinking about how fulfilled you are in respect of the issue being asked about.

For each emotional need, give yourself a score of between 0 and 5 (0 = emotional need completely unmet and unfulfilled, and 5 = emotional need completely met and fulfilled). Watch out for the tendency to rush this exercise or to score yourself too highly. Ask yourself once you have a score in mind, 'Does this score feel accurate?'; if it does, great, write it down; if it doesn't, reassess and score again.

QUESTIONNAIRE: unmet emotional needs

For each emotional need, give yourself a score of between 0 and 5 (0 = emotional need completely unmet and unfulfilled, and 5 = emotional need completely met and fulfilled).

To what degree:

1. Do you feel safe? ☐

2. Do you receive enough positive attention from those around you? ☐

3. Can you attain privacy when you need to? ☐

4. Do you give positive attention to those around you? ☐

5. Do you have a sense of autonomy and control in your life? ☐

6. Do you feel emotionally connected to others? ☐

7. Do you feel part of the wider community? ☐

8. Are you able to experience friendship and intimacy? ☐

9. Do you have a sense of competence and achievement? ☐

10. Do you live your life with meaning and purpose? ☐

11. Are you respected and acknowledged by your peers? ☐

12. Are you respected and acknowledged by your family? ☐

13. Are you respected and acknowledged by your partner (if applicable)? ☐

Having completed the questionnaire, go through it again and check with yourself whether the score you have given yourself truly reflects the facts of the situation as it currently stands. Generally, the lower the score, the greater need for some action to be taken in order to start meeting that need. For those emotional needs that you have scored 3 or less, highlight them with a marker pen, and, starting with the need that you scored lowest with, follow the suggestions below in order to start meeting that need.

Meeting your emotional needs

This is not a Human Givens exercise, but one that I have adapted for use with my own patients. It's more effective if you write down your answers as you proceed through the questions. To demonstrate how the process works I've shared with you a real-life example of the dialogue that took place with Mike:

Step 1

Identify your lowest scoring unmet emotional need and write down its opposite.

Mike's example: *I feel safe [for which he scored 2] becomes I feel unsafe.*

Step 2

In as much detail as possible, describe what this means to you.

Mike's example: *I don't like the area I live in; I get very nervous walking down the streets at night. I feel intimidated by, and uncomfortable around, most people. I don't have enough money in my bank account to feel financially safe.*

Step 3

When you think about this situation, how does it make you feel?

Mike's example: *Scared, vulnerable, sad and isolated.*

Step 4

How does this impact on other areas of your life?

Mike's example: *I am reluctant to invite people around to my house, I* *don't look forward to the start of the day, I am reluctant to change my job, which doesn't pay well, but it is secure.*

Step 5

Now take ten minutes to do this visualisation exercise. This will help you find solutions to your unmet emotional need:

Exercise: visualisation

1. Close your eyes and imagine that upon waking tomorrow morning a miracle has occurred, you are now living a life in which in your unmet emotional need is fulfilled completely.

2. Take three deep breaths and allow your imagination to create a movie of how your new life looks. Where are you living? How are you feeling and looking? Who is with you, how are they acting? What does your home look like? What work are you doing? (Give yourself plenty of time to do this).

3. What is it about this new life that confirms your emotional need is now being fulfilled? When you start to feel as though you are really living this new life of yours, imagine the 'new you' meeting the 'old you'. Tell your old self exactly what he or she needs to know and to do in order to make this new life a reality. Give this time, be patient and something will come.

4. Once the insight(s) have been revealed to you, open your eyes, take a deep breath and notice how different you feel.

Mike's example: *the insights revealed to Mike were for him to apply for a job in a seaside town (a place he had always wanted to live in) that he had heard about through a friend and for him to register with some recruitment agencies. In the meantime he was going to ask for the sum of money back that he lent to a friend, and give notice on his current flat.*

Step 6

Make a list of the actions that were revealed to you, along with a time schedule.

Mike's example:

1. *Phone a company based in a seaside town and request an application form (Monday).*

2. *Go online tomorrow (Saturday) and register with a minimum of five recruitment agencies.*

3. *Phone my friend tonight at 7 pm, explain the circumstances and ask for my money to be repaid within four weeks.*

4. *Contact the estate agent on Monday and give notice.*

Step 7

What could stop me from implementing these changes, and how can I overcome those barriers?

Mike's example: *I might get home and start worrying that it might all go wrong. I can prevent this by getting the support of my best friend Tom, using the instant stress release* [see page 368] *and visualising my new future each day for at least five minutes.*

Step 8

The final step is to implement the plan and to follow the strategies to overcome the barriers to its success. I have found that keeping the vision and 'new life' in mind is very effective in helping someone to make the change that is necessary. Plus, getting the support of your friends, family and a practitioner also helps. Once you've made the necessary changes and started to meet the emotional need upon which you are working, reassess your emotional needs again with the questionnaire and start working on the next lowest-scoring need. I've had patients successfully meet an emotional need within hours of leaving the consultation room, although the average time taken is nearer to two weeks. You'll also find that successfully fulfilling an emotional need tends to improve the scores of many of the others, because most are interrelated.

Now that you have reached the end of this chapter, my advice is to reread it one more time. While doing so highlight those sentences (using a highlighter pen) that you feel are important to you. Once you've done this write down at least five steps or actions that you are going to take, and spend a moment visualising yourself implementing them. Once you have completed this, move on to your next barrier.

MIND–BODY ESSENTIALS

- Each of us has innate emotional needs that are as important to total health as physical needs. These emotional needs include the need for attention, respect, safety, intimacy, social connection, competency, status, meaning and purpose.

- A failure to meet these emotional needs causes stress, and for some people this can lead to anxiety, depression and psychosis.

- Resolving any health challenge that is related to unmet emotional needs involves identifying which needs are not being met, and using visualisation exercises and other means to help identify what action needs to take place in order to fulfil them. In addition the use of tools to reduce emotional arousal and manage emotions is important.

- Recommended mind–body tools to accompany this chapter: emotional freedom technique (page 332), focusing (page 356), Bach Flower Remedies (page 298), tame the inner critic (page 395), meditation (page 376), conscious breathing (page 314) and relaxation (page 380).

- For recommended reading see Resources, page 427.

barrier

Psychological stress

It's not often my patients come into see me with complete clarity about what their underlying challenges are, but Barry was different. Barry was a senior executive of a multinational company. His life was a blur of meetings, international flights, hotel rooms and more meetings. He'd been 'running on adrenaline' for the last six months, and was feeling absolutely exhausted. His sleep was 'erratic', his diet 'awful', and the relationship with his wife 'in jeopardy'. In a nutshell he said, 'I'm stressed.'

We've all experienced stress at one time or another in our lives, but what determines whether stress becomes good or bad for us, and what action can we take to increase our ability to withstand stress and recover from the ill effects caused by it? How do we even recognise that we are stressed? For some people it's easy, they just know they are stressed. For others – mainly people who are unable to make contact with or accept their emotions – the stress tends to express itself through the body: muscle tension and tightness, headaches, back pain and irritable bowel syndrome can all be symptomatic of a stressed mind, downloading into a stressed body. Bear this in mind as you read this chapter; give some thought as to how you experience stress and what evidence there is that your body is being involved.

What is stress?

That's not actually an easy question to answer, because so many people have so many different ideas about what stress is. When someone says they are stressed or that they are finding something stressful, they will often find it very hard to describe exactly what the problem is. What does it mean to you to be stressed? My own experience and understanding is that when someone says they are stressed, they are referring to it in a negative light, in that the pressure of a situation is causing them to experience emotional distress.

Here are two other stress definitions:

- Stress is the adverse reaction people have to excessive pressure or other types of demand placed on them.[1]

- Stress occurs when pressure exceeds your perceived ability to cope.[2]

For the purpose of this chapter I'm going to divide stress into:

- **Positive stress**, also called eustress, which enables you to access your maximal creativity, enthusiasm and performance. When you experience positive stress you feel competent, able to adapt to change and will be motivated in what you do. It enables you to get the most out of yourself and it makes for a much more exciting life. An example would be an athlete experiencing eustress just minutes before taking part in a competition. The positive stress response is the fuel to drive him or her to successfully achieve their goal.

- **Negative stress**, also called distress or chronic stress, which is stress that no longer has a positive purpose and is in some way contributing to the deterioration in the health of the person experiencing it. It has the exact opposite effect to positive stress. It reduces creativity, enthusiasm and performance, makes you feel incompetent, unable to adapt to change (therefore stuck) and depletes you of all motivation. An example would be someone stuck in a job or marriage that they don't want to be in.

Each of these two types of stress involves a three-part process:

1. **The stressor** The situation that triggers the emotional and physical response.

2. **The perception** The interpretation of what the stressor means to you.

3. **The stress response** The emotional and physical response.

What determines whether something is positively or negatively stressful is mainly your perception – your perspective on the situation in which you find yourself. For example, you could have two people lose their jobs (the same situation), with one of them seeing it as a catastrophe because of loss of income and the new lack of security, whereas the other person might see it as an opportunity to leave a job they weren't enjoying and find a job that they do want to be in. Because of the way they have perceived the situation, the first person will experience negative stress and the second positive stress.

Your reactions to stress

Any threat to your physical, emotional or psychological state of balance triggers an inbuilt protective mechanism called the fight-or-flight response, or acute stress response. This primitive survival mechanism triggers a firing of the sympathetic nervous system (a branch of the autonomic nervous system that controls automatic functions such as breathing and blood pressure) and a flooding of the body with the stress hormones adrenaline and cortisol. In the short term this is exactly what you need. These stress hormones:

- Speed up your heart rate and rate of breathing in preparation.

- Provide a quick burst of energy so that you can take action.

- Increase your alertness and narrow your attention so that you can focus one what is happening.

- Shunt blood to your muscles and away from non-essential parts such as your gut and reproductive system.

- Boost the immune system, so that it can respond to any injury.

- Lower sensitivity to pain, in case you get injured.

The difference today, compared with thousands of years ago, is that many people have lost touch with their own gut feelings telling them that they are stressed. This lack of awareness prevents any appropriate action from taking place and they get stuck in the high arousal, fight-or-flight state.

Your reactions to chronic stress

Prolonged activation of the sympathetic nervous system and ongoing secretion of the stress hormones eventually start to take their toll and can have a dramatic and negative effect on the body, including:

- Reducing nutrient absorption

- Raising cholesterol and triglyceride levels

- Inhibiting the immune system

- Raising blood pressure

- Adversely affecting memory and concentration

- Suppressing thyroid function

- Reducing wound healing

- Decreasing bone density

- Decrease in muscle tissue

- Higher blood pressure

- Lowered immunity

- Increased deposition of fat around the abdomen

These changes in biochemistry are only part of the story when it comes to chronic stress. Chronic stress also leads to a whole variety of changes in behaviour, some of which are designed to alleviate the sensations associated with stress (such as muscular tension, headaches, tremors, sexual problems and butterflies in the stomach), the distressing emotional states associated with stress (such as depression, anxiety, anger, shame and embarrassment) and some of the distressing psychological consequences (such as unpleasant images, nightmares, negative thinking and a strong inner critical voice). These behaviours include:

accident-proneness	nervous cough
addictions	overeating
aggression	poor diet
alcohol abuse	poor driving
avoidance/phobias	poor eye contact
checking rituals	poor time management
compulsive behaviour	restlessness
decreased/increased sexual activity	sleep disturbances
eating/walking/talking faster	stuttering
eating disorders	sulking behaviour
frequent crying	teeth grinding
increased absenteeism	tics or spasms
irritability	unkempt appearance
loss of appetite	violence/abuse
low productivity	withdrawing from relationships

It is the total combination of these behaviours, biochemical and hormonal changes that is believed to be the mechanism behind which stress contributes to so many different diseases, such as multiple sclerosis, depression, irritable bowel syndrome, obesity, peptic ulcers, diabetes, anxiety, sexual dysfunction, heart disease, arthritis and high blood pressure.[3]

One particularly interesting study from King's College, London, claims to have found the link between a past history of childhood emotional trauma/stress and an increased risk of heart disease and diabetes. The researchers monitored 1,000 people in New Zealand from birth to the age of 32, noting any factors that were particularly stressful, and recording each partipant's level of CRP – a marker of inflammation. They found that the people who reported physical or sexual abuse, or being rejected by their mother at a young age, were twice as likely to have significant levels of CRP in the blood compared with those who reported no abuse. The hypothesis put forward is that psychological stress directly triggers inflammation, and also reduces a child's ability to produce glucocorticoid hormones, one of the main mechanisms the body uses to turn off inflammation. Inflammation, as we discovered in Barrier 5, is a significant contributor to more than 100 different diseases. [4]

Identifying whether you are stressed

Part of the challenge in managing your stress is to realise that you are stressed. Stress is a rather insidious creature that creeps up on you, and it's surprising how long someone can be experiencing stress without even knowing.

Ask yourself

By far the easiest and simplest way to know whether stress is affecting you is to ask yourself the question 'Am I stressed?' The perception of ourselves as being stressed, once we are ready to admit it, is a very accurate indicator that we are stressed. Levels of stress as perceived by an individual are closely correlated with the health problems I mentioned earlier.

Take the stress questionnaire

If you haven't already filled in the questionnaire on page 27, please do so now. A score of 10 or more is suggestive that you are stressed.

Measure your cortisol and DHEA levels

One of the most accurate ways to assess the effect of stress on your body is to measure the levels of the hormones DHEA and cortisol in a saliva sample taken at four different times during the day. The levels and ratios of each are then measured and compared with what would be expected in a healthy person. For more information about this test visit the website of Individual Wellbeing Diagnostic Laboratories (see Resources, page 418).

Managing your stress levels

If you feel stressed, or scored 10 or more on the stress questionnaire and/or your saliva test indicates you are stressed, follow the five steps below:

Step 1 • Get to the heart of the problem

This really is the key to managing your stress. Whereas exercising, meditation and some supplements might help with your stress, if your biggest source of stress is the fact that you're in debt, that's what needs to be addressed. To get to the heart of the problem you really need to start facing reality (see Barrier 12).

What's causing you to be stressed?

Make a list of all the things that are stressing you out; include things relating to your work, home, relationships, finances, health, appearance – the works. Now, go through each in turn and decide which one of the following three options you are going to use to reduce the stress that you are under.

1. **Option 1** is about action. List in very precise and realistic terms what action you can take to change the situation. If you get stuck, imagine a friend of yours is in exactly the same circumstances as you – what advice would you give them? Write it down.

2. **Option 2** is about perspective. Changing the way you see the problem, and the meaning you give it, is a very powerful way of reducing the stress that it triggers. Again, imagine that you are helping a friend with the same problems to come up with three different perspectives – what advice would you give them? Write it down.

3. And finally, option 3 is about acceptance. If you truly can't change the situation or your perspective on it, then the way to release any stress is to stop resisting the situation and accept the reality of it as it is now. Interestingly, doing this often frees up creative ideas and invites new possibilities.

Once your list is finished for each source of stress, implement the options. Get a friend or therapist to help if you get stuck.

Are you meeting your physical needs?

Neglecting any of your body's needs, such as the need for fresh, nutrient-rich whole foods, water, exercise, touch and sleep, can put a strain on your body and be a significant contributor to your experience of stress. As a general rule the body thrives when it's fed mainly fresh fruits, vegetables, high-quality protein, 1 litre (1¾ pints) of water a day, and when it is exercised aerobically for 30 minutes three times a week, and put to sleep for at least seven hours a night.

Are you meeting your emotional needs?

Emotional needs are as important to your health as your physical needs. They include the need for positive attention, respect, safety, intimacy, social connection, competency, status, meaning and purpose. A failure to get one or more of these met can result in stress arising in the bodymind. To work out what action needs to take place, close your eyes and imagine that you are now living a life in which all of these emotional needs are being met. Give yourself some time to experience this new life, then once you really feel it as a possibility, tell yourself what you need to do in order to make it happen. Often you'll get some great ideas. It's then up to you to implement them.

Is there a hormonal or biochemical imbalance?

Blood-sugar imbalances, nutrient deficiencies, toxicity, alcohol, caffeine, nicotine, drugs, sex hormone imbalances and, particularly, adrenal fatigue can result from the behaviours caused by psychological stress, and can also be a source of stress to the bodymind themselves. If you've been feeling stressed for some time, the most important starting place is to check the health of your adrenal glands (see Barrier 6). Eating a healthy diet, getting adequate sleep, some exercise and taking supplements such as a multivitamin–mineral and Siberian ginseng to support the adrenal glands can produce a considerable improvement in your ability to cope with stress. The total-health questionnaire on page 21 will help you decide which of these factors are relevant.

Step 2 • Increase your emotional resilience

Emotional resilience is the ability to withstand pressure – the body-mind's inbuilt psychological buffer system, which enables you to withstand various potentially stressful situations. Learning how to increase your emotional resilience and your coping threshold is an important part of coping with stress. Here are some ideas:

Take control

Feeling that you have some degree of control in the events of your life, or controlling the way you choose to respond to those events is a panacea for stress. Whenever you feel stressed, identify at least three ways in which you can take control of the situation. For example, you've been in the same job for over ten years, you're fed up with having no say in decision matters, and everything about it is starting to stress you out. Taking control, for example, could involve you in: (1) telling your supervisor how you feel and asking for more responsibility, control or a different role; (2) looking for a new job; and (3) changing the meaning you give to the job, by seeing your job as a source of income that allows you to do the things you enjoy.

Take the challenge

Labelling a situation as a problem is itself a problem, as it implies that there's no way around it and that it's a dead end. Try to get into the habit of seeing the situations that you are in as challenges – invitations to explore different options by finding creative solutions. Taking this attitude keeps you much more empowered and focused on the solutions than the problems. It also decreases your stress considerably.

Get connected

Close relationships, committed partnerships, a supportive family and involvement within the local community are a powerful antidote to stress. The more connected we feel (and the less isolated we are) the greater the ability to cope with life's situations. Being able to share challenges with others and draw upon other people's suggestions and support can often be the difference between coping well and depression. I'm not suggesting that you suddenly get married, or go into the streets and find yourself a partner, but actively making the most of the people you do have in your life, getting involved in a community-based project and even volunteering for one or two days, can have a large, positive effect on your life and health.

Break out of the mould

A lot of what we do and say is out of habit, conditioned responses we learnt often from early childhood. Make today a day when you break out of this mould and start to run your life the way you want to. Try this: when you are faced with a situation and you would normally respond in a certain way (perhaps with a certain phrase or when answering the telephone), change it and see how good it feels to say and act in ways that are new and fresh!

Get creative

Make a commitment right now to doing something creative for at least one hour a week. Choose something unrelated to work that allows you to get into the flow – this could be anything from learning to play an instrument or playing chess to writing or taking a dance class. Notice how good and free it makes you feel afterwards.

Start journaling

Keeping a daily diary in which you can write down your thoughts, reflect on the day's activities and put into words your worries and problems is a great stress reliever. Use the diary as an opportunity to write down at least five things that you are grateful for. See the journaling mind–body tool on page 372 for more information.

Organise yourself

When you feel overwhelmed by the number of things that you have to do, stand up, pick up a pen and paper and sit down somewhere else. Now ask yourself, what are my priorities? Once you've written the list, return to your workplace and start with number one on the list. If you organise yourself this way you'll get through them much quicker and more effectively.

Keep a pet (and care for it)

Pet therapy is widely used in nursing homes, prisons, hospitals and schools to reduce stress levels and improve health. Stroking a cat or dog or watching fish in an aquarium have all been found to lower blood pressure. The results long term are even more impressive. Owners of pets are more likely to survive a heart attack, make fewer visits to their GP, experience less loneliness and suffer less from depression. However, there is a caveat with pet therapy, you have to make time to spend with the pet and you have to take care of it.

Practise appreciation

Change your life and those whom you meet today by telling them what you appreciate about them. Be genuine and sincere. Watch their faces light up.

Step 3 • Try some relaxation techniques

It's one thing to realise that you are stressed, and another thing actually to do something about it. Stress, worry, anxiety, indeed any negative emotional state, has a magnetic pull about it, sometimes it's so strong that people feel as though they've been completely caught up by it. Here's how to get out of the whirlwind of stress and into your calm centre.

Take a series of deep breaths

This is the simplest and most effective stress-management technique of all. When you catch yourself feeling stressed, take ten long, deep breaths, and notice how much calmer you feel.

Change your posture

Your body posture has a direct link into the way you feel. Try this: think of something that has happened to you recently that you found upsetting, allow yourself to feel those emotions. Now, sit up straight, look up, relax your shoulders, smile softly with your eyes and mouth and, while keeping that same posture, think about the same event. Notice how the intensity of the emotions has been greatly diminished. Next time you are stressed, stand or sit tall, look up and relax your shoulders and breathe deeply – it's a great stress reliever.

Switch your attention to your feet

This sounds like a strange thing to do, but whenever we worry or get stressed about something, we accumulate a lot of emotional charge around the head area. By switching your attention to your feet and breathing in and out of that area, this head charge diminishes considerably and you will start to feel calmer almost immediately.

Reconnect with nature

Nature has a wonderful calming effect, if you allow it to work its magic on you. Try to spend at least 30 minutes each week in some area of natural beauty. Find a local park, forest, river or ocean and go for a walk, but rather than going up into your head and worrying about problems (watch how often you do this) allow your attention to turn to nature – observe it, listen to it, feel it and smell it. Allow yourself to become connected to whatever it is you are observing – the sky, the trees, the animals. Notice how natural and effortless nature is, breathe it in and notice how much calmer you feel. Nature is a great teacher.

Learn to meditate

Meditation is a great way of getting more in touch with your body, and a very effective way to relax. There are many different methods to choose from, but a simple one is to close your eyes and to be aware of your breath as you breathe in and out of your nose. Do this for five to ten minutes and notice how you feel.

Use your imagination

Using your imagination to relax your bodymind is an effective and proven method of inducing the relaxation response. Although you can imagine yourself lying on a beach somewhere or having a hot bath, I find most of my patients prefer to listen to someone on a CD guide them through a relaxation than to actually do it themselves (see Resources page 423).

Listen to some relaxing music

Music has a powerful effect on the biochemistry and well-being of the body. Listening to some relaxing music that you enjoy can help you enter a deep state of relaxation in just a couple of minutes. Everyone's taste is different, so choose something that works for you.

Step 4 • De-stress your body

Your body mirrors your emotional state. Whenever you get tense or stressed, your body mimics those emotions, whether you realise it or not. You can think you're covering it up with a smile, but to the trained eye subtle signs of the underlying emotions are always visible. In the long term this stress and worry builds up as tension within your musculature. You just have to give a stressed person a massage to see that. So de-stressing the body is about helping to relieve the body of that tension, but also because the body is a gateway into the mind, body-based approaches can also help reduce your stress levels as well. Here are some ideas:

Scan your body for tension

Get into the routine of spending a couple of minutes – this could be on waking in the morning or even when visiting the bathroom – to scan your body from head to toes for any feelings of tension. When you come across some, contract and tense that part of your body and then let go completely while breathing out. Repeat this until all of the tension disappears. Now continue down your body.

Get physical

Physical exercise is a great way to de-stress and release pent-up emotions. If you sense things are getting on top of you get yourself down to the gym and really go for it on the treadmill or take your anger out on the punch-bag. Alternatively, go for a long run or swim – either will make you feel a million times better.

Soften your gaze

Next time you are stressed about something or are facing a problem, notice how narrow your focus of attention has become. For example, you could be walking down a street and literally notice nothing else. Next time you find yourself caught up in a problem, try this: look up, eyes open and soften your gaze so that you take in everything in the periphery of your vision. This defocusing instantly de-stresses the body and mind.

De-stress your face

Next time you're feeling out of sorts, go into your bathroom and look at your face, observe the tension, the stress and the way it looks. Now take two deep breaths in and out and then make exaggerated movements of your forehead, your cheeks, your mouth and your jaw, make ugly monster-like faces – really go for it! Do that for 30 seconds, then close your eyes, and give your face a loving massage, while thinking of a past happy and enjoyable experience – allow the feeling of that experience to arise within you. Open your eyes and look at the transformation.

Release your tension

We carry a lot of repressed emotions as tension in our muscles (particularly our legs) and this tension can prevent our creative energy from being available to us and significantly reduce our energy levels. Book yourself in for session with a practitioner who can help you release these tensions – some of the best therapies are deep tissue massage, Rolfing (deep manipulation of the body's soft tissue to realign and balance the body's structure), core energetics and rebirthing/breathwork. The result is that you feel more alive.

Enjoy a hot bath

Treat yourself at least once a week to a nice hot bath. If you live with others, ask them not to disturb you. Put on your favourite relaxing music, use bubble bath, incense or whatever else works for you, and allow yourself to let go – you deserve it.

Practise smiling

Next time you're feeling down or stressed, try this: make yourself smile, not only with your mouth but also, and most importantly, with your eyes. Even though it feels unnatural to do so, just do it. As you keep smiling, deliberately soften your mouth and the area around your eyes, keep softening and softening, while breathing deeply from your belly. Notice how after 30 seconds, you start to feel much better.

Treat yourself

Treat yourself once a fortnight to some form of relaxation therapy. It could be a massage, a session in a flotation tank or even a manicure – something that allows you to rest and relax. If you feel you haven't got time for this, then you definitely need to do it.

Get intimate

Sex and intimacy tends to take a back seat when you are stressed, but if you make time for it, sex can be a potent source of stress relief and enjoyment. It's not just the release of energy in the orgasm that helps, it's also about giving and receiving touch, connecting to the person you love (or fancy), coming into the moment and allowing your body to release its natural supply of endorphins.

Step 5 • De-stress your relationships

Your relationships with people have a tremendous impact on your stress levels and your well-being. A supportive social network can help buffer you from the effects of events that would otherwise knock you for six, whereas the presence of just one person who is causing you stress can be enough to send your health plummeting down.

Give up being right

One way to lower your stress levels instantly and raise your energy levels is to stop being right all the time. Next time you start defending yourself, take a deep breath, smile to yourself that you can see what's happening and let go of the argument – notice how good it feels.

Protect yourself

Are you the kind of person who gets easily drained in the company of certain people or certain situations? If so, try this next time you find yourself in that situation: imagine an egg-shaped ball of light around you, then imagine or feel a layer of green light surrounding it and then violet light. Do this whenever you find yourself in this situation and you'll find that you no longer get negatively affected by people.

Use the bell-jar technique

Next time you find yourself getting stressed by noise, visualise a glass bell jar being placed over the people or situation and notice how the noise suddenly doesn't seem to bother you any more.

Redesign your enemy

If there's someone you work with who winds you up or constantly annoys you, try this to change the way you react to them: imagine that person as a small kid, wearing a big over-sized nappy – smile at how ludicrous it all looks. Now, next time you see that person, see them in their nappy and I guarantee that you'll feel differently about them.

Make someone's day

One day a week do something for someone else, without expecting anything in return. This could mean turning to a stranger who looks lost and offering your help, smiling at someone you've never smiled at before (for example your boss) or buying your receptionist some flowers to say thank you for the work that they do for you.

Now that you have reached the end of this chapter, my advice is to reread it one more time. While doing so highlight those sentences (using a highlighter pen) that you feel are important to you. Once you've done this write down at least five steps or actions that you are going to take, and spend a moment visualising yourself implementing them. Once you have completed this, move on to your next barrier.

MIND–BODY ESSENTIALS

- Stress is part and parcel of life; positive stress enables us to tap into our creative energy, it empowers us and allows us to achieve our potential. Negative stress, on the other hand, disempowers us and disengages us from our creative energy.

- Managing stress can involve one or more of the following: identifying the underlying cause of stress, increasing emotional resilience, using relaxation techniques, de-stressing your body and de-stressing your relationships.

- Keeping to a routine, eating healthy foods, exercising regularly, getting enough quality sleep, meeting your emotional needs and developing a social network are the foundations of creating an emotionally resilient life.

- Recommended mind–body tools to accompany this chapter: exercise (page 350), instant stress release (page 368), meditation (page 376), conscious breathing (page 314) and relaxation (page 380).

- For recommended reading see Resources, page 427.

Addictions

Lucy loved chocolate. Her joint favourite was Cadbury's Twirl and Flake, although Green & Black's dark chocolate ran a close second. Unlike most people who have a passion for chocolate, hers was a large part of her life: on an average day she would eat at least ten chocolate bars. If she was having a 'stressful time' that number would increase twofold, and at its worst she once ate 30 bars in one day. Lucy came to me because of her considerable weight and the fact that this passion for consuming chocolate was now starting to consume her.

Lucy was addicted to the pleasure and excitement generated by the thoughts and images she had about chocolate. The power of those thoughts and her emotions were in fact so strong they had held her to ransom for over two years, destroyed her marriage and were slowly destroying her emotional, and now her physical, health. Of course, Lucy is not alone; addictions are very common, so much so that it is rare in my experience to come across someone who does not have an addiction of some sort. Whether it be to the obvious addictions such as alcohol, caffeine, food, cigarettes, sugar, exercise, drugs, gambling or sex, to the not so obvious ones such as certain behaviours, experiences and even thoughts. Addictions are endemic in our population and they represent a large barrier to our total health.

So what's the solution? In my experience and having worked with hundreds of people with some form of addiction, the key to overcoming addictions is to set yourself free using the different ideas and techniques that I am going to be sharing with you, while addressing the underlying reason for the addiction in the first place. Having the support of a trained healthcare professional as well as family and friends while this is going on will also make a big difference.

What is an addiction?

There are quite a few different definitions, but the one I prefer to use describes an addiction as a pattern of behaviour driven by a psychological and/or physiological dependence on a particular addictive substance or situation. The feature that makes something an addiction is the powerful and sometimes overwhelming emotional compulsion to experience the addictive substance or situation. It becomes the centre of a person's life and will persist despite the detrimental effects on the physical, financial, emotional and social aspects of their life.

Why do we become addicted?

There are many reasons why we become addicted to substances or situations. These include:

- **To change the way we feel** Feelings of emptiness, frustration, unhappiness, depression, anger, guilt, remorse and loneliness are of course unpleasant, especially when they are the dominant underlying emotional state. Temporarily shifting these feelings through the use of addictive substances or situations is a good, short-term strategy.

- **To experience highs and an altered state of mind** Caffeine, for example, prevents the breakdown of dopamine, to give an energised lift; heroin mimics the body's supply of opiates leading to the feeling of euphoria.

- **To dissolve cravings** and alleviate withdrawal symptoms, such as low blood sugar and allergies.

- **To avoid facing some aspect of reality** by covering over feelings that are alerting us to some problem. Addictions can 'buy' time.

- **To increase energy levels** Nutritional and hormonal imbalances due to poor diet and lack of exercise lead to a tired, lethargic body. Addictive substances can provide a temporary energy boost.

- **Genetic factors** There is some evidence that some people with addictions are predisposed because of variations in a gene that controls the levels of dopamine receptors, which allow us to experience pleasure. People with variants of these genes have less receptor sites and therefore need more stimulation, with drugs or caffeine for example, in order to achieve the same degree of pleasure as someone without the gene variant.[1]

- **Histadelia** is a genetic condition in which high levels of histamine are produced. Symptoms include compulsive and obsessive behaviour.[2]

The cycle of addiction

In the very early stages of addiction the addictive substance or situation gives a high that feels great, but is usually followed by a low. As time passes these highs decrease as the body accommodates to the addiction, and the lows deepen. To deal with this the person needs to increase the amount of the addictive substance in order to get the same high, this leads to the cycle of addiction. The classic example of this is the person with alcoholism who needs to drink increasing amounts in order to numb his or her emotional and physical pain. While caught in this psychological trap the only solution appears to be to drink more. This either leads them down a path of ill health or even death, or, if they are fortunate, they are able to seek help before they spin too far out of control.

Why are addictions a problem?

Addictions represent a serious barrier to total health for many reasons:

- **They are a direct trigger or cause of disease** For example, excessive and regular *caffeine* intake is linked to blood-sugar imbalance, irritability, anxiety, insomnia; *sugar* to immune suppression, dental decay and cancer; *alcohol* to liver disease, chronic inflammation and nutritional deficiencies; *smoking* to cancer, chronic degenerative diseases and nutritional deficiencies; *drugs* to infection, cancer, inflammation and mental health problems.

- **They create mood difficulties** Underlying problems such as depression and anxiety are frequently a contributor to addictions, but also a consequence of addictions for many reasons. These include failing to have the person's emotional needs met, nutritional deficiencies and hormonal imbalances.

- **They cause mineral and vitamin depletions** For example, chronic alcohol use can reduce the body's levels of B vitamins, leading to problems with memory and concentration, and tryptophan and omega-3 leading to depression.

- **They have social effects** Addictions can have a profound effect on personal relationships, alienating loved ones and friends, and can lead to antisocial behaviour such as abuse, violence and burglary.

- **They create a distraction from facing some aspect of reality** Addictions are a very effective short-term strategy for distancing ourselves from feelings that are trying to draw our attention to some aspect of reality that we need to face.

- **They prevent you from reaching your total health potential** Addictions can be so consuming mentally and physically that they leave little time and energy for meeting your emotional and physical needs or for growing and developing as a human being.

Are you addicted?

Scoring more than seven on the addiction questionnaire on page 28 suggests that addictions might be a problem for you. Part of the challenge for you might be actually admitting to yourself that you are addicted to something. We tell ourselves stories that justify the way we are, and if you have a rather elaborate story, and most people do, then you might not think that there is a problem. One way to tell if your mental story is covering up an addiction is to stop the suspected addictive substance, such as coffee or cigarettes, and see if it generates an anxiety. If it does it is a clear sign you are addicted.

Are you ready to change?

One of the most challenging and frustrating aspects of addictions for the friends and family of someone with an addiction is that change happens only when the person is ready for change. What that means generally is that forcing someone into counselling or a treatment programme when they are not ready to do it will rarely be successful. People tend to change the way they live their life only when they reach rock-bottom. There are exceptions of course, but this rule tends to be true. To help understand why this is the case, a model called the Stages of Change, describes the six stages that people go through when change occurs.[3]

1 The pre-contemplation stage

This is where the person with the addiction is unwilling or unable to contemplate seeking help or making any changes to their life.

2 The contemplation stage

The person has some awareness of the problems that they have and they are starting to think about making some changes. This stage can last a long time.

3 Preparing to change

The person is now willing to make some changes to their life. Of importance in this stage is the need to provide continuous support and encouragement and the need to reinforce feelings of self-belief and self-worth. This can be a difficult period, as the person is torn between the old, familiar ways and lifestyle and the new ways of living that will set them free. One of the critical factors at this stage is whether the person believes the benefits of the new changes outweigh the benefits of the old way. If they don't they will probably revert back to stage 2. Adequate planning, preparation and support is essential during this stage.

4 Making the change

This stage is about action. It's about taking steps towards the new life, while being aware of and overcoming the inevitable resistance and anxiety that will arise. Again, support and encouragement are essential.

5 Maintaining the change

Once the person is no longer taking the addicted substance or engaging in addictive behaviours the next challenge is to prevent a relapse. This is why addressing the underlying reasons for the addiction is so important. This stage needs to focus on helping the person meet their physical and emotional needs, while also helping the body and relationships recover, and finding their own authentic sense of self (see Barrier 14).

6 Relapse stage

If the person is unable to maintain the changes, then relapse is possible. Life's circumstances, low self-esteem and self-defeating beliefs can all put someone back a couple of stages. The way forward during this stage is to focus on the progress that has already been achieved and the changes that have occurred.

This model is useful for many reasons: it allows us to understand the well-trodden path of change and to become aware of the different types of challenges that we might encounter at each stage. It also gives some structure to the recovery process. Most people move backwards and forwards, spending varying amounts of time at each stage, but generally most will progress from one stage to the other. I've seen it many times with my own patients; when someone rushes through (or is rushed through) a stage – for example, stage 2: contemplation – then the chances of success are considerably reduced. If you are presently experiencing addictions, identify which stage you are at, and familiarise yourself with the other stages. This will help to orientate you as you move through your programme.

How to overcome addictions

If you have an addiction and want to overcome it, here are some suggestions. I do realise how hard it can be to follow through on what I am about to share, and it is for this reason that I would encourage you to work alongside an integrated medical doctor who has experience in helping people overcome addictions. The first part of the total health addiction programme focuses on addressing the underlying causes of addictions, and the second provides specific approaches that you can use to overcome addictions.

Step 1 • Address the underlying causes

Meet your emotional needs

Failing to meet certain emotional needs, such as the need for security, meaning, intimacy and challenge, creates an empty feeling inside. This lack of inner fulfilment is a major contributor to addictions and a common reason why addictive substances and experiences are used to fill 'the space' within. Barrier 8 will walk you through the process of identifying which emotional needs are not being met in your life and make suggestions as to how you can start meeting them.

Face reality

Facing reality is tough. Most of us have a natural innate tendency to avoid things that generate pain and discomfort inside, yet if we are committed to growth and total health, facing reality and using the emotional distress as your barometer and source of energy to change is essential. Barrier 12 will show you how to identify what is causing you distress and how to work through it. One word of caution though: you should only face reality if you feel ready to do so, and/or if you have the support and resources to help you do so. One of the main reasons we avoid pain and reality is because our bodymind knows that facing the truth would simply be too overwhelming.

Manage your psychological stress

The pace of life and the demands placed on us, and by ourselves, inevitably lead to the experience of stress. As I've discussed before, that's not intrinsically a bad thing. We need stress to grow and develop, but when it becomes too much it becomes a threat to our health, and it's often then that we turn to addictive substances, such as cigarettes, alcohol and coffee, to manage our feelings relating to our life situation. There are, however, plenty of alternative and effective strategies for stress management. I've outlined a few in Barrier 9 and I would encourage you to read them.

Treat any physical imbalances

Whereas it might not at first glance be apparent that someone's addictions might be related primarily to a physiological problem, they should definitely not be missed, because they are so easily treatable. That makes sense when we acknowledge that diet, nutrients, hormones, and so on, all impact on our feelings, and therefore influence our propensity to addiction. Here are just a few examples that I have encountered in my own clinical practice:

- **Candida overgrowth and blood-sugar imbalance** can contribute to addictions to carbohydrates and sugars. See Barrier 7.

- **Adrenal stress and low functioning thyroid** can contribute to addictions to caffeine, speed and cocaine. See Barrier 6.

- **Zinc deficiency** can contribute to eating disorders such as anorexia and bulimia.

- **5-HTP deficiency** can contribute to obsessive compulsive disorder (OCD), depression and eating problems.

- **Histadelia,** a genetic condition, causes a range of symptoms including OCD, poor pain tolerance, depression, frequent infections, high libido, frequent headaches, itchy/warm skin, and a high level of perspiration.

If the questionnaires on pages 21–32 suggest that these might be an issue for you, I would encourage you to seek the help and support of a nutritional therapist or integrated medical doctor.

Step 2 • Use specific techniques

Once you have started to address the underlying issues, you can use the following in parallel to help overcome addictions:

Use a nutritional approach

Diet and nutritional supplementation have a big role to play in the treatment of addictions. Good nutrition not only helps to correct the nutritional and hormonal imbalances that can underlie addictions but it can also support the process of recovery and repair, and considerably reduce withdrawal symptoms. As a bare minimum, I start all of my patients on a healthy-eating plan (Barrier 1), a high potency multivitamin–mineral and antioxidant, and extra omega-3 fish oil and evening primrose oil. In addition to these you could also add:

- **A daily dose** of 800mcg of the mineral chromium polynicotinate and 5g of l-glutamine powder to help alleviate sugar and carbohydrate cravings.

- **The amino acid l-tyrosine**, 500–1,000mg three times daily in between meals for coffee addiction. Tyrosine converts to the energising neurotransmitter noradrenaline.

- **The amino acid taurine** 3g daily to help reduce alcohol cravings.

- **Zinc** 50mg daily to help with anorexia and bulimia.

- **5-HTP** 50–100mg twice daily can help alleviate low mood and depression.

- **Calcium and magnesium** can help alleviate the cramps associated with opiate withdrawal.

- **Just taking a daily multivitamin** and mineral supplement (along with a healthy diet) can keep 81 per cent of alcoholics off booze after six months compared to 38 per cent who are left to their own devices.[4]

- **L-theanine**, a green tea extract, can help to alleviate underlying anxiety and worry.

- **Niacin vitamin B3**, can be used in conjunction with a sauna to help speed up the release of toxins from the body. This is especially good for people undergoing drug detoxification. Take 30 minutes before entering a sauna, or on an empty stomach.

- **Alkalising minerals** such as Higher Nature's Alkaclear, can help to alkalise the body and help it recover quicker from withdrawal.

- **A dose of 500mg of calcium** and 500mg of methionine twice daily, and 50–100mg of vitamin B_6, zinc 15mg, manganese 5mg and vitamin C 2,000mg once daily, can help alleviate the symptoms of histadelia.

Change the image you have of the addictive substance

One of the many reasons we choose to continue with an addiction is because the image we have of it in our mind generates pleasurable feelings in the body. So we think of, say, a cup of coffee, then an image comes up, pleasurable feelings arise and before we know it we are off to our favourite coffee house. For most people this is an unconscious cycle; that is, something triggers the thought, feelings are generated, and before you know it you find yourself ordering a cup of coffee. Fortunately this cycle can be broken. I started using mental imagery techniques to break addictive cycles with patients over four years ago, and it is definitely one of the most powerful tools at your disposal. The essence of this approach is to replace the pleasure-generating image with an image that evokes a consistently strong, negative response – the stronger this response, the more effective. It can work almost immediately for addictions to specific types of foods or drink. But if the addiction has had an impact on the physiology of your body you will also need to follow the dietary and nutritional changes as well. I'll now share with you the exact process that put an immediate stop to Lucy and her chocolate addiction. Even I was surprised at how powerful and quick this was.

1. Choose the specific item that you want to no longer crave or be addicted to (for example a cup of coffee, bar of chocolate, slice of cake, bottle of wine or a cigarette).

2. Close your eyes and notice the feelings inside your body that arise when you think of the substance that you are focusing on.

3. Now we are going to alter that image. How you do this is entirely up to you and your fertile imagination, but your goal is to create an image that makes you feel sick and revolted. An image so upsetting that no part of you wants the addictive substance. Here's what I asked Lucy to imagine: 'See the chocolate bar in front of you. Now notice how it's actually been made of human excrement, look at the maggots in it and flies surrounding it. Breathe deeply and allow yourself to feel the nausea. [I did warn you this is not pleasant!] Now pick it up in your hands and force it down into your mouth and swallow it [as she did this she started gagging, I nearly did as well]. Now open your eyes. 'Do you want some chocolate?' Her answer was 'No bloody way!'

4. With Lucy we just had to do this visualisation once. In her follow-up session some six weeks later, not only had she not eaten any chocolate but because she had been addressing the underlying emotional reasons for the addictions in the first place, her emotional and physical health had improved considerably. This process doesn't always work after just one session, however, sometimes it takes a couple more. The real key to its success lies in finding an image that generates a powerful negative response.

5. Once you've used it successfully you can start applying it to other parts of your life as well.

Tap your way to freedom

The emotional freedom technique (EFT) (page 332) provides details of a very simple and effective process for overcoming barriers to total health – this includes addictions. By tapping on various acupuncture points while being emotionally connected to the feel-ings associated with the addictive substance, you can change the hold it has over you and, importantly, address the underlying beliefs that might have contributed to it. Once you've read about EFT, try using the set-up phrases below. Of course it's much better to use your own version:

- 'Even though I have this addiction to coffee, I deeply and com-pletely accept and forgive myself.'

- 'Even though I have this craving for cigarettes I deeply and com-pletely accept and forgive myself.'

How many times you will need to use EFT will depend on you and your addiction. Having used EFT with numerous patients, I tend to find that as you start using it you discover the underlying causes, rather like the layers of an onion peeling away, so eventually you use EFT on the core underlying issues, which could be anything from 'I am unlovable', to 'I am unworthy'. On average one or two 10–30 minute EFT sessions a day for a week appear to be suited to most people. If you get stuck or are unsure as to what you should focus on, I would encourage you to work alongside an EFT therapist – see Resources, page 421 for more details.

Rediscover your authentic self

One of the most common reasons someone turns to addictive sub-stances or addictive behaviours is because they have lost touch with their real sense of self. This is very common. Barrier 14 on low self-esteem provides an overview as to how you can start to recon-nect with your authentic sense of self. This is a process that often takes many years, but it is one that ultimately leads to what most people desire: a real sense of who they are and what they are here to do.

Putting it all together

Whereas all of the suggestions have the potential to help you over-come an addiction, it can be a bit daunting trying to work out which you should do and when. To simplify the process, my advice would be to:

1. Get established on a healthy eating and exercise programme and start taking your supplements straight away.

2. Choose a day in which you are able to dedicate to tackling your addiction.

3. In the morning of that day use EFT and the imagery technique – either do these by yourself or find yourself a practitioner.

4. In the afternoon go through the chapters on emotional needs (Barrier 8), psychological stress (Barrier 9) and facing reality (Barrier 12). Create a plan of action, visualise your future goals and take the first step on this day to implement that action plan.

5. Share your new vision with someone you trust, and ask them to support and help you by providing you with motivation. If you don't have anyone close to you who can help you with this, you could consider working alongside an integrated medical doctor (see Resources, page 413).

6. If you step back into your addiction, just return to number 1 on this list. Remember: the more times you attempt to overcome an addiction, the more likely you are to overcome it once and for all.

Please note: if you feel unable to follow my recommendations, or if you are unwell with your addictions, you should seek the help of an integrated medical doctor.

Now that you have reached the end of this chapter, my advice is to re-read it one more time. While doing so highlight those sentences (using a highlighter pen) that you feel are important to you. Once you've done this write down at least five steps or actions that you are going to take, and spend a moment visualising yourself implementing them. Once you have completed this, move on to your next barrier.

MIND–BODY ESSENTIALS

- Overcoming addiction starts by being ready to change, not because you feel you have to because of demands that have been placed upon you.

- Addictions are really a symptom of some underlying problem. If these imbalances are not resolved, there is a high probability that you will relapse, or one addiction will be replaced by another.

- For more significant addictions, such as drugs and obsessive–compulsive disorder, I would recommend you work alongside an integrated medical doctor.

- Recommended mind–body tools to accompany this chapter: emotional freedom technique (page 332), symptom dialogue (page 391), creative visualisation (page 319), Bach Flower Remedies (page 298), meditation (page 376), conscious breathing (page 314) and relaxation (page 380).

- For recommended reading see Resources, page 427.

Disconnection

Brian came to my workshop so that he could learn ways of connecting to others. He had felt like a loner for all of his life, and despite being in a relationship with a woman whom he described as 'perfect and loving', he couldn't feel her love. He felt numb inside.

In my experience Brian's problem is very common. In Brian's case the desire to be connected emotionally, interestingly also reflected a quite profound disconnection from his own body. He treated his body as though it was a hindrance, and because of that he had little or no respect for it. His diet was appalling: crisps and ready-made meals made up 90 per cent of what he ate. The last time he exercised was when he was at school some 40 years ago and he found it excruciatingly hard to even look at himself in the mirror. He didn't like his body. In Brian's case the solution for him was not only to learn the skills that I am about to share with you in this chapter but also to reconnect to his own physical body by nourishing it in a way that valued and respected it. Brian identified unhealthy diet, body acidification and hormonal imbalances as barriers relevant to him, and, despite a shaky start, after 12 months he declared himself as being 'connected'. His wife was over the moon, and as for Brian, he was shining. It was an honour to help him.

The prevalence of people feeling disconnected probably shouldn't come as a surprise. We are social creatures designed to be in relationship to others. Thousands of years ago our family would have consisted of mum, dad, uncles, aunts, grandparents and trusted friends, all of whom played an active role in bringing us up. But in some parts of the Western world, the social unit has been reduced to a handful of often distracted people. More and more people are feeling isolated, fearful of the community they live within, caught up in the circumstances of their life and without the skills or awareness to do anything about them. In my work as an integrated medical doctor, I have seen how disconnection contributes to the sadness, misery and suffering of my patients. But on the positive side I also see how patients who discover ways of connecting with others in a mutually meaningful and fulfilling way can turn their health and life around. Life is, after all, made of special moments, often shared with those you love and care for. In our final days and moments before departing these shores, I am convinced that many of us will not look back at our achievements, but at our relationships. I believe it is through relationships that we can heal ourselves, mature as human beings and find the fulfilment that we mistakenly believe can be found through the pursuit of power, money and prestige. Relationships, whether they are bringing up a child, entering into a marriage, or spending time with parents, can, and are perhaps the greatest of challenges, but the riches and memories they hold far outweigh the inevitable pain and challenges. Getting and staying connected is one of the golden tickets to total health.

How being connected benefits your health

Some of the most compelling research as to the health benefits of being in a caring relationship come from researchers who have investigated the health benefits of marriage.

- One study found that a married man with heart disease can be expected to live, on average, nearly four years longer than an unmarried man with a healthy heart. The advantages for women are similar.[1]

- Research from Yale University found that a married man who smokes more than a pack of cigarettes a day can be expected to live as long as a divorced man who does not smoke.[2]

• Other studies have highlighted the multiple benefits of feeling emotionally supported.

• Children who tend to work by themselves, are not very well liked by their peers, or are otherwise socially isolated may have a higher risk of cardiovascular disease in adulthood. In one study researchers tracked the health of 1,037 children from birth to 26 years old. At age 26 the subjects were considered socially isolated if they had no social or emotional support or close relationships and had not dated at all or been involved with a partner in the past year. Those subjects with signs of social isolation in childhood had a 37 per cent increased risk of poor health at 26 years old.[3]

• In a study of 194 heart-attack patients, those who reported lower amounts of emotional support in their lives were nearly three times as likely to die within six months as those with higher levels of emotional support.[4]

Deepening the connection with others

The desire to connect with others is a genetically programmed need, but the degree to which we need to do so, and with how many people really depends on you. Temperament plays a big part in this. Extroverts get their energy through interacting and connecting with other people. Introverts energise themselves through time spent alone. So whereas it's important to feel connected, we need to find ways of connecting that are right for us. An introvert might experience sufficient levels of connection through just one intimate relationship and meditation, spending time in nature or even through a pet. An extrovert, on the other hand, might find fulfilment through community projects, a busy social life and having numerous friends. So, bear this in mind as you read the following suggestions, and choose those recommendations that fit in with your own personality and preferences.

Visualise yourself connecting to others

Mentally rehearsing meetings and creating rapport with others is a simple and effective way to improve your relationship skills. Try the following:

1. Think of someone that you know you will be meeting within the next seven days.

2. Take a couple of deep breaths, then close your eyes and set an intention to connect with this person.

3. Create a mental movie of your interaction starting with just before you meet to just afterwards.

4. Step inside that movie and play your new self. What do you see, hear and feel that tells you that you are connecting with this person? Make those senses bigger, brighter and bolder. Really feel what it is like to be in rapport with this person.

5. If the person you have in mind usually intimidates you, reduce the size of their image and imagine a big smile on their face – that will help!

6. Once you've finished this exercise get a feel for your new-found confidence.

7. Practise a couple of times prior to the meeting, and notice after the meeting what a positive impact this made.

Be attentive

Think of the last time when someone was paying you genuine positive attention. How did it make you feel? Probably pretty good? The truth is that most people savour positive attention. We are hardwired to seek attention as a means of being able to connect with others and have our needs met. Learning how to tap into this need and make it happen for others is a great skill that, when learnt, can make being connected with others all the much easier.

1. Have a genuine intention to listen to the person that you are with.

2. See this as an opportunity to learn something from them.

3. Breathe deeply and allow your body to naturally mimic theirs. Orientate your body towards them, keep relaxed eye contact, nod your head gently, and match their physical movements and tonality of voice. This might seem awkward initially, but it will come naturally with time.

4. Ask questions that get them to go deeper into the subject that they are talking about. There's a couple of ways of doing this, either by repeating the last sentence; for example, 'I have a lot of respect for what he did.' You reply, 'So you respect him?', or by simply saying something open-ended such as 'Tell me more.'

Be appreciative

Genuine appreciation is the quickest and most effective way of opening the floodgates of connection. You don't have to agree with what a person is saying but you can appreciate them for saying it. If you appreciate someone when they least expect it, that holds even greater power. For example, a patient of mine told me about her boss with whom she had been working as a PA for over 20 years. Although they had a good working relationship, he had never once verbally appreciated her – until a week ago. Out of nowhere he came into her office and said to her 'Alice I just want you to know how much I appreciate all of the hard work that you have done for me and this company. You are an asset and I'm lucky to have you working with me.' He smiled and then left the room. She said 'That moment will live with me for ever. It felt like all of the hard times were suddenly worth it. I felt like I had truly been appreciated at last.' She was telling me this with such a radiant smile, I couldn't help but smile along with her – such is the power of appreciation. Here are some suggestions:

• Practise appreciation. As you go through your day, offer random acts or remarks of appreciation to people you meet. Keep them short, to the point, relevant and, most importantly of all, genuine.

• Choose a friend whom you have known for some time, and either tell him or her in person or phone them up and say how much you have appreciated their support and friendship.

- Next time you see your postman, milkman or dustbin man, tell them how much you appreciate the work they do.

- If you have a shop that gives you particularly good service, tell them or write a letter to their manager.

Deepen the connection with your partner

It doesn't matter whether you've been in a relationship for one week or ten years, every relationship can benefit from the following exercises. Committed relationships offer an unprecedented opportunity to grow and develop as human beings and to experience extraordinary levels of intimacy and connection. But to do so you need to work on your relationship. A relationship is a separate entity formed of your energy and that of your partner. To stay alive and grow it needs constant attention and nourishment. Failing to do so, by assuming it will take care of itself, is a sure way for it to fail. Relationships need to be tended to, developed and constantly infused with creativity and aliveness. The degree to which you both consciously contribute to your relationship will determine its future. If your partner isn't up for this process, don't worry too much, your awareness and willingness to do some of this work yourself will automatically change the relationship. With time, hopefully your partner will also come on board.

Step 1 • To what extent are you nourishing your relationship?

There are numerous well-defined behaviours within relationships that will both contribute to and help grow a relationship, or destroy intimacy, trust and connection.[5] The following exercise is designed to help you and your partner shine light on your relationship as it stands, as well as giving you a flavour of how you can deepen your connection through modifying your behaviours.

Read through the following list of behaviours. If you are doing this exercise by yourself think of a time when you displayed this behaviour.

If you are doing this exercise with your partner, talk through them in turn, identifying times when you experienced those behaviours. The amount of time you spend in nourishing and toxic behaviours will tell you a lot about the health (and prognosis) of your relationship.

Nourishing behaviours	Toxic behaviours
Appreciation	Criticism
Positive attention	Negative attention
Listening	Ignoring/Interrupting
Joking	Character assassinations
Intimacy	Withholding
Fun	Lack of fun
Respect	Disrespect
Keeping promises	Breaking promises
Compromising	Refusing to compromise
Supporting	Ridiculing
Encouraging	Putting down
Treating as equals	Parenting
Compliments	Insincerity
Offering advice	Forcing unwanted advice
Confronting	Attacking
Facing reality	Denial or avoidance of reality
Openness	Defensive
Flexibility	Rigidity
Authenticity	Lack of honesty
Turning towards your partner during stress	Turning away
Solving problems together	Solving problems separately
Giving/receiving love	Closed to love
Balanced closeness/separateness	Separateness/enmeshed
Appreciating their differences	Resisting their differences

Once you've been through the list, use the nourishing behaviours list to help create your relationship vision.

Step 2 • Create your relationship vision

One way to help you fulfil your relationship potential is to be clear about what you want from it. Having a vision gives you something to work towards together. This exercise takes about 45 minutes.

- Working separately at first, each write a series of statements beginning with 'we' to describe the kind of relationship you would like to have – this can include qualities you already have and want to keep.

- The statements should be framed in the present tense as if it were already happening, such as, 'we have fun together', 'we have great sex', 'we enjoy being affectionate with each other'.

- Score each statement with a number 1 to 5: 1 = very important; 2 = important; 3 = it matters, but not too much; 4 = take it or leave it; 5 = totally unimportant.

- Circle the three items that are most important to you and then share them with your partner.

- Once your partner has shared their list, create a common vision by writing a combined list starting with the items you both agree are most important.

- Put a cross beside the items you both think would be most difficult to achieve.

- Where you have any differences try to compromise, but if you can't, leave them off the list.

- Place the list where you can see it, and refer to it at least twice a week.

This is the list that was provided by two of my workshops participants:

- We have fun together
- We meet each other's needs
- We are sexually faithful

- We trust each other

- We settle our differences peacefully

- We are healthy and physically active

- We communicate easily and openly

- We share our secrets with each other

- We enjoy parenting

- We are growing in intimacy everyday

- We talk and laugh a lot together

You can revisit your list for updates any time, and discuss how you think you are doing as a team in creating the relationship you both want together.

Step 3 • Use the appreciation exercise

One of the most effective ways of avoiding stagnation, and keeping intimacy and aliveness in a relationship, is to appreciate the other person in ways they recognise as appreciation. For example, one woman might be over the moon when she receives some flowers whereas to another woman flowers mean nothing. However, for the second woman being told that she is beautiful in a genuine and caring way might mean everything to her. The only way to know for certain with your partner is to ask them what they consider to be signs of appreciation – this exercise provides a useful framework for doing that.

1. Write a list of what your partner is already doing that pleases you. Be specific and positive, focusing on items that happen fairly regularly.
   For example, I feel loved and cared about when you . . . *hug me when I am upset, make me a cup of tea without me asking for one, compliment me on the way I look, call me from work just to see how I am etc.*

2. Write a list of any specific caring behaviours that you used to receive

from your partner in the romantic stage of your relationship, or any that you would like to receive but have never mentioned.

For example, *buying me flowers, cooking a special dinner, sleeping naked, reading to me, giving me a massage, holding my hand when we're walking, buying me a small surprise gift, having breakfast in bed together.*

Now exchange lists and read your partner's list. Put a cross beside any item that you are not willing to do at this time. The remaining items are now your personal guide to appreciating your partner. Using your list for inspiration, aim for appreciating your partner on at least two separate occasions each day. This might feel 'false' initially, but do persist, the rewards will be worth it.

In addition to these gestures and gifts, one of the most potent ways to feel connected in relationship is through genuine verbal appreciation. We all know how wonderful it is to receive appreciation. Try the following as an exercise for the next two weeks. While it might seem artificial initially, it will soon become natural, and when it does your relationship will improve considerably. Appreciation combined with full attention is the quickest way to get connected to someone.

When you start this exercise, the key is to be sensitive to ways in which your partner can be appreciated. It is important not to go overboard with this, as too much appreciation loses its sincerity. Aim for genuine appreciation between one and three times a day. Here's some ideas to get you started:

- Become more sensitively aware of yourself and your partner.

- Focus on a positive aspect of your partner and communicate it directly: 'I appreciate you for . . . ', 'Thank you for . . . '

- Women tend to prefer to receive appreciation with more detail; men like short, direct appreciations.

- Experiment: you can give appreciation through hugs, caresses, surprises, and helping gestures, as well as verbally.

- If in doubt, ask! 'Could you think of something I can do today to express my appreciation of you?'

Areas of focus for appreciation

- Essence/qualities: tune into your partner's special unique qualities and say a few words about them.

- Helpful actions: what does your partner do that makes life easier that you may be taking for granted?

- Appearance: what do you appreciate about the way your partner looks?

- Accomplishments: what has your partner achieved or helped you achieve that you're grateful for? What do you admire about them?

- Learning opportunities: what have you learned from your partner or from being in a relationship with them?

Try to find specific ways to communicate your appreciation a minimum of three times a day for one month and monitor any changes in your partner – the results may well convince you to continue developing this skill until it becomes second nature to you both.

Step 4 • Learn to argue more effectively

The Four As exercise is a really good exercise that I use myself and have recommended to be used by my patients. It allows tension between two people to be defused and addressed, before the energy and upset spills out into a full-blown argument. To make this process work, you should have practised it (before a conflict arises) with your partner and agreed on a sentence that indicates to the other that you want to use this technique. For example, something along the lines of 'I need you to sit down and listen to me' is fine.

EXERCISE: four As

A = Awareness

1. Become aware that you are stressed, tense or upset with your partner.

2. Say to them your sentence such as 'I need you to sit down and listen to me', then ask 'Is now a good time?'

3. If it is, move on to the next step, if it isn't, agree exactly when would be a good time. As a general rule of thumb it is best to do this exercise in the moment.

A = Active Listening

1. Both of you should sit down opposite each other.

2. The person who has called to do this exercise should take a few deep breaths and then start talking, while the other person listens.

3. The person who is listening is going to use active listening. This, as the name suggests, means actively listening to the other person without interruption. Your goal is to understand what is going on for the other person, by listening to them, and trying to see things from their perspective.

4. The person who is speaking needs to explain what is going on for them. One very effective and relatively non-threatening way to communicate is to use 'I' statements that communicate your feelings about some aspect of their behaviour. Stay clear of character assassinations.

For example:

You have absolutely no respect for all of the hard work I do around the house. You just sit there and treat me like a slave. You are arrogant and selfish.

Becomes:

I feel taken for granted and unappreciated at the moment. I'm really tired and exhausted with doing all of this housework myself. If you could help me for just 20 minutes twice a week that would make me feel so much happier. It would demonstrate to me that you really care for me.

5. Once the message has been communicated, the listener needs to feed back the message in a way that demonstrates that he or she has genuinely understood the other person. At this stage you don't have to agree with what has been said, but you are validating and acknowledging what has been said. The receiver then asks whether he or she has correctly understood everything. The first person either says yes or communicates the areas that have been left out. The listener once again provides feedback.

6. Now you reverse roles, so that the other person shares their feelings.

A = Action

Once you have both communicated your feelings to each other, and if it has been done effectively and genuinely, you should notice a shift in the energy between you. The focus is now on what specific action, if any, needs to be taken. Using the example above, Mary and John agreed:

1. John will help with the housework for 20 minutes every Saturday morning and Wednesday evening.

2. When John gets home from work, rather than watching television, he will spend 15 minutes with Mary so that they can talk about their respective days.

A = Appreciation

Once you've agreed on a plan of action, then it's time to reconnect to each other. This could be anything from hugging, going for a walk, to kissing or making love. Whatever works!

When arguments cross the threshold

From time to time, arguments might get out of hand, by that I mean:

- Verbally abusive

- Potentially physically abusive

- One of you feeling emotionally overwhelmed

If any of these rear their head, then TIME OUT can be called. Calling time out is a clear signal that the situation has gone too far and that you can't cope.

1. On calling time out, all exchanges and communication must stop instantly.

2. The person who called time out must leave the room.

3. Each person then must use whatever tools they want to calm them down. I recommend: emotional freedom technique (page 332), conscious breathing (page 314), venting your anger into a pillow, journaling (page 372).

4. Once the person who called time out feels calm enough, they return to the room with the other person and ask if he or she is ready to talk.

5. If the other person is ready, use the four As exercise.

Step 5 • Allow yourself to receive love and experience connection

It's one thing to give positive attention and be appreciative, but another to allow yourself to receive it. There are many reasons why we don't allow compliments in: they might not fit with the belief that we hold about ourselves; for example, a belief of 'I am unlovable' or 'I am not worthy' will filter out any events in your environment that don't fit in with those beliefs. You might have had a childhood in which you rarely, if ever, received compliments. So receiving them feels unnatural or uncomfortable. If you experienced abuse as a child, you would have learnt that being vulnerable and open equals emotional pain; quite understandably you might have erected barriers around yourself to prevent yourself from feeling the same pain again. Alter- natively you might not recognise that you are being complimented. We each experience compliments and love in different ways; for one person a bunch of flowers equals appreciation, for another person love might mean leaving a card in a surprise place saying how much you love and care for that person. Whatever the reason might be, we can all learn skills for opening ourselves to deeper levels of intimacy.

Using a score of between 0 and 10, with 0 = completely disagree and 10 = completely agree, to what extent do you agree with the following statement:

'I allow myself be congratulated, appreciated, nourished and loved by others completely and totally without any resistance whatsoever.'

A score of 9 or less suggests you would benefit from the following:

The 'I Love You' exercise on page 288 will take you through a process in which you can remove some of the shields to receiving love and compliments. An alternative exercise, or one that can be used along-side this one, is a process developed by Silvia Hartmann, the developer of EmoTrance (see Resources, page 422).

EXERCISE: receiving love and compliments

With a partner try the following. You will need between one and three hours to do this.

- You and your partner should separately write down a list of compliments that you find hard to receive and experience. For example: 'I love you', 'I am really proud of you', 'You are incredible', 'You are beautiful'.

- Stand opposite one another, and decide who is going to receive the compliments/love/appreciation and who is going to give them.

- The receiver should choose which of the compliments that they would like to receive most. The giver should then say that compliment to them in a sincere and meaningful way.

- The receiver will experience one of two things. Either they will feel it in their body, or they will feel nothing. If you feel it in your body, use EmoTrance (on page 344), to remove that blockage, until that compliment energises and uplifts you. If you feel nothing, and the compliment was said with meaning and emotion, that suggests that you have erected a shield around you, to protect yourself. This is quite common.

- The interesting thing with shields is that the receiver will actually get a sense of where this shield is located around them, and what it is like, by just simply holding an intention to feel it.

Quite often the shield will be a couple of inches or feet in front of the receiver.

- The next step is for the receiver to imagine making a progressively larger hole in the shield so as to allow the compliment to come through. Most people start by putting a pinprick in the shield. Once this is done the giver of the compliment should say the compliment again. Because this compliment can now be received, because of the hole, the receiver should feel it impacting in their body. If so, use EmoTrance as usual, and then repeat the process after making the hole bigger – for example the size of a grapefruit. You repeat this process of compliment–EmoTrance–bigger hole, until the receiver feels safe to remove the entire shield.

- Once the shield is removed, use the EmoTrance to accept and experience the compliment.

- Then swap over, repeat the process and work through each compliment in turn.

Of all the processes that I use in my workshop it is this one that I love most. It's an incredible honour to witness people experiencing love and appreciation, sometimes for the first time in their lives. This is a profound and life-changing process.

Other ideas for connection

- Nutritional and hormonal imbalances, toxicity, digestive health problems, indeed any physical body imbalance can affect your ability to experience connection. Use the total-health questionnaire (on page 21) to identify any particular areas that might be affecting you.

- Keeping a pet and taking care of it can provide an invaluable source of connection. Pets don't tend to judge us and answer us back, unlike humans. Keeping a pet has been found to reduce blood pressure, cholesterol levels, alleviate some of the symptoms of depression and reduce loneliness.

- Phone or email a friend that you haven't connected with for some time, keep in regular contact and enjoy some good memories with them. People with a network of friends and support boost their chances of surviving life-threatening illness, have stronger, more resilient immune systems, improve their mental health and live longer than people without social support.

- Having at least one person that you can share everything with, someone who acts as a witness to your inner world, is one of the most important people you can have in your life. If you haven't got someone, set an intention for the universe to send you someone, and see what happens!

- Spending time in nature and allowing yourself to appreciate and connect with what you can see and feel can for some people provide a powerful form of connection and emotional nourishment.

- Join a social, sports or special interest club to meet like-minded people. Support groups for people going through illness or a life crisis can provide an invaluable source of support and help. There is also some good evidence that they can improve recovery, and in the case of cancer, help extend people's lives.

- Develop a spiritual practice. People who have a faith or belong to some kind of religious or spiritual group enjoy better health and greater support than those who don't. Meditation and mindfulness are very effective tools for developing a deeper connection with the divine, which you could call God. See the mind–body tool on meditation for more information (page 376).

Now that you have reached the end of this chapter, my advice is to re-read it one more time. While doing so highlight those sentences (using a highlighter pen) that you feel are important to you. Once you've done this write down at least five steps or actions that you are going to take, and spend a moment visualising yourself implementing them. Once you have completed this, move on to your next barrier.

MIND–BODY ESSENTIALS

- To improve your connection with others, try visualisation, attentive listening and active appreciation.

- Connecting through committed relationships can be enhanced by identifying whether your existing behaviours are nourishing or toxic towards the relationship. Creating a relationship vision, actively appreciating one another, learning how to argue more effectively and how to receive love and compliments are skills that can be learnt and used to improve intimacy and honesty within relationships.

- Regular contact with friends, keeping pets, being a member of a club or group, spending time in nature and having a spiritual practice can all increase the degree to which you feel connected.

- Recommended mind–body tools to accompany this chapter: emotional freedom technique (page 332), emotional trauma release (page 341), journaling (page 372), goal setting (page 362), creative visualisation (page 319), Bach Flower Remedies (page 298), meditation (page 376), conscious breathing (page 314) and relaxation (page 380).

- For recommended reading see Resources, page 427.

Denial of reality

Bernadette absolutely point-blank refused to admit that the lump in her breast was anything to worry about. It was only three years later when she fractured her hip following a fall that the consequence of her decision become apparent. The X-ray of her hip found that it had become weakened because of a cancerous lesion. Her breast lump was in fact cancer, and because of her refusal to admit that there was a problem, as well as growing in size, it had spread throughout her body and was now inoperable.

Bernadette's story is of course an extreme and rare case, but nonetheless a powerful reminder of how important it can be to face reality. When I spoke with Bernadette, she said that part of her always knew it was cancer, but another part, the part she decided to believe, simply wasn't brave enough to face the consequences of it. As Bernadette put it in her own words, 'You cannot escape reality, you can kid yourself that there is not a problem, but life has a mysterious way of making you face your truth – eventually.'

Most of us, to differing degrees, deny reality – it's part of being human. It is so easy to get caught up in the drama and whirlwind of life (and life's challenges and pressures) that the idea of stepping back from it all and taking stock of what we are doing, and whether what we are doing is bringing us fulfilment and allowing us to enjoy good health, actually seems like quite a hard thing to do. And it is! Life events have a magnetic pull about them, our awareness gets sucked into our worries, our fears, our relationships and career; so much so, that it's the events and people in our life that determine the course of our life, not ourselves – and that's a problem. When we live life reactively, and without awareness, we make the same old mistakes, repeat the same patterns and never truly feel fulfilled. What's the solution?

Well, part of the solution is to step back from your life and check in with yourself as to whether life is working for you or against you. Life certainly appears simpler when you can cruise on automatic pilot; I've met many people who are OK with feeling sad or frustrated, because that's how they've always felt and it's what they know best. They sustain their life situation by ignoring or denying those aspects of reality that threaten their comfort zone. That's OK, if you truly are content with your life. However, if you are committed to achieving your total health potential, it is necessary and absolutely essential to open your eyes and face reality.

What is reality?

Reality, for the purpose of this chapter, refers to the facts of your life's situation as it is right now. This encompasses everything that is happening in this moment, particularly your health, finances, career and relationships, as it is usually one or more of these that is holding you back from total health. Although facing reality can also involve looking at past events and memories, we're going to stick with what is happening in your life now. Why? Because the most significant influence on the quality and appearance of your life in the future are the choices and actions that you take today. And what is the most powerful determinant of the quality of those choices? It's your level of awareness, and to be aware requires you to open your eyes and face reality.

What is denial of reality?

If facing reality is about taking a look at the facts of life as they are for you right now, denying reality is refusing to look at the facts of some aspect of your life right now. Denial is a conscious or even subconscious refusal to admit that something is occurring or has occurred. Most people when they deny some aspect of their life, such as poor financial health or relationship problems, have a degree of awareness of the issue but are refusing to keep their attention or focus on it. So why would you want to do that?

Why deny reality?

We deny reality for a very good and valid reason, because if we did look at a certain aspect of our reality, such as the state of our finances or relationships, it would trigger some pretty unpleasant and uncomfortable feelings. Denial therefore is effectively an emotional analgesic: it temporarily numbs us to a certain aspect of life that has the potential to cause emotional upset. From a short-term perspective you could argue that denial of reality holds a positive function and purpose. Let's see if this holds true for you.

EXERCISE: denying reality

Think back to a recent event, in which you now know, on reflection, that you were avoiding facing some situation. What was the situation? What were you doing? What were you feeling and thinking? Why did you not want to face reality? The answer for the last question is that nine out of ten times it's because it would have felt uncomfortable to do so.

We deny reality in order to avoid the feelings of discomfort, anxiety or emotional distress, which you would feel if you did face reality. Tied up with that is the belief that you don't know how, or don't have the confidence, means and resources to cope with the issue. That makes sense, because if you did know how to cope with the situation, you'd have no problems facing it.

Here are some typical examples of why you might not want to face reality:

- You don't want to know certain things; for example, by ignoring the payment demands of your credit card company you are avoiding the reality of having to find the money to pay it off.

- You don't want to feel a certain way; for example, by pretending that you do still love your partner, you are avoiding the reality of knowing that you do not want to be with them any more.

- You don't want to become aware of something; for example, by ignoring people's concerns that you might be an alcoholic you deny the reality that your need to drink a bottle of wine every day confirms that you are an alcoholic.

So, if denying reality can let us off the hook emotionally, why would we want to start facing reality?

What is the benefit of facing reality?

So far, denying certain aspects of reality appears to make sense, it reduces your experience of anxiety and emotional pain, it appears to make life simpler and you get to feel that you are in control of your life experience. If you don't like the look or feel of something, you just need to turn your attention away and the problem is no longer there. So why would you want to face reality? Well, to start with, denying reality is actually quite tiring. Deliberately turning your attention away from an issue, suppressing and ignoring thoughts and feelings, and going out of your way to avoid situations consumes a fair amount of your creative energy. Secondly, when you deny reality, you deny part of your experience, and in doing so you disconnect part of yourself from reality. This in turn generates a lack of fulfilment and deep dis-ease. Thirdly, the temporary relief from the emotional stress that denial offers often comes at a price in the long term. That is exactly what happened with Bernadette, whose story I mentioned at the very beginning of this chapter.

Contrary to what you might believe, and as long as you have the support and resources available to you, facing reality can be a liberating experience. Here are just some of the benefits that I have personally experienced and witnessed with my own patients when they start to open their eyes and face reality:

- You feel better able to go with the flow and respond more effectively to life's challenges.

- Life appears to start working for you rather than against you.

- You feel more connected to life.

- Your energy levels go up.

- You experience greater clarity on issues and challenges.

- You have more honest and open relationships.

- You have an improved sense of intuition and knowing.

- Life becomes simpler, less complicated.

- You experience less suffering and worry.

- You feel better able and more likely to achieve your goals.

Now you know some of the benefits of seeing reality, what do you need to do?

Facing reality

Opening your eyes and facing reality is a life-long process, a skill that takes time and perseverance. I recommend you share your experiences and seek support from a counsellor or life coach, or even a good friend, as you go through this process, because it can make you feel quite disorientated, temporarily. Switching on the light, so to speak, is an exciting moment, particularly because it signifies a commitment to getting real and a positive first step in redesigning your life to one that meets your emotional and physical needs. The process of opening your eyes and facing reality involves four parts:

Step 1 • Commit yourself to seeing reality

Before you take stock of what's going on in your life, see if you can come up with some good reasons to start seeing reality. This will help to keep you motivated, particularly in those moments when you are tempted to turn a blind eye to what is happening in your life. Take a few moments to write down in a notebook at least three reasons why you and your life would benefit from facing reality. If you get stuck, refer to the list above for inspiration.

Here's an example of one of the lists of benefits given to me by a patient:

When I start facing reality I will:

1. *Start to get my life back on track*

2. *Feel freer and happier*

3. *Enjoy a closer relationship with my husband*

Step 2 • Give up the need to be right

Are you one of those people who just has to be right? When was the last time you said to someone, 'I'm sorry, I made a mistake'? Think of a time when you refused to back down, or failed to admit that you were wrong, despite knowing that you were wrong? A person who feels they need to prove themselves by being 'right' is really, underneath the façade, someone who is terrified of being 'wrong'. As to why that might be really depends on the person, but a core belief of 'I'm not good enough' or 'I'm stupid' is often the culprit. Being 'right' is a very subtle and effective way of compensating for a lack of inner strength and self-belief by stealing power away from the person you are making wrong.

If you are the kind of person who needs to be right, take a few deep breaths now and ask yourself, 'What thought about myself am I trying to cover up and disprove when I fight to be right?' The answer you give yourself will tell you a lot about why you need to be right. Bearing that in mind, next time you find yourself needing to be 'right', notice what you are doing, take a deep breath and stop what you are saying. Be with whatever it is you are feeling and ask yourself (particularly if you are arguing with your partner), 'Do I want to be right or do I want to be in a relationship with this person.' Giving up the need to be right can have an instant and positive effect on your relationships. Give it a try!

Step 3 • Open yourself to other people's perspectives

How good are you at listening to and acknowledging other people's perspectives? How much flexibility do you have in adapting your own beliefs and worldviews when you learn something new or gain insight into something? Your ability to listen and consider other people's perspectives tells you a lot about the degree to which you are currently embracing reality. Reality, remember, consists of everything. If you therefore refuse point-blank to even consider that some of the beliefs of Islam, for example, might have some validity or that acupuncture might be able to help you recover from back pain, then what you are in effect doing is blanking out part of reality. Doing so denies you the opportunity to learn and grow in understanding and awareness. Part of being committed to total health is a willingness to explore other people's worldviews and perspectives. It doesn't mean you have to make them your own beliefs or agree with them, it just means you are humble enough to acknowledge that you do not know everything. When you open yourself to other points of view, several things happen. Firstly, you gain insight and feel more connected to that person. Secondly, you feel lighter and more energised, because you are no longer investing your energy in resisting the reality of another perspective. And thirdly, you become more humble, as you start to realise that opening yourself to another person's perspective (remember you don't have to believe in what they are saying) is one of the greatest acts of respect that you can make. Give these two exercises a go:

EXERCISE: other people's perspectives 1

Next time you catch yourself automatically rejecting another person's worldview or perspective, rather than ignoring it or arguing against it, breathe deeply and listen deeply. The point of this exercise is not to judge what is being said, but simply to practise allowing another person's right to have a perspective. If you want to go one step further ask yourself, 'What can I learn from this person?'

EXERCISE: other people's perspectives 2

1. Think of a person who upsets you in some way. (The stronger the upset, the greater potential for you to get something out of this exercise!)

2. Now close your eyes and imagine yourself in their shoes. Imagine

what life has been like for them, see yourself living their life, and get a real feel for their worries, fears, concerns and perspectives. The idea of this exercise is not to pass judgement on what they are doing but simply to experience an alternative perspective on life. Take your time with this and, if you can, allow yourself to develop some understanding as to why they are the way they are.

3. Once you've completed the exercise write down at least three new insights or perspectives that you have learnt. Take a moment to give thanks for this.

Step 4 • Take a reality check

Now it's time to take an honest look at the various components of your life, and to start identifying what issues specifically you are in denial about. A simple way of doing a reality check is to fill in a chart such as the one below. Choose one issue for each category that you know you are in denial about. To make sure that you don't fall into the trap of glossing over an area of your life that does need to be faced, check in with the feelings within your body when you think about a specific area, such as relationships or finances. For example, a patient of mine, Karen, told me that the relationship with her partner was great, and that things couldn't be better, yet her body language, her eyes and her tone of voice didn't mirror that. When I asked her to check in with how she felt when she said those words, she realised that there was heaviness in her heart area. Watch out for this. It's really easy to kid yourself that things are OK when they aren't. So when you look at the following aspects of your life, pay attention to your feelings. A feeling of peace and lightness tends to indicate that there is no problem, heaviness and discomfort a problem – and an invitation to open your eyes and face reality.

Aspect of your life	Specific issue that needs addressing
Health	
Finances	
Career	

Aspect of your life	Specific issue that needs addressing
Relationships (family)	
Relationships (friends)	
Relationship (partner)	
Any other	

Here's an example of a chart drawn up by a patient of mine:

Aspect of your life	Specific issue that needs addressing
Health	Stomach pains that have been coming and going for two years
Finances	Credit card bill of £8,000
Career	I don't find my job fulfilling any more
Relationships (family)	My dad still treats me like a child even though I am 45 years old
Relationships (friends)	Peter runs me down in front of my mates and I hate it
Relationships (partner)	I do everything I can to get out of having sex
Any other	The batteries in the smoke alarm need replacing

Once you've identified the various issues that need facing, the next step is to spend a few seconds, or even a couple of minutes, focusing on each one in turn. Breathe deeply and allow yourself to feel and embrace the feelings that come up. If you sense yourself wanting to escape them, which you might well do, just turn your attention back to your feelings and continue breathing. Eventually, usually just after a couple of minutes, you will feel calmer, more energised and even more at peace. This happens because you have stopped resisting your emotions and have accepted the reality of their presence. Not only does this feel better, but you should now be able to think more clearly and experience greater clarity of insight as to what action needs to be taken. If you struggle to get to that calm emotional state, either do this exercise with a friend who can support you, and/or turn to page 344, it will guide you through a process called EmoTrance, which will help.

When you embrace reality – firstly by identifying the issues that you are resisting, and secondly by allowing yourself to feel your emotional response fully to those issues, you free your creative energy and that gives you the power and insight to either make positive change in your life or accept deeply the circumstances of your life. Opening your eyes and facing reality has the potential to be one of the most liberating experiences of your life.

Now that you have reached the end of this chapter, my advice is to reread it one more time. While doing so highlight those sentences (using a highlighter pen) that you feel are important to you. Once you've done this write down at least five steps or actions that you are going to take, and spend a moment visualising yourself implementing them. Once you have completed this, move on to your next barrier.

MIND–BODY ESSENTIALS

- Facing reality requires us to acknowledge 'what is': the facts of our life as they are right now.

- No one is obliged to face reality. However, denying reality can prevent you from growing and living the life that you desire. It can stifle your creativity, drain your energy and, the worst-case scenario, lead to a problem that is far worse and more serious than the situation you were originally faced with.

- Being clear about the positive benefits of facing reality and taking a reality check on your life as it is right now will quickly get you started on the pathway to seeing reality.

- Recommended mind–body tools to accompany this chapter: journaling (page 372), symptom dialogue (page 391), focusing (page 356), creative visualisation (page 319), Bach Flower Remedies (page 298), meditation (page 376), conscious breathing (page 314) and relaxation (page 380).

- For recommended reading see Resources, page 428.

Emotional mismanagement

Frances was intellectually sharp – the kind of person who was articulate, smart and quick to grasp new ideas. But beneath this controlled exterior was a very unsettled emotional world. She had never been shown how to manage her emotions as a child and, because of that, emotions were 'things to be scared of'. Whenever she felt herself getting emotional she would either distract herself or rationalise them away. Either way, she felt deeply uncomfortable with her emotions, and she suspected that this might be contributing to her health problems. She was right. Frances had been suffering from back pain on and off for three years. Despite numerous trips to the doctor, injections into the back, physiotherapy and constant painkillers, her back pain was continuing to get worse. It was also interfering with her work, she couldn't exercise more, and her social life was 'near to zero'. She even thought that her back pain was a big factor in her splitting up with her long-term boyfriend. Even though they parted company over a year ago, she thinks about him daily, and it was still difficult for her to even talk about him. Her inner life, in her own words, 'was a mess'.

I meet a lot of people like Frances, people who are psychologically sound but emotionally under-developed. It's very common. In the case of Frances, I explained to her how stuck and unexpressed emotions can be a major contributing factor in pain of any kind. Learning how to release those emotions, and developing the skills to manage subsequent emotions, would hopefully provide her with a way out of this difficult period in her life. I shared with her what I am about to share with you. After three weeks of using my five steps, she phoned me elated. Her back pain had disappeared four days previously. She dared not call me in case it came back, but so far it hadn't. She sounded like a new women. Since that call she has moved forward in leaps and bounds in her life. She found a new man, changed her job (which she had previously described as 'a pain in the back') and she started to enjoy her emotions. This is the power of emotional management.

If you identified emotional mismanagement as one of your barriers, then learning about the nature of emotions is your first step to greater emotional well-being.

What are emotions?

Emotions are messages from your bodymind telling you something that you need to hear. They are information, a source of wisdom and guidance. Emotions add richness and depth to our lives, they make the body come alive with energy and in some circumstances they invite us to discover more about ourselves. Avoiding emotions, just as Frances did, denies a part of what it is to be human. To read about emotions and the mind–body connection please see Appendix I.

What are the different types?

There are a lot of different flavours of emotions, and many ways of categorising them, but the simplest one uses just four major categories. I came across this form of categorisation in an excellent book called *The Emotional Toolkit* by a clinical psychologist called Dr Darlene Mininni.[1] She places all of the emotions under the following subheadings:

Happiness	Anger	Sadness	Anxiety
joy	frustration	grief	fear
pleasure	resentment	shame	nervousness
gratitude	upset	inadequacy	dread
contentment	irritability	hurt	concern
love	rage	guilt	insecurity

There are a lot more emotions than these, but this list gives you a taste of how emotions can be categorised.

What do the different emotions mean?

Whereas the specific underlying meaning of the emotions will depend on you and your circumstances in any given moment, some general rule-of-thumb conclusions can be made about different emotions:

- **Happiness**, or one of its variations, arises because we have gained something positive. The question is *what have I gained?*

- **Anxiety**, or one of its variations, arises because of some threat to us, combined with a belief that at some level we can't cope. The unanswered question is *what am I afraid of?*

- **Sadness**, or one of its variations, arises because of some kind of loss. The unanswered question is *what have I lost?*

- **Anger**, or one of its variations, arises because of some threat. The unanswered question is *how am I being threatened?*

Think back to events from the past when you experienced each of these four emotions. For each one in turn ask the relevant question and find your answer. Here are some responses provided by one of my workshop attendees, Pam:

Happiness

Situation *My husband announcing that we are going on holiday to the Maldives (I've always wanted to go there).*

Gained: *A sense of being appreciated and cared about.*

Anxiety

Situation *One hour before having to do a presentation at work.*
Afraid *Of being laughed at.*

Sadness

Situation *Finding out that the house purchase has fallen through.*
Lost *My dream of living in that house.*

Anger

Situation *Husband not listening to me.*
Threat *He loves football more than he loves me.*

The emotions we experience

What determines which emotions we experience? This is an important question to answer, because doing so helps to explain why the same event can result in different people experiencing very different feelings. Here are just some of the factors at play:

Meaning

The emotions and the strength of the emotions that we have in any moment are closely related to the meaning we have attached to whatever it is we are experiencing. For example, you get a letter through the door saying you've won £1,000. One person, who maybe doesn't have that much money, might attach a meaning along the lines of 'Wow, that's fantastic. I'm going to be able to buy the kids their Christmas presents, or buy some new clothes.' Her emotions will probably be one of joy or excitement. Another person, who is a millionaire, might attach a meaning along the lines of 'Oh, I wish I had won the bigger prize of £100,000.' His emotions might be of disappointment or frustration. Same situation, but with different meanings = different emotional response.

Temperament

Each of us has certain behavioural and emotional patterns hard-wired into us from conception.[2] These are heavily influenced by our genetic inheritance, although fortunately they can be modified using emotional management skills. Some people, for example, are predisposed to excessive amounts of worry, self-criticism or over-sensitivity. This increases the likelihood of them experiencing anxiety and sadness-related emotions, when compared to someone with a calmer temperament.

Pattern matching

Have you ever overreacted to a situation and felt emotions that were disproportionate to what the situation warranted? Or have you witnessed yourself automatically and predictably reacting to a situation, just like you have done a hundred times before? I'm sure you have, we've all had moments when we've been surprised and sometimes shocked by what came out of us, or surprised at how the way someone looked at us or said something could trigger such a strong emotional response. So what's going on?

It's called pattern matching and it's happening all the time. Our brains have a pattern-matching technology built in to them. It's a very clever survival and learning mechanism that loosely compares your current experience (including events going on around you and your own thoughts and images) to similar past experiences. At one level that's very useful, it allows you to get inside a car and know, without having to think, how to drive it. It also explains why certain smells can remind you of someone or a certain place, or how seeing someone with long blonde hair can instantly bring up the memory and feelings associated with a friend. There is, however, a significant downside to the process of pattern matching, one that can cause significant distress and stop you from learning and growing from experiences. For example, if you grew up in a household where your mother or father criticised you (the past), part of you will automatically be primed to look for any evidence of being criticised by those around you now (the present). So if your partner says something that you interpret as having even the slightest hint of criticism, the event will be pattern-matched, and you will immediately feel the emotional load from the past (anger/frustration) arising inside you. Because this process is so quick and automatic, it's easy to see why you would wrongly attribute the way you feel to your situation, whereas, in truth, your situation has simply re-awakened the past. For more information on this fascinating subject I encourage you to read *Human Givens* by Joe Griffin and Ivan Tyrell (see Resources, page 429).

Perceptions

I mentioned earlier how the meaning we attach to something influences what we see. So what influences meaning? The answer is: beliefs. Beliefs are assumptions that we hold about ourselves and everything to do with the world we live in. They are like filters through which information and our experiences are passed, and because of this they distort reality. Most of us tend to see our beliefs rather than the reality of any given situation. For example, Marcus, a medical doctor, had a belief that complementary and alternative medicine doesn't work. That was his belief. Because the mind is designed to prove beliefs right, he only ever read information and research literature that backed up his case, and ignored those that didn't. This selective bias is usually unconscious, so the person, and in this case Marcus, isn't even aware that it is going on. Beliefs therefore distort the way we interpret and perceive reality, which in turn influences the feelings that we feel. Every time I mentioned the words complementary alternative medicine you could see his body tense up, and feel his anger rising. That's the power of beliefs!

Biological factors

The health of your body also has a big influence on your emotional well-being. Just think back to the last time you had a full-blown cold. Do you remember how miserable you felt? Those emotions weren't just because you weren't happy about having your cold, it's because your immune system released chemicals in your body that alter the way you feel. It's actually a very clever way of forcing you to rest and recuperate. All of the following biological factors can also influence the way you feel:

- **Diet, exercise and sleep.**

- **Nutritional deficiencies**, particularly omega-3 and omega-6 essential fatty acids, vitamin C, B vitamins, folic acid, chromium, magnesium and zinc.

- **Food and chemical sensitivities**, particularly to gluten (found in rye, oats, wheat and barley), casein (dairy products), caffeine, egg white, chocolate, aspartame (a sweetener) and moulds.

- **Toxicity**, due to lead, mercury, cadmium and aluminium.

- **Blood-sugar imbalance**, due to excessive consumption of refined carbohydrates and sugar.

- **Hormonal imbalances** Thyroid, adrenal and sex-hormone imbalances.

- **Diseases** Anaemia, diabetes, chronic fatigue syndrome, chronic pain, cancer, arthritis, premenstrual syndrome, insomnia, stroke, multiple sclerosis, any chronic disease.

- **Prescription drugs**, such as atorvastatin, amlodipine, atenolol, diltiazem, ibuprofen, propanolol, captopril, cimetidine, diazepam, levodopa, prednisolone, indomethacin and opiates.

- **Recreational drugs**, such as alcohol, marijuana, tobacco, caffeine, and cocaine.

An essential step in resolving any kind of emotional or psychological challenge is to make sure that biological factors are not playing a major role.

When emotions become a problem

Most people like to divide emotions into two groups, positive and negative, and then further subdivide them: joy, happiness and peace (positive), and anger, rage, sadness and fear (negative). This polarisation of emotions is unfortunate because all contribute to the experience of being human, being real. Denying or negating any of these emotions blunts our ability to experience the full spectrum of emotions. This in turn disconnects us from a valuable source of insight and information. Emotions are, therefore, not inherently bad. Anger is not bad, rage is not bad, sadness is not bad; what determines whether they are healthy or unhealthy or not is our relationship to them. These are the five main relationships:

1. Feel fully, accept them as they are without wanting to do anything with them and allow them to pass through and out of your awareness – HEALTHY.

2. Discharge them, through physical activity, sharing your thoughts – HEALTHY.

3. Allow yourself to be overwhelmed by them and act them out – UNHEALTHY.

4. Suppress them: when emotions come up, you consciously resist them which often involves distracting yourself/or chemically changing the way you feel through behaviours, such as eating, alcohol, smoking, and so on – UNHEALTHY.

5. Repress them: emotions are automatically prevented from coming up into the awareness – VERY UNHEALTHY.

I use the term 'emotional mismanagement' to describe someone who hasn't yet developed the awareness and skills to deal with their emotions effectively and in a healthy way. When emotions are mismanaged in an unhealthy way, they always interfere with our quality of life, and can put us at risk of disease.

How emotions cause disease

Dr Candace Pert, pioneering researcher and psycho-pharmacologist, discovered and brought to the public awareness through her book *Molecules of Emotions* a revolutionary understanding and theory of how emotions influence the body.[3] She suggests:

• **Emotions** are the bridge between the mind and the body.

• **Peptides** are the physical correlates of emotions; they are the carriers of information between the brain and body, body and brain.

- These peptides enable every system of the body to be in a constant state of dialogue. This includes the immune system, brain, skin, muscles, endocrine system, digestive system and nervous system.

- All of the systems of the body upon receiving their messages via the peptides have the capacity to answer back – to generate their own peptide response. There is no system in the body that is unaffected by emotions.

- Each type of peptide represents a particular type of emotional tone. For example, endorphins are the correlates of bliss; vasoactive intestinal peptide the correlates of self-love, and prolactin the correlates of bonding.

- Every change in our physiological state is mirrored by a shift in our emotional state, and every change in the emotional state is mirrored by a change in our physiological state. Happy emotions generate health-promoting peptides; unhappy emotions generate disease-promoting peptides.

Dr Candace Pert's own understanding is that the act of blocking or repressing emotions clogs up the peptide receptors, leading to a malfunction in the cell to which it is attached, and a breakdown in communication and the flow of chemicals and information. This sets up the conditions for disease to take place and the process of healing to be impaired. To enjoy full and total health, emotions need to be brought into awareness and allowed to flow.

Improving your management skills

Learning how to manage your emotions is an essential skill that you need if you are committed to total health. It's a process that can take quite some time, given that you will have to undo your existing habits in how you deal with your emotions. But it is hugely worthwhile and the rewards are many. They include being in touch with your intuition, experiencing deeper levels of intimacy and connection to others, enjoying much higher levels of emotional and psychological health, and reducing the risk of developing health problems relating to emotional mismanagement. The five-step approach that I'm about to take you through is similar to the one that I use in my workshops and retreats.

Step 1 • Identify your approach to emotions

In my workshops I talk about four different approaches to dealing with emotions: the proactive approach, the open approach, the closed approach, and the anti-emotion approach. Each has a different philosophy, spoken or unspoken, about emotions. Read through the descriptions below and see if you can identify which group you belong to at the moment:

The proactive approach

Someone with a proactive approach:

- Understands that emotions are information and are there to be experienced and harnessed.

- Feels comfortable with experiencing the full range of emotions.

- Knows how to express and use their feelings in ways that are appropriate to the situation.

- Is more understanding of other people when they are experiencing emotions – they won't try to close people down, rather they will help them move through their emotions.

- Knows how to use emotional management skills to limit any detrimental impact of emotions such as anger and sadness.

The open approach

Someone with an open approach:

- Also understands that emotions are an invaluable part of being human.

- Will allow themselves to express their emotions; that is, become angry or sad, but unlike those who use a proactive approach, they are more likely to surrender to the emotion, rather than actively managing or soothing their emotions. They will just wait for the emotion to pass.

- Will tolerate other people being emotional, but will not know how to help them move through their emotions.

- Is unlikely to investigate and take action to address the underlying reasons for their emotions.

The closed approach

Someone with a closed approach:

- Keeps their feelings hidden and out of sight.

- Will be aware of the emotions inside of them, but are fearful of expressing them. Common reasons include: fear of being criticised (from a parent, for example), fear of losing control, fear of being weak (if they have a belief that showing emotions are a sign of weakness) and fear of upsetting others.

- Will find it difficult to experience intimacy and connection because of their struggle to reveal and share their inner experience.

- Will be upset, intimidated and/or overwhelmed by those who do show their emotions.

- Will dismiss others who are emotional; for example, by saying 'you really shouldn't be upset', or 'it's not that bad'.

The anti-emotion approach

Someone with an anti-emotion approach:

- Will be similar to someone with a closed approach: they also prefer to keep emotions hidden.

- However, unlike a closed approach, they respond to other people's 'negative' emotionality with hostility. For example, a mother might say to her child, 'If you don't stop crying, I'll give you something to cry about', or 'You can stop that now, you ungrateful little so and so.'

- Is constantly involved in power struggles and knows only how to 'feel in control' by putting other people down.

- Will 'blow hot and cold', and be emotionally unstable. This can be very intimidating for people close to them.

You can probably guess, given the descriptions that I have provided, that when it comes to achieving total health a proactive approach is more effective than an open approach, which is more effective than a closed approach, which is more effective than an anti-emotion approach. However, these are not fixed levels. Regardless of which approach you use at the moment everyone can move up the emotional ladder using the suggestions below:

Step 2 • Develop your emotional awareness

Noticing your feelings, without actually doing anything with them, is a useful way of familiarising yourself with your emotional landscape.

EXERCISE: emotional awareness

1. Select a day on which you are going to do your emotional awareness exercise. On that day make a commitment to noticing your emotions.

2. Every time you interact with someone, or go for a walk, notice what you feel, and label the category that those feelings belong to: sadness, happiness, anger or anxiety.

3. Once you get the hang of this, you can repeat the exercise, but this time see if you can further refine the emotions that you are feeling. For example, rather than labelling sadness, use hurt, guilt or grief instead. Once you get good at this, start noticing how you behave and act when you experience different types of emotions. What do you do when you are angry, sad or anxious?

4. Continue with this for at least another week or so, until you become quite proficient and confident at noticing your emotions and reactions.

If you get to this stage well done – you are doing great!

Step 3 • Choosing and using your core emotional-management tools

Being aware of our emotions is one thing, but proactively doing something with them is another. Of course, most of the time you won't have to because emotions, by their very nature, come and go. However, if you are experiencing any of the following, then you would almost certainly benefit from selecting some tools from the Mind–Body Toolbox:

- You find it hard to feel emotions, or you feel numb inside.

- You are stuck in your emotions; for example, grief, anxiety or depression.

- Your behaviour is affecting your health, relationships or quality of life.

- You have an open, closed or anti-emotion approach to emotions.

- You use alcohol, food, nicotine or any other distractions to manage your feelings.

Most of the core emotional tools are in Part 3 of this book. My advice is to read through them all and see which ones appeal to you. Different people like different tools. For example, one of my workshop attendees, Mary, found journaling, Bach Flower Remedies and focusing to be beneficial, whereas Josephine liked EFT, exercise and meditation. The emotional tools I recommend are:

Appreciation	Instant stress release
Bach Flower Remedies	Journaling
Conscious breathing	Meditation

Emotional freedom technique   Relaxation

Exercise   Tame the inner critic

Focusing

I usually recommend that everyone finds two or three favourites that they use regularly and become proficient in. Try not to fall into the trap of learning them all and not using any of them!

Step 4 • Release any emotional trauma

One of the biggest barriers to successful emotional management can be unresolved emotional hurt and trauma from the past. Getting to the heart of an underlying issue, such as heartbreak or abuse, and then using one of the simple and safe processes in the emotional trauma release section (page 341) can make a dramatic and immediate shift in the way you feel. If you think this might apply to you then I would recommend you read through this chapter.

Step 5 • Learn how to communicate more effectively

Being able to communicate your needs and feelings without getting a verbal battering from the person you are speaking to is not easy sometimes, but it is a skill that can be learnt. Here are some ideas to get you started:

1. Mentally rehearse your communication skills. Close your eyes, and allow an image of a confident and assertive you to appear. See yourself engaging in the types of situations that would normally make you upset. Watch yourself keep calm, but acting firmly and appropriately. Once you've got the hang of it, become one with this new you, and imagine yourself as an assertive, confident person. Get a real experience of how it feels to be this way. What things would you be saying that are new? If you looked in a mirror how would you look? What would your friends and family say? Allow yourself as much time as you need to experience and make real this new you. Muster as much energy as you can to allow yourself to feel alive and confident. Experience yourself managing situations effortlessly and enjoy the experience! Repeat

this exercise as often as you want – I suggest at least once a day for 14 days.

2. If you are being overrun with emotions, before you say anything, take three deep breaths. Breathe in for the count of five and breathe out to the count of seven. This will help to calm your mind and reduce the intensity of the emotions that you are feeling.

3. Use 'I' statements. One way to make a person feel that they are not being criticised is to start a sentence with 'I'. For example rather than saying 'you never help with the kids' the 'I' approach would be 'I am really struggling to cope with the kids by myself, it makes me feel overwhelmed, would you be able to help me by putting them to bed tonight?' You can see what a difference starting with 'I' makes.

4. Try role playing. With a trusted friend or even a practitioner, recreate a typical scenario that would lead to you becoming emotional. Practise different ways of asserting yourself. Remember to breathe deeply. Tell your friend what it is you want. Practise changing your voice, your posture and your body language. Work out between you what works and rehearse it until this becomes your new way of relating.

5. If you are in a relationship, take a look at Barrier 11, which has some further suggestions on how to communicate more effectively.

Now that you have reached the end of this chapter, my advice is to re-read it one more time. While doing so highlight those sentences (using a highlighter pen) that you feel are important to you. Once you've done this write down at least five steps or actions that you are going to take, and spend a moment visualising yourself implementing them. Once you have completed this, move on to your next barrier.

MIND–BODY ESSENTIALS

- Emotions are messages from your bodymind telling you something that you need to hear.

- Emotions are not intrinsically good or bad; it's how to relate to our emotions that determines whether they are healthy or unhealthy.

- The five steps to improving emotional management skills are: identifying your approach to emotions, emotional awareness, choosing and using your core emotional tools, releasing emotional trauma and learning how to communicate more effectively.

- Recommended mind–body tools to accompany this chapter: all of them! (See pages 291–402.)

- For recommended reading see Resources, page 428.

Low self-esteem

At first glance, Maria, a young business executive attending one of my workshops, appeared to have it all. She came across as being confident, fun and sociable. At face value all was well. But as the morning progressed and the focus of the workshop turned to the way we feel about ourselves, she revealed, to the surprise of the group, that she was in fact desperately unhappy and lonely. Despite being in a loving relationship and having a well-paid job, she said, 'I have been living a lie for as long as I can remember. I have been covering up this feeling of inadequacy for so long now, I no longer know who I am. The pain of this is too much to bear, I can't go on like this any more.'

This was the first time in her 32 years of existence that she had revealed her pain, her truth, to someone. Maria had just given voice to a secret that many people carry around with them. She was speaking of her low self-esteem. She revealed how she had 'managed' her feelings of low self-esteem for years through binge drinking and eating. This had lead to her gaining a considerable amount of excess fat around her middle, which, she believed, exacerbated her asthma. She was absolutely convinced that all of her physical ailments had their root cause in her low self-esteem. I think she was probably right. However, unlike the majority of people, she was courageous enough to have taken a major leap forward to changing the way she felt. In admitting to herself and others her truth, she had started the process of transformation that I am going to share with you in this chapter. In my opinion, this is some of the most profound and important work that someone can take – the raising of self-esteem.

What is self-esteem?

Self-esteem is an energy and power source that emerges from the depths of ourselves, to the degree that we accept and value who we are. Unlike confidence, which is a skill that can be learnt and developed, self-esteem is controlled by our internal relationship – the relationship that we have with ourselves.

High self-esteem

Someone with high self-esteem has a real and authentic sense of self. They genuinely accept, value and appreciate themselves, and they believe in themselves and their worth. They have a realistic appreciation of their own strengths, talents and limitations and, despite life's challenges, they will not lose sight and sense of who they are. A person with a high level of self-esteem is therefore authentic – they are true to themselves and the situation they are in. They will not try to be someone they are not.

Low self-esteem

Someone with low self-esteem is yet to access the sense of self and authentic power that comes from complete self-acceptance. This failure to connect with their inner power source has left them feeling weak and vulnerable on the inside, and scared that anyone should discover what lies beneath their confident persona. Maria, like millions of other people, had devised a series of strategies to fill this hole inside. Her strategy was to make people laugh, pretend to be confident, drink alcohol and take the occasional drug. David, another person in the same workshop, used bullying and intimidation of others, the thrill of driving fast cars and the acquisition of wealth as his hole filler. Mary used emotional dramas and binge eating to fill in the hole within. All of them had lost sight or failed to connect with who they are; instead they had become someone deep down inside that they knew they weren't.

My job as an integrated medical doctor and workshop facilitator is to re-orientate people like Maria. By showing her how to raise her self-esteem she was, within just two weeks, able to make a significant and positive shift in the way she felt about herself. Not only did she feel happier and calmer but also her relationships started to blossom. In her own words she 'felt like a new women'. As she continues her work, she will benefit in many other ways as well.

Why is self-esteem important?

Self-esteem is intrinsically connected to our level of fulfilment, happiness and success. People with a high level of self-esteem are:

- Less likely to experience anxiety, stress, loneliness, depression and engage in destructive social behaviour, such as crime and abuse.

- Generally healthier, happier and naturally more confident.

- Less likely to experience addictions, take drugs, and have problems with friendships and relationships.

- Able to adapt to life's challenges more creatively and proactively.

- More likely to treat other people with respect, care and kindness.

A high level of self-esteem provides an undercurrent of power, clarity and knowing that enables them to shine in the world.

How is your self-esteem?

This might appear to be a very straightforward question, but most people will answer it so quickly that they don't allow a true answer to rise within them. It's tempting to give a response in alignment with how you would like to be rather than how you actually, truly are. Although this is rather a crude way to assess someone's overall self-esteem, take a couple of deep breaths and say out loud the following:

I DEEPLY AND COMPLETELY ACCEPT MYSELF

Continue with a couple of slow, deep breaths and bring your attention to your body. How true does this statement feel? Score yourself between 0 and 10; 10 = this statement is absolutely 100 per cent true, 0 = this statement is 100 per cent false. If you score less than 10, read on.

How to lift your self-esteem

Raising your self-esteem is not something that's going to happen overnight. It's an ongoing process that requires a sincere commitment to changing the way you are with yourself. If this is something that you are serious about I would encourage you to come along to one of my retreats or workshops.

Step 1 • Accept yourself

Accepting yourself as you are is the single most potent strategy for allowing your self-esteem to rise. When I first started working on my own issues of non-acceptance, one of the fears I had was that self-acceptance would result in me losing my drive, ambition and enthusiasm. In fact it did the exact opposite. What I found, and have seen in many of my patients who follow these steps, is that when you totally and completely accept yourself, the energy and clarity of insight that emerges from within actually enables you to make better decisions and take more action. This is the self-acceptance process that I teach in my workshops:

EXERCISE: self-acceptance

1. List the ways in which you do not accept yourself. Then rank them in terms of how important they are to you. The first will be your most important.

For example (the following examples were given by my workshop attendees):

1. *I give myself a hard time and beat myself up when things go wrong.*

2. *I criticise myself.*

3. *I hold back for fear of making a fool of myself.*

4. *I hate the way I look.*

5. *I feel embarrassed by my nose.*

6. *I don't feel confident in my abilities.*

7. *I wish I were taller and better looking.*

8. *I should be a better mother.*

9. *I don't know how to relate to people.*

10. *I should be married by now.*

You get the idea? It's important to be really honest with yourself; try not to hold back. One of my workshop attendees identified 55 ways in which he didn't accept himself!

2. List at least ten events and experiences from the past in which you were not accepted for who you were.

For example:

1. *My mother told me that she always wanted to have a boy, rather than me.*

2. *I was told by my parents that I was an accident.*

3. *I was sent home from school for wearing make-up.*

4. *My parents never listen to me.*

5. *My husband ignores what I say.*

6. *The other children didn't want to play with me at school.*

7. *I was told by my parents that crying was a sign of weakness.*

8. *I wasn't allowed to go to art school.*

9. *I was abused by my uncle.*

10. *My dad said he was embarrassed by me when I came last in a swimming race.*

3. List at least five reasons why you shouldn't accept yourself.

For example:

1. *Self-acceptance will stop me from being motivated.*

2. *It is wrong to accept myself; I can only be accepted in the eyes of God.*

3. *It will make me arrogant.*

4. *I am not worthy of self-acceptance.*

5. *I am scared of what might happen.*

4. Starting with those at the top of your list, use the emotional freedom technique on page 332 to reduce the power that these statements have over you.

It's important when using EFT that you use a set-up statement that feels right for you. It should capture the essence of what you are feeling. Here are a few set-up statements to get you started:

- Even though I am not accepting myself, *when I give myself a hard time and beat myself up when things go wrong*, I deeply and completely accept without judgement that I am not accepting myself.

- Even though *my mother told me that she always wanted to have a boy, rather than me*, I deeply and completely accept this and myself without judgement.

- Even though *self-acceptance will stop me from being motivated*, I deeply and completely accept this and myself without judgement.

As you start to tap on these issues, you should find that your perspective on the other issues will also change. If so that's a good sign that progress is being made. And while it might be tempting to tap on all of the issues in one day, people who do this tend to rush through EFT and don't get the full benefit. My advice is to spend a couple of days, or even a week, on this exercise. The most important thing is to make sure that when you do tap on a statement that you reduce the score to zero.

5. Watch out for when you are not accepting yourself.

From now on, when you catch yourself putting yourself down, write down the issue and then, when you get a chance, use EFT on it.

Step 2 • Change your self-image

The way you see yourself – the mental picture that you have of yourself – has a powerful influence on the way you feel and behave. Its influence is much stronger than objective fact. For example, a young woman might be incredibly beautiful in the eyes of other people, but if her mental self-image is distorted, she will take that as truth, not other people's opinions. If you say to her that she is beautiful, or clever or talented, she simply won't believe you because the information from her own self-image says she is not. This is how powerful images are! An observation made by a plastic surgeon called Dr Maxwell Maltz, in his book *Psycho-Cybernetics* illustrated this point very well. He noticed that many of his patients undergoing plastic surgery experienced a transformation in the way they felt about themselves. They felt more confident, happier and attractive. But this wasn't always the case. For some patients despite the fact they looked better, they didn't feel better on the inside. The positive changes on the outside, for some reason, were failing to translate into a positive change on the inside. His conclusion as to why this was so was that these patients had a distorted self-image. And the solution? To use visualisation to change the self-image, in combination with plastic surgery to change the outside appearance. When he did this the self-esteem of his patients soared.

By changing the image we hold of ourselves we transform the way we feel and act. It's that simple. Here's the process that I have used, based on Dr Maxwell Maltz's work to help hundreds of my own patients and workshop attendees experience a higher level of self-esteem.

EXERCISE: your self-image

1. Find some place where you won't be disturbed for at least ten minutes.

2. Sit down, make yourself comfortable and take a couple of long, deep breaths.

3. Now close your eyes, and picture yourself living to your potential. This new you is your authentic self. What do you look like? How confident, healthy and happy is your authentic self? How would your authentic self act? What effect would it have on people?

4. Once you get a real sense of what your authentic self looks like, imagine watching your new self going about its life.

5. Now step inside your authentic self, and allow yourself to become that authentic self. Breathe deeply.

6. Look through the eyes of your authentic self and experience yourself living life to its full potential. How does it make you feel, how would you interact with people, how would you respond to life's challenges, and what quality of life would you have? Give yourself plenty of time and allow yourself to enjoy the authentic you.

7. Once you have a real sense of this authentic part of you, open your eyes and take a deep breath.

I really like this exercise. It gives you a taste of your own potential and allows you to experience new possibilities as a distinct reality. To get the most out of it try using it once a day for a minimum of ten days.

Step 3 • Change your self-talk

The way you talk to yourself, and whether you believe or don't believe that talk, also has a big impact on your self-esteem. Most of us have a running commentary going on inside our heads. We're constantly evaluating and interpreting experiences, trying to work things out, worrying, hypothesising, going over the past. For some people this mind chatter can be quite exhausting. Of course, the ability to think is an essential tool enabling us to navigate and make sense of the situations we encounter, it's part of what makes us human. However, when the content of our self-talk pulls us down and keeps us from fulfilling our potential for total health, it becomes a problem. If you are experiencing negative self-talk, try the following:

Address any underlying imbalances

If the negative self-talk is coming about because of some underlying biological or biochemical problem, such as a nutrient deficiency, hormonal imbalance or toxicity, then that's where you need to take action. I've had many patients with depression try and fail to control their negative self-talk with psychological techniques, because their underlying problem was biological. Taking a fish oil supplement, a natural mood lifter, eating a healthy diet, detoxing your body of heavy metals and even exercising, might be the answer for you. To work out which you need to do, fill in the total-health questionnaire on page 21 and let it guide you to the relevant chapters.

Tame the inner critic

I came across the work of Hal and Sidra Stone, two American psychologists, two years ago and it transformed my understanding of the human psyche. They believe that we have not just one personality but tens, if not hundreds, of different and distinct personalities within us. For example, there is the *pleaser subpersonality*, who tries to please everyone, the *perfectionist subpersonality*, who has extraordinarily high standards, the *inner judge subpersonality*, who judges things, and the *inner critic subpersonality*, who criticises us. While all of our subpersonalities contribute to our sense of self, it is this latter one – the inner critic – that has a particularly potent effect on our self-esteem. Mind–Body Tool 16 (page 395) has a couple of suggestions as to how you can manage this one.

Use enquiry

A spiritual teacher, Bryon Katie, developed a process of enquiry called The Work to help people transform their relationship to their thoughts and beliefs. Her understanding is that our most intimate relationship is with our thoughts and that the way we relate to them has a considerable influence on the way we feel. Because most people habitually believe their thoughts, if those thoughts are negative and disempowering they will become trapped by them. Her process is a method of turning down the power of a particular thought to the extent that alternative possibilities are revealed. I love using this process and have witnessed many of my patients experience a positive shift when they've applied it to a self-limiting thought or belief. I would encourage you to visit her website www.thework.org or buy her book *Loving What Is*. The exercise below gives you a flavour of the work. I have modified it slightly, but I would encourage you to refer to her original work.

EXERCISE: enquiry

Next time you have a self-limiting thought such as 'I am useless, there is no way I can do this', try the following. For the best results write your answers down.

1. Ask yourself: is this true? Usually the immediate response is yes or no.

2. Now ask yourself: am I absolutely 100 per cent certain that this is true? This time don't rush to answer it, breathe deeply and allow an honest answer to rise in your body. Whatever answer you get is fine. *If you answer no, notice how this shifts the energy in your body.*

3. Now notice what happens when you believe your thought; how does it make you feel? How do you treat others when you believe this thought? How does this thought influence your actions? *This gives you some insight into the power this thought is currently having on your life.*

4. Now, ask yourself: 'if this thought no longer existed, how would I feel?' Give yourself plenty of time to become aware of the new feelings that arise. You need to breathe deeply and give them plenty of space to come up. Now ask yourself 'if this thought no longer existed, how would it change my life?' Again, breathe deeply and give yourself time to see and think about how your life would be different.

By following these four steps you are shifting the power from the thought to you. Thoughts are just perspectives, and by becoming wrapped up in a particular thought it prevents us from accessing other insights and our own intuition. By going down the steps you are progressively separating yourself from the thought, so that you can decide yourself what is true for you.

Step 4 • Love yourself

OK, this is going to sound a bit wacky and off the wall, but bear with me on this. Of all the processes I use with my workshop attendees it is the 'I Love You' exercise that tends to leave a lasting and most meaningful impression on them. I've always found it a little curious that most people have no problems working on issues of anger, fear and depression but really feel uncomfortable when talking about love and self-acceptance. I deliberately leave this exercise to last, by which time most people are just about ready for it.

EXERCISE: I love you

1. Find a time when you will be completely alone and undisturbed for at least 30 minutes.

2. Stand in front of a mirror – preferably a full length one – and say to yourself out loud while looking at yourself: I love you. Don't worry if you don't mean it – this will still work!

3. Do this again, but this time breathe deeply and slowly and say it slower: I – love – you.

4. As you say these words become aware of your body. Where in your body do those words feel blocked? Where can you feel some discomfort? Most people feel it in their heart, stomach or throat area – but it can be anywhere. What you are feeling is the location of a block that is preventing these words from flowing through and energising your body.

5. To release the block, say out loud: I LOVE YOU. Now close your eyes, and breathe slowly in and out through the area that is blocked – what you are feeling is energy that wants to flow.

6. Now speak to that energy and tell it to soften and flow. If it helps, massage the area gently. Eventually you are going to notice that the energy is moving. This can take a minute or two.

7. Now sense which direction the energy wants to move to – it will be up, down, to the side, backwards or straight out of the body. This energy knows which way it wants to go.

8. Now ask yourself: 'If this energy could exit my body, where would it choose to leave?' You should get a sense of it. The first time you do this you'll be quite surprised because there will be a definite exit route – such as the top of the head, out through the ears, eyes, mouth or nose, or maybe out of the hands or feet. Whichever way, allow the energy to flow out of your body, telling it gently and lovingly to 'soften and flow' as you go.

9. Eventually you'll sense that the energy has moved out of your body. This can take anywhere between a couple of seconds and 20 minutes. If it takes longer, just be patient, breathe deeply and 'soften and flow.' If you get to this stage, well done you are doing really well.

10. Now repeat the process, saying: I LOVE YOU. This time the block might be in the same location, or somewhere else completely different. Do exactly what you did before until the energy has flowed out of your body completely. Then keep repeating until you get to the stage when saying the words I LOVE YOU completely energises and uplifts you. When you feel those words, when you know in your heart that those words are true then you have successfully completed this exercise.

The power of self-acceptance and self-love is extraordinary. I never cease to be amazed and humbled by its profound impact on people's lives. If you find this exercise difficult, I would encourage you to come along to one of my workshops or to contact a practitioner of EmoTrance through the website www.emotrance.com.

Now that you have reached the end of this chapter, my advice is to reread it one more time. While doing so highlight those sentences (using a highlighter pen) that you feel are important to you. Once you've done this write down at least five steps or actions that you are going to take, and spend a moment visualising yourself implementing them.

> ## MIND–BODY ESSENTIALS
>
> - Self-esteem is an energy and power source that emerges from the depths of ourselves, to the degree that we accept and value who we are.
>
> - The level of self-esteem experienced within us is controlled by our internal relationship: the relationship that we have to ourselves. The key to raising self-esteem is to transform the inner relationship that we have with ourselves from one of resistance and denial, to one of complete and total acceptance and love.
>
> - When we completely accept ourselves, creative energy, clarity of insight and intuition is liberated. This source of power and guidance provides an authentic sense of self and the foundations for fulfilling our total-health potential.
>
> - Recommended mind–body tools to accompany this chapter: emotional freedom technique (page 332), emotional trauma release (page 341), creative visualisation (page 319), Bach Flower Remedies (page 298), meditation (page 376) and relaxation (page 380).
>
> - For recommended reading see Resources, page 428.

PART THREE

The mind–body toolbox

Introduction:
how to use the toolbox

Wouldn't it be useful to have a toolbox that contained specific techniques and approaches for overcoming health challenges and improving your well-being? Well there is, it's called The Mind–Body Toolbox, and it consists of the 16 most popular and effective of the mind–body tools that I teach to my patients. One of the many benefits of having mind–body tools at your disposal is that as you encounter the various challenges that life will throw at you, you will have something to help you respond in a more effective health-orientated way; for example, the emotional trauma release (page 341) or creative visualisation tools (page 319).

To work out which ones will be of most benefit to you, follow the guidelines below:

- If you have a particular health challenge, such as infertility or angina, then use Option 2: Health Condition Guide on pages 33–44. It will tell you which of the tools will be of greatest help to you.

- If you have already identified which barriers are relevant to you, the best tools for overcoming the barrier are suggested in the summary box at the end of that chapter.

- Alternatively, read through them all and see which ones resonate with you!

On average I give my patients two to four tools to learn and use. It's a good idea to have at least this number so that you can turn to them as and when you need them. Some of the tools, such as relaxation (page 380), exercise (page 350) and meditation (page 376), should ideally become habits, by incorporating them into your everyday routine. Others, such as tame the inner critic (page 395) or instant stress release (page 368), need only to be used when appropriate.

chapter 1

Appreciation

Feeling appreciation is the fastest and most powerful way to experience the flow of connection between you and the person, object or issue that you are appreciating. It dissolves barriers, lifts your spirits and it does wonders for your relationships. Research has found that those people who practise appreciation not only enjoy better health and experience less mental illness but they are also better equipped to ride out life's challenges and stresses. Appreciation is great for your health!

Heart intelligence

When you appreciate something with sincerity, you access heart intelligence, a powerful source of information and intelligence originating from the heart.[1] Like a conductor of an orchestra, heart intelligence brings order and coherence to the workings and functioning of the bodymind. It sends out information that not only affects the physiology and health of the body but also the way we perceive situations, the way we feel, the decisions we make and how we behave. When the heart is in charge, you literally see the world in a different light.

Learning appreciation

Appreciation, like any skill, can be learnt and developed. If practised until it becomes a habit, this usually takes a couple of weeks; it then becomes a natural way for us to be. That's when we start reaping the rewards of being bathed in heart energy. The key to the skill of appreciation is focus and how we interpret what we see. You and I could both look up at the sky, and whereas you might remark on a beautiful bird flying by, all I might see is the grey cloud in the distance. We could be leaving a restaurant and the waiter comes out after us and hands us the briefcases we left behind; I might think nothing about it, whereas you offer your sincere gratitude, realising all of the hassles that would have been caused had the waiter not returned the case to you.

Try this exercise. Think back over the last 24 hours and count how many missed opportunities there were to be grateful for something. When you get to 30, stop. I'm sure you are getting my idea. Life is full of missed opportunities for appreciation. Here are some tips to help you start experiencing the benefits of appreciation.

EXERCISE: the benefits of appreciation

Identify a situation that is troubling you. Write down your perspective as you see it, and notice how it makes you feel. Now write down three reasons to be thankful for the situation and notice how they make you feel. You don't have to believe that these new perspectives are correct for this to work. When our thinking gets stuck in a rut, issues and problems can appear to be insurmountable. However, by deliberately exploring different perspectives through appreciation, we gently rock ourselves out of the rut, until we are free.

Example: *Karen did this exercise in one of my workshops and here's what she wrote:*

Situation
I don't get on with my new boss, she doesn't value anything I say.

Blessing one
This gives me a kick up the backside to change my jobs – I've been thinking of doing this for five years!

Blessing two
It's made me realise that I do exactly the same to one of the girls who works in the office – what a hypocrite I am!

Blessing three
One of the other girls is treated the same way as me, but she doesn't get upset by it – I can therefore choose whether I let this get to me or not.

At the start of each day and in the final moments before going to bed, give thanks for five things in your life – they can be anything. The temptation is to list them quickly. The benefit comes, not from identifying what we are appreciated for, but from allowing ourselves to feel and experience appreciation. This means focusing on each thing in turn, breathing deeply and allowing appreciation to rise within in us.

Make a habit of appreciating people, especially your partner. While this might seem a bit false at first, if it comes from a genuine place, it will be warmly received. With practice it will start to feel right for you as well. For example, when you get home from work, take a moment to appreciate the dinner that's been prepared or the fact that your clothes have been ironed or washed. Taking others for granted is a sure way to quash the spark in any relationship.

The next time you feel out of sorts, breathe deeply in and out of your chest area and find something to appreciate. It could be something that's happening around you, something you've seen or even something from the past – the important thing is to keep focused, breathe deeply and to allow yourself to experience appreciation.[2]

Start appreciating yourself – this is very difficult to do for a lot of people. Write down 15 things that you appreciate about yourself. If you can't do it, you're not trying hard enough, everyone's got 15! Take a few seconds each day to appreciate and give thanks for your body – if you struggle or feel uncomfortable with this, take a look at Barrier 14 on low self-esteem.

MIND-BODY ESSENTIALS

- Appreciation is the fastest and most powerful way to experience the flow of connection between you and the person/object/issue that you are appreciating.

- Appreciation can be learnt and practised as you would develop any skill. If we can practise it until it becomes a habit, then it becomes a natural way for us to be.

- Whenever you feel down or stuck in a situation, take a couple of deep breaths and find two or three things to appreciate about your circumstances. Try seeing then through the eyes of someone else.

- Try not to take people for granted – look for ways that you can appreciate who they are and what they do, in ways that they recognise as appreciation.

- For recommended reading see Resources, page 428.

chapter 2

Bach Flower Remedies

'There is no true healing unless there is a change in outlook, peace of mind, and inner happiness.' Dr Edward Bach, 1934

Edward Bach, British medical doctor and pioneer of mind–body medicine, dedicated his life to discovering a system of natural healing that would comprehensively address the emotional and mental roots of disease.[1] Rather than treating people on the basis of the disease they were experiencing, he came to the conclusion that by treating people on the basis of their personality characteristics – including attitudes, belief systems, emotional states and behavioural patterns – deep healing and even spiritual transformation would occur. He believed illness came about because of the conflict between the soul (which wishes to realise its full potential) and certain aspects of the personality (which holds back its full expression). This failure to blossom spiritually was, he believed, responsible for depleting the body of its natural life force and making that person susceptible to disease and suffering.

Flower essences

His solution, and the heart of his emotional-healing approach, was to give his patients specific flower essences, according to the personality characteristics that were imbalanced. These remedies were prepared by boiling the flowers in spring water for 30 minutes, or by floating the flowers in a shallow bowl of spring water and then exposing the flowers and water to unbroken sunlight for several hours. He believed that this remedy, when correctly matched to a person with certain personality traits, would dissolve the limiting emotional frequency patterns and in doing so help that person's true nature – or essence – to shine. This return to wholeness brought health, peace of mind and inner happiness. These flower remedies are still used today and many people claim to benefit from them. They are simple to use and harmless to take. Read below to find out which ones might be helpful for you.

Which essence should you take?

I've used Bach Flower Remedies with my patients for over six years and I never cease to be amazed at how well some people respond to them. However, it can sometimes take a couple of months to see a significant change, although it is often less. There are a number of ways of selecting which remedies are suited to you;[2] dowsing, kinesiology and the assistance of a trained Bach Flower Remedies practitioner are all options, but I find using the following self-help questionnaire seems to work well. It takes about five minutes to fill in, and requires you to identify which of the personality traits are true for you right now.

QUESTIONNAIRE: Bach Flower Remedies

As you go through the questionnaire tick only those questions that you gave a definite 'yes' answer to. Each 'yes' answer equals one point. Add up the scores as you go along and then use the key at the end to make up your remedy.

Agrimony

1. When worried or in pain, do you tend to hide it behind a cheerful and smiling face?

▶

2. Do you 'give in' so as to avoid arguments and conflicts? ☐

3. When stressed do you find yourself drinking alcohol, or using stimulants or drugs to help you cope? ☐

Total score ☐

Aspen

1. Do you worry that something bad might happen to you? ☐

2. Do you often find yourself distressed and anxious, but without knowing why? ☐

3. Do you wake with a sense of fear and anxiety of what the day might bring? ☐

Total score ☐

Beech

1. When assessing people and situations, do you look for what you can find wrong? ☐

2. Do you prefer to work or be alone because others irritate you? ☐

3. Are you critical and intolerant of the habits and shortcomings of others' standards or expectations? ☐

Total score ☐

Centaury

1. Do you find it difficult to say no to those who impose upon your good nature? ☐

►

2. Are you easily influenced by those with a stronger personality than yourself? ☐

3. Do you deny your own needs, in order to please others? ☐

Total score ☐

Cerato

1. Do you lack confidence in your ability to judge things on your own and make decisions? ☐

2. Do you change your mind often? ☐

3. Do you constantly question your own judgement and decisions? ☐

Total score ☐

Cherry plum

1. Do you have a tendency to act irrationally and violently, exploding into unexplained fits of rage? ☐

2. Do you fear losing control of yourself? ☐

3. Do you fear losing control and hurting yourself or others? ☐

Total score ☐

Chestnut bud

1. Do you find that you don't learn from past experiences? ☐

2. Due to lack of awareness, do you find it necessary to go over things already done? ☐

▶

3. Is there a recurring theme, situation or condition in your life that you would like to overcome? ☐

Total score ☐

Chicory

1. Are you possessive of those close to you, and do feel you know what's best for them? ☐

2. Do you need to be needed? ☐

3. Do you often feel unloved or unappreciated by people despite what you have done for them? ☐

Total score ☐

Clematis

1. Are you absentminded, or do you feel spaced out? ☐

2. Do you tend to daydream, wishing you were somewhere else? ☐

3. Do you find yourself dozing off frequently, regardless of where you are? ☐

Total score ☐

Crab apple

1. Do you find yourself preoccupied with small physical problems such as pimples, small blemishes or rashes while overlooking more serious conditions? ☐

2. Do you feel there is something wrong with, or there are some things you would like changed in, your physical appearance? ☐

►

3. Are you obsessed with cleanliness? ☐

Total score ☐

Elm

1. Do you feel inadequate when it comes to dealing with the tasks ahead of you? ☐

2. Do you find yourself overwhelmed by your responsibilities? ☐

3. Do you become despondent when faced with the size of your commitments? ☐

Total score ☐

Gentian

1. Are you easily discouraged when faced with difficult situations? ☐

2. When setting out to accomplish a task, do you become oversensitive to small delays or hindrances, which may lead to self-doubt, and at times to depression? ☐

3. Is it hard for you to start over again once you've encountered difficulties? ☐

Total score ☐

Gorse

1. Have you lost hope that you will recover from or be helped in overcoming an illness or difficulty? ☐

2. Do you feel it is a worthless task to seek further help for your problem? ☐

▶

3. Do you believe nothing can be done to help relieve your situation? ☐

Total score ☐

Heather

1. Do you talk incessantly and take little interest in what others have to say? ☐

2. Do you dislike being alone and prefer to be seeking the company of others? ☐

3. Are you self-absorbed, concerned only about yourself and your issues? ☐

Total score ☐

Holly

1. Are you suspicious and mistrusting of other people's motives and intentions? ☐

2. Are you full of jealously, envy or hate? ☐

3. Do you find yourself lacking compassion or warmth towards others? ☐

Total score ☐

Honeysuckle

1. Do you find it difficult to change your present circumstances because you are always looking backwards and not into the future? ☐

2. Are you dissatisfied with your accomplishments? ☐

▶

3. Do you find yourself reminiscing about the good old days, wishing you were able to live your life over again? ☐

Total score ☐

Hornbeam

1. On rising in the morning, do you feel too tired to face the day? ☐

2. Do you lack enthusiasm; do you tend to procrastinate? ☐

3. Do you feel bored with your life? ☐

Total score ☐

Impatiens

1. Do you find yourself losing patience, becoming tense and irritable with people and things that move too slowly for you? ☐

2. Do you do things with a sense of urgency, always rushing to get through? ☐

3. Do you prefer to work alone? ☐

Total score ☐

Larch

1. Do you lack self-confidence? ☐

2. Do you not try things for fear of failing? ☐

3. Do you feel inferior, and that others are more capable and qualified than you? ☐

Total score ☐

►

Mimulus

1. Do you have fears of known things, such as spiders or heights? ☐

2. Are you shy, overly sensitive and often afraid? ☐

3. When faced with situations or things that frighten you, do you become too paralysed to act? ☐

Total score ☐

Mustard

1. Do you ever become depressed for no obvious reason? ☐

2. Does this depression descend and then lift quickly? ☐

3. Do your moods swing back and forth? ☐

Total score ☐

Oak

1. Are you exhausted but nonetheless struggle on against all odds? ☐

2. Can you always be depended on to complete what you set out to do, regardless of the challenge? ☐

3. Do you tend to throw yourself into your projects, neglecting your own needs? ☐

Total score ☐

Olive

1. Do you feel completely physically and mentally drained? ☐

▶

2. Do you tire easily with no reserve energy to complete your tasks or to enjoy the day? ☐

3. Is everything an effort? ☐

Total score ☐

Pine

1. Are you full of guilt and self-reproach? ☐

2. Do you blame yourself or feel responsible for everything that goes wrong? ☐

3. Are you hard on yourself when you fail to live up to the standards or expectations you've set for yourself? ☐

Total score ☐

Red chestnut

1. Are you excessively concerned about your friends and family? ☐

2. Do you fear that something may happen to those close to you? ☐

3. Are you distressed and disturbed by people's problems? ☐

Total score ☐

Rock rose

1. Do you feel terror and panic? ☐

2. Do you tend to panic and become hysterical or freeze in the face of fear? ☐

▶

3. Do you suffer from nightmares? ☐

Total score ☐

Rock water

1. Do you have an inflexible approach to life, always striving for perfection? ☐

2. Do you deny yourself the simple pleasures in life? ☐

3. Do you feel it's important to make an example of yourself by living up to your ideals, so that others may follow? ☐

Total score ☐

Scleranthus

1. Do you suffer from indecision, uncertainty or hesitancy? ☐

2. Do you lack concentration; are you fidgety and anxious? ☐

3. Do your moods change from one extreme to the other? ☐

Total score ☐

Star of Bethlehem

1. Have you suffered a shock in your life such as an accident, serious illness or assault? ☐

2. Do you feel a past surgery or accident is responsible for your present condition? ☐

3. Have you recently, or in the past, suffered a personal loss or grief, which you haven't quite recovered from? ☐

Total score ☐

►

Sweet chestnut

1. Do you feel that the future holds nothing for you? ☐

2. Do you suffer from mental anguish and deep despair? ☐

3. Do you feel that you have reached the limits of what you ☐
   can endure?

Total score ☐

Vervain

1. Do you have strong opinions, but ones that you are ☐
   convinced are the right ones?

2. Is your over-enthusiasm so strong it is almost bordering ☐
   on being fanatical?

3. Are you highly strung, at times tense and over-enthusiastic, ☐
   always teaching and philosophising?

Total score ☐

Vine

1. Do you tend to take charge in circumstances and ☐
   situations you're involved with?

2. Are you domineering and overbearing? ☐

3. Do you feel the need to be always right? ☐

Total score ☐

Walnut

1. Are you experiencing a major change in your life right ☐
   now?

▶

2. Are you finding it hard to let go of certain attachments? ☐

3. Are you distracted by outside influences? ☐

Total score ☐

Water violet

1. Do others find you aloof, overly proud and at times condescending? ☐

2. Do you bear your grief and sorrow in silence? ☐

3. Are you self-reliant? Do you prefer spending your time alone? ☐

Total score ☐

White chestnut

1. Do you find you can't sleep because your thoughts go round and round? ☐

2. Do you find your head full of persistent, unwanted thoughts that prevent concentration? ☐

3. Do you relive unhappy events or arguments over and over again? ☐

Total score ☐

Wild oat

1. Are you displeased with your lifestyle and feel dissatisfied with your achievements? ☐

2. Have you tried many different directions in life, but nothing seems to bring satisfaction? ☐

▶

3. Do you have ambition, but feel that life is passing you by? ☐

Total score ☐

Wild rose

1. Do you find you are indifferent and apathetic towards life? ☐

2. Are you resigned to your current circumstances? ☐

3. Do you lack motivation to change and improve your life? ☐

Total score ☐

Willow

1. Do you feel that life has been unfair or unjust to you? ☐

2. Do you feel resentful and bitter? ☐

3. Do you have difficulty forgiving and forgetting? ☐

Total score ☐

Make up your remedy

Once you've completed the questionnaire, go through the list again and select all of the flower essences for which you scored three points. Record them below. You can have a maximum of six remedies in your formula, although you can have as few as two. You can also, if you wish, make up the number to six by using those that you scored two for. The ones that you have selected will be used to make your formula. If there is only one remedy that you have identified, this can be taken alone.

Flower essence 1: _____

Flower essence 2: _____

Flower essence 3: _____

Flower essence 4: _____

Flower essence 5: _____

Flower essence 6: _____

Ordering the remedies

Contact Crystal Herbs on 01379 642374 or visit www.crystalherbs.com for your essences. If you have identified more than one flower essence, remember to order an empty 25ml mixer bottle as well.

Preparing your own formula

Once you receive your flower essences fill your 25ml empty dropper bottle to the halfway point with pure spring or filtered water. Add two drops from each flower essence bottle that you have selected. A teaspoon of brandy or apple cider vinegar can be added as a preservative. Then fill the bottle to the top with more spring or filtered water. Rescue Remedy, which contains five Bach Flower Remedies (and is excellent at stabilising your response to acute trauma), counts as one remedy if used.

Rescue Remedy

The most popular and well-known Bach Flower Remedy is Rescue Remedy. It is often used as and when needed and is especially beneficial in bringing a sense of calm when you find yourself in stressful situations.

How often should you take it?

The minimum suggested dosage for mixed remedies is: four drops under the tongue, four times a day. If your Bach Flower Remedy comes with instructions, however, follow those instead.

Is it working?

If you start to feel better and your symptoms start to resolve that suggests the Bach Flower Remedies are working. You should continue taking them until the emotional imbalance is fully resolved. If you have experienced no improvement after two to four weeks, you should reassess your formula or see a trained practitioner.

A word on safety

Because Bach Flower Remedies are completely safe they can be taken by babies and children. They are free from side effects, and any addictive influence.

MIND–BODY ESSENTIALS

- Bach Flower Remedies were developed by Dr Edward Bach, a holistic medical doctor and a pioneer of emotional healing.

- His approach is based on the matching of personality traits to specific remedies containing the essence of a flower, whose vibrational character is able to restore balance to that person.

- Dr Bach saw his 38 remedies as tools that would help us overcome the limiting programmes and behaviours of the personality so that we could connect with the true essence of ourselves.

- You can select your remedy combination by using the self-help questionnaire provided here or by consulting a trained practitioner.

- For recommended reading see Resources, page 428.

chapter 3

Conscious breathing

Take a moment to tune into your body right now. What can you sense? Are you relaxed and tension-free? Do you feel a heaviness or any discomfort? Now take a couple of long, slow, deep breaths and recheck your body. How does it feel now? The chances are that those couple of deep breaths have made a real and noticeable difference to the way you feel. Most people, having taken those deep breaths, report feeling lighter, calmer and more grounded. All from just a couple of breaths!

The value of conscious breathing

Learning to regulate your breathing consciously is a valuable skill to learn.[1] We all know from our biology lessons at school that breathing enables us to bring nutritive oxygen into our body, and breathing out expels waste carbon dioxide. This helps to stop toxicity from building up and it supplies the cells of our body with oxygen so that they can function optimally. But there's more to breathing than that. Taking control of our breathing rate and depth also allows us to stimulate the body's brakes: the parasympathetic nervous system. This in turn switches the body into the repair and regeneration mode that is necessary for healing.

Breathing also controls the flow of energy or life force through our body. And because movements of energy through us are registered as feelings, breathing rate and depth provide us a thermostat for controlling emotional intensity. Most people intuitively already know this. You just have to watch how a child holds his or her breath, or breathes very shallowly, when upset; this reduces the intensity of their feelings. I've had many patients quite convincingly tell me that there is little worry or stress in their lives, and yet when I asked them to deepen and slow their breathing, and focus inwards, they are shocked to find tension and emotional upset in their bodies. Paradoxically, when I ask them to keep breathing like this while feeling the tension in their bodies, the tension will release. Because emotions are such a powerful source of insight and wisdom, not breathing deeply and slowly prevents us from accessing them fully. On the one hand this is useful if those emotions are unpleasant; on the other hand if we are committed to total health and want to grow in awareness, then we need to make contact with them in order to receive the message that they hold for us. (The focusing mind–body tool on pages 356–361 goes into this in more detail.)

One final thing, slow, deep breathing can also calm a busy and chattering mind. Try it next time you have thoughts whizzing around.

A key component of creating total health, relaxing, and bringing balance and harmony to the bodymind is therefore to learn how to breathe consciously and effectively. The following exercises will help you achieve this.

EXERCISE: breath awareness

1. Find a quiet, warm place where you will be undisturbed. Sit relaxed and close your eyes lightly.

2. Turn your attention to your breathing, breathing in through the nose and out through the mouth. Observe it for a full minute without interfering with its rate, rhythm or depth. If your mind wanders, simply return your attention to your breathing.

3. Now place one hand on your chest and the other over your stomach. Continue breathing as normal and observe with your open eyes whether your chest hand or stomach hand moves up

and down most. Chest-hand dominance suggests that you are presently breathing inefficiently and therefore restricting the benefits to be experienced with breathing. Stomach-hand dominance suggests that you are diaphragmatic breathing, which is one of the most efficient means of breathing. This is the preferred method of breathing.

4. If you were a chest breather, practise the exercise below, if you are already a diaphragmatic breather proceed to either the connected, cleansing or healing breathing exercise.

EXERCISE: diaphragmatic breathing

1. Following on from the exercise above return your attention to your breathing, place your hand on your stomach and breathe as though you are drawing oxygen in and out of the stomach area. This automatically enables you to breathe effectively and fully.

2. You can make this exercise even more powerful by doing the following: when you breathe in, touch the tip of your tongue on the point where the roof of your mouth meets the upper front teeth. The Chinese believe that this forms a connection between two of the body's main meridians (energy pathways in Chinese medicine) that allow you to bring in vital energy to balance the whole of the body.

3. When you breathe out, open your mouth slightly, gently dropping the tip of the tongue. Continue taking deep breaths, bringing air in as deeply as possible and letting it out as slowly as possible without force. With further practice you will be able to breathe in and out in this way at a rate of between four to six breaths per minute. Practise this exercise on wakening in the morning, before eating, when stressed and before retiring to bed.

The connected breath

Many of the popular forms of breath work use a technique called connected breathing, meaning that the in-breath and the out-breath are connected without pause, unlike normal unconscious breathing, in which there is typically a gap between the exhalation and inhalation. The purpose of connected breathing is to allow the continuous uninterrupted flow of life force through the whole body so as to create harmony between the body, mind and soul. You start by simply breathing in and out without a pause or effort. This should be practised for a minimum of ten minutes each day.

The cleansing breath

This advanced breathing exercise involves taking a deep, abdominal breath, holding it and sticking your tongue out. Next, you bring up the air as though you're going to exhale, but, instead, prevent it from doing so by placing a throat lock on it causing a gag. You don't necessarily have to make the gagging noise. This ancient technique is used to dissolve mental and emotional blockages and help access states of happiness and bliss.

The healing breath

Healing breathing is specifically designed to bring the mind, body and soul back into alignment, particularly when you are feeling 'out of sorts'.

EXERCISE: healing breathing

1. Sit relaxed in a chair and close your eyes. Slowly take a deep breath in until you can hold no more air.

2. Now exhale slowly until all the air is exhaled. Next, inhale ten consecutive deep diaphragmatic breaths while pulling in your stomach on the exhalation.

3. Now start breathing rhythmically using the following as a guideline. Inhale to the count of 4; hold it to the count of 4; exhale to the count of 4; and pause to the count of 4. Repeat this three times. Inhale to the count of 6; hold it to the count of 6; exhale to the count of 6; and pause to the count of 6. Repeat this thee times. Do the same thing to the count of 8. Repeat this three times.

4. Practise the healing breath daily – early morning or late at night is usually best.

MIND–BODY ESSENTIALS

- Conscious breathing – that is, deliberately controlling the rate and depth of our breathing – is a powerful tool for creating total health.

- Learning to breathe consciously and deeply increases your connection with reality, and allows you to receive the wisdom of your emotions.

- Practising breathing techniques such as the ones offered in this chapter, or through learning yoga for example, can improve your health, calm your mind and help accelerate healing.

- When you want to know truly how you feel about any given situation, breathe deeply and slowly.

- For recommended reading see Resources, page 428.

chapter 4

Creative visualisation

Think of someone who you have a problem with, or don't like. Take a couple of deep breaths, and notice how this makes you feel. I'm guessing you feel upset, stressed or tense. Now turn your attention to someone who you really respect or care for. Notice how you feel now and note the contrast between the two experiences.

So what caused you to feel so differently? In a nutshell it's the stored images you have of these two people. Your mind stores information as images. When you access these images by turning your attention towards them, your physical body reacts to them as changes in physiology (hence you experience muscle tension or a fast heart beat) and to your vital body as feelings. The nature of those feelings and bodily reactions depends on the content of the image. For example, if you've just walked into a room and spotted someone that you used to go to school with, how you feel will depend on the image that your mind throws up. If the content of your image is positive, you'll experience positive feelings. However, if you have a negative image (maybe because that person bullied you), unpleasant feelings will arise and you'll feel very uncomfortable. In that moment your entire state of well-being is at the mercy of an image. However, if you knew how to modify that image, you could instantly change the way you feel and subsequently behave. This is the power of creative visualisation and the skill that I am going to show you how to develop.

What is creative visualisation?

Visualisation is the conscious and deliberate use of imagery to change and improve your life and health. Rather than being subservient to the images generated automatically in response to your worries and concerns, visualisation puts you firmly in control of the way you feel and your body's physiology – and even your future! What's more, visualisation is not limited to just seeing pictures, you can also imagine tastes, sounds, smells, sensations and feelings. The most effective forms of visualisation combine and use all of these.

What are the benefits?

There are a number of studies that have shown the positive effects of specific visualisation techniques in helping people to manage symptoms and recover from disease. Indeed, with the correct training, each of us has the ability to influence most of our body's major control systems, including heart rate, temperature, blood flow, immune function, and even wound healing. Other uses include reducing complications associated with childbirth, encouraging new behaviours, reducing allergic symptoms, decreasing pain and the need for medications, reducing the side effects of treatment, increasing confidence, reducing stress, worry and fear, and helping prepare for surgery or a forthcoming event.[1]

Harness the power of your imagination

Leaning to visualise is like riding a bike. Initially it can be quite daunting; when you start, you fail to get going for the first few times (and can get very frustrated in the process), but with patience and persistence, eventually you are up and running. It took me at least two weeks to get the hang of visualisation; even now my images are a little blurred, but I am convinced that it has positively influenced my health and life. My recommendation is to start with the first three exercises, as these will help you prepare for the creative visualisation exercises that follow.

EXERCISE 1: experience the power of imagery

This is the classic exercise for demonstrating how the images we hold in our mind trigger strong bodily reactions.

1. Close your eyes, breathe deeply and imagine yourself to be holding a big juicy lemon.

2. See yourself placing it on a chopping board, then carefully cut it in half with a sharp knife.

3. As you cut the lemon, watch its juices pour on to the board. Lift it up to your nose and smell its tangy flavour. Now bite deeply into its rind all the way through to the juice.

4. Taste the sharpness on your tongue as you suck the juice into your mouth and swish it slowly around for a few moments.

5. Become aware of how you feel, and notice whether you are salivating.

Were you surprised at how real the experience seemed? Remember the body cannot distinguish between real and imagined reality. This exercise gives you experiential proof of that.

EXERCISE 2: develop your ability to concentrate

To use visualisation successfully – that is to help you get the results you want – you need to be able to hold your attention on the image that you are focusing on. That's easier said than done, of course, and, in my experience, most people's ability to concentrate is pretty poor. However, help is at hand. The following exercises are designed to improve your powers of concentration.

A. Close your eyes and imagine a blackboard in front of you. Now count from 1 to 100, imagining each number appearing in white on the blackboard as you count forward. When your mind wanders, start again at one. After a couple of minutes doing this, record the maximum number that you reach. Next time you try the exercise see if you can beat your previous score.

B. Get yourself a watch or clock, with a second hand that indicates how many seconds are going by. Sit down, hold it in front of you and keep your full attention on the second hand as it goes around. The moment your attention goes elsewhere – as it will – return back to the second hand. Most people when they start this can manage just a couple of seconds, but with a little practice, you should be able to hold your focus for at least 60 seconds.

The secret of mastering concentration is regular practice. The more time you devote to these exercises the quicker and better at visualisation you will become.

EXERCISE 3: develop your ability to visualise

If you really are struggling to visualise, you can take heart that you are not alone. Some people are more in tune with their feelings or with what they hear than with images. However, given the right amount of practice, everyone can visualise successfully. Try this:

1. Look around the room you are in. Focus on a particular area and try to memorise what you can see.

2. Close your eyes and try to build up an image that matches what you've just been looking at.

3. Give yourself plenty of time to do this, breathe deeply and then open your eyes again.

4. Keep repeating the exercise so that you remember more and more detail.

Like a muscle that hasn't been used for some time, effective visualisation requires you to practise whenever you can. Try using this exercise when travelling on a bus or train – it doesn't take long to do and you should find you improve very quickly, normally after just a few days.

Healing visualisations

There are a lot of different visualisation techniques on offer for anyone who is interested in visualisation. The four that I've selected are the ones I have most experience with, and the ones that my patients and workshop attendees report greatest success with.

1 Transform the way you feel

As we've learnt, the way you feel about someone or something has a lot to do with the quality, content and type of images you have relating to that someone or something. An image that is big, bold, bright, close up and in colour, will generate the most intense emotional experience. An image that is dull, far away, blurred and in black and white, however, will have much less emotional intensity. Knowing this, gives you a very powerful tool for changing the way you feel. Try this quick exercise so that you can experience this for yourself.

EXERCISE: imagining

1. Imagine in two hours' time you are going to give a presentation to a group of people. Imagine yourself being there – feeling nervous, stuttering over your words, with people laughing at you – basically, imagine it not being a success! On a scale of 1 to 10, how much are you looking forward to the speech?

2. Now imagine yourself feeling calm and confident – see the people smiling at you and nodding in agreement with what you are saying. Now score yourself again, using the same scale, and notice what a difference the type of pictures you made about the event had on the way you feel.

Before you put this technique to use on something more personal, I want to introduce the idea of association and disassociation. When you identify and associate with an image – that is, you see, hear and feel the contents of the image as though you were in it – then those feelings will become much stronger. When you detach from the images, they become weaker. There are various different ways to detach from an image. For example: seeing the image through a window, floating above yourself and seeing yourself in the image, and watching the image on a television. If at anytime you get upset or stressed when doing the following visualisations, just disassociate using one of these methods.

EXERCISE: association and disassociation

1. Make a list of five different things that make you *feel* uneasy, distressed or upset. List them below:

1 _____

2 _____

3 _____

4 _____

5 _____

2. Taking each one in turn, notice what picture or image comes up when you think of that person or situation.

3. Step out of the image (so that you are now looking at it from a distance, rather than being in it) – this is disassociation.

4. If the image is moving, make it still.

5. If the image is large, make it very small and distant.

6. If the image has colour in it, drain it, and make it black and white.

7. If the image is bright, make it dull.

8. If the image is in focus, make it out of focus.

9. And if you can hear sounds, make them quieter, muffled and more distant.

Once you've done this notice how you feel differently about the issue you were working on. This works a treat. If you want to, you can take it to the next level by reprogramming a more positive image in its place. Here's an example:

Helen was a rather nervous 24-year-old woman who came along to one of my workshops. She was searching for more confidence and wanted help controlling her anxiety. When I asked her to think of a particular situation that triggered her anxiety, she immediately mentioned her 'bullying boss', who was always running her down. The image she had of her was of a powerful, angry woman who made her feel small and scared.

She used the above process, and I also asked her to imagine her boss wearing a nappy and speaking with a quiet, squeaky voice. This brought some humour into an otherwise very serious situation, and had an immediate calming effect on her.

Next, I asked her to create a positive image of herself that would replace the old one. This is essentially the reverse of the process above. I asked her to get inside the image of her looking at her boss, and told her to see and feel herself being confident. I got her to sit up straight, relax her shoulders and adopt the posture of a confident person – this works really well. When she opened her eyes, she felt 'really calm – and confident'! I left her with instructions to repeat this visualisation anytime she felt disempowered and overwhelmed.

2 Heal your body

This is one of the visualisation exercises that I teach in my workshops. I personally like it because I feel calm and centred afterwards. Other people, particularly my patients with cancer, have found it very useful to use on a daily basis, as an empowering means of supporting their bodies' healing and recovery.

EXERCISE: healing

1. Sit down, make yourself comfortable and take three deep, long breaths. Bend both arms at the elbow, raise them to the height of your shoulders and turn your right palm up and your left palm down. Now imagine energy (in whatever way feels natural) running from the universe down into your right hand, through the entire length of the body and then returning to the earth via your left hand. Keep breathing deeply throughout and give yourself at least one minute to do this. You may or may not feel energy running through your body when you start this.

2. The next step is to breathe in a silvery or white light through your solar plexus (the area around your stomach). As you inhale, allow this light to flow into and fill up your entire left leg.

3. Breathe in again, and now fill up your right leg. Breathe out. Breathe in again and fill up your pelvis. Breathe out. Breathe in and fill your abdomen. Breathe out. Breathe in and fill your chest. Breathe out. Breathe in and fill your neck and shoulders. Breathe out. Breathe in and fill your head. Now breathe in and allow your entire body and the area surrounding it to be filled with this white, rejuvenating energy. Allow yourself to enjoy this experience.

4. Now imagine all of this light and energy creating a spiralling vortex. Using your intention, direct it into those parts of your body that need healing and repairing. Breathe deeply and continue this for a few minutes, until you feel that the work has been done. If you are enjoying it, allow yourself to do this for as long as you like.

5. Once you have finished, ask for innocent energy to fall upon you. Innocent energy is like a fine mist. It will feel extremely pleasant and make you tingle – breathe deeply.

6. When it feels right, give thanks for your experience and open your eyes.

3 Accelerate your recovery

If you have a particular issue such as stress, pain or cancer, using a visualisation technique that is more focused on dealing with those issues can be a very easy and effective way of instructing the body's healing wisdom to speed your recovery. There are no fixed rules here, so play around with the images that you use. At the end of the day it's all about finding something that works for you. Here are a few ideas to get you started.

Depression/anger/anxiety

Imagine your emotions forming a ball of energy attached to a big helium balloon, which then floats up and out of your body.

Infections

Imagine millions of white blood cells armed with vacuum cleaners going around your body clearing and removing any infection and debris.

Smoking

Imagine yourself smoking a cigarette and then maggots, or some unpleasant thing, coming out of it into your mouth. Hold the vision, breathe deeply, keep associated and intensify the feelings and images, keep focused on the experience and allow yourself to be repulsed by it. When you've finished, repeat this until you feel unsettled every time you think about a cigarette.

Upset with a person

Imagine whoever it is that you are upset with. Make them much smaller than you, give them a squeaky voice, put them in clown boots and swap their clothes for a nappy. Breathe deeply.

Cancer

Imagine a vortex spinning furiously and sucking up all the cancer cells in your body. If you are using chemotherapy or radiotherapy, imagine a red laser destroying all of the cancer cells.

Wounds

Imagine the cut or wound healing over perfectly. See yourself touching it, and notice how pleasing it feels to know that it is completely healed.

Stress

Imagine yourself on a beach or somewhere that you feel relaxed, allow the rays of sun to soothe and calm you. Alternatively, imagine all of the stress that you are carrying draining out of your feet.

Heart disease

Imagine your blood flowing effortlessly through the clean pipes that make up your vascular system.

Pain

Imagine that the pain is controlled by a dial with the numbers 1 to 10 on it. Gradually turn the dial from 10 to 1 and, as you do so, experience the pain decreasing in intensity. If inflammation is a problem, imagine a fireman hosing the area down with cool, fresh glacial water.

4 Enter your healing sanctuary

This is one of my favourite visualisation exercises. It was inspired by the work of Silvia Hartmann and her Project Sanctuary.[2] The healing sanctuary is a very creative exercise in which you mentally construct an inner healing sanctuary, a place of healing and relaxation that enables you to gather different perspectives on your life situation and also experience different types of healing treatments. It can also be used as a place in which you can meet your inner adviser – a wise and loving part of us that is available to ask questions of, and to seek help and advice from. Take a few minutes to read the description of the process, and when you are ready find somewhere quiet where you won't be disturbed. This takes at least ten minutes to do.

EXERCISE: healing sanctuary

Step 1 • enter the healing sanctuary

1. Sit or lie down and make yourself comfortable. Bring awareness to your breathing, observe the in and the out breath and allow yourself to relax both physically and mentally (the relaxation mind–body tool will help you with this – page 380). If you wish to, put on some gentle music in the background and allow that music to help you relax.

2. Now imagine a golden heart, located just behind your own physical heart. Observe it shimmering with bright white light. Make it bigger and bigger, until it is at least seven foot tall, seven foot wide.

Now create a doorway in the centre of the heart. This is the gateway to your sanctuary. Open the doorway and step through.

Step 2 • explore the area

1. Having stepped inside, say the words 'healing sanctuary' and notice what images come up for you. If nothing comes, just repeat the word 'healing sanctuary' with a calm reassurance that your sanctuary is there and that it will present itself to you. As you wait, your sanctuary will start to form around you. It might at first appear a little hazy; that's OK, things will get clearer with time.

2. Once you can see some images, start exploring your healing sanctuary. Are you indoors or outdoors? Are you in a building, a forest, or next to mountains or water? Is it sunny or overcast? Is it raining or snowing? Can you see animals or people? Can you see any objects of interest? Can you hear any sounds? Go for a walk and explore the area. At this stage try not to analyse what's happening, just go with the flow of the experience.

Step 3 • meet your inner adviser

1. To find your inner adviser is easy, just look around. Your adviser will be there. He or she might seem very familiar to you.

2. Walk towards them. As you do so, ask yourself these questions. Is your inner adviser male or female? How are they dressed? Are they young or old? Do they have any distinguishing features?

3. As you approach nearer, introduce yourself and ask their name and anything else you would like to know – they will provide it. The inner adviser is a great sounding board, and someone who is always willing and very able to give feedback and offer perspectives on situations. If it feels right, allow them to accompany you as you continue with the visualisation.

Step 4 • create your healing sanctuary

1. In this part of the visualisation you are invited to create specific features within your sanctuary. If it helps, turn to your inner adviser and ask, 'What do I need to do to make my sanctuary just right for

me?' You will be told or shown, through insights and impressions. Some ideas that you might consider include:

A dwelling: castle, palace, mansion, futuristic building, and so on.
Rooms within that dwelling: healing room, meditation room, spa room, dream analysis room, music therapy room, relationship counselling room, library, play room, body sculpturing room, behaviour transformation room, problem-solving room, relaxation room, time travel room, channelling room, bedroom, cellar, and so on.
Objects within those rooms: plants, pictures, crystals, sculptures, art, animals, people, flooring, decorations, pets, toys, family members, friends, music, instruments, treasures, chimes, furnishings.
Grounds around that dwelling: gardens, trees, orchard, greenhouse, secret garden, wildlife, flowers, butterfly garden, moat, well, fish pond, roads, Jacuzzi, waterfalls, mythical animals, sculptures, pyramids, farm, wood, swimming pool, beach, and so on.

2. As you explore each of these areas, be creative and inspired, turning to your adviser whenever you feel the need to do so.

For example, in the meditation room, you could have cushions, curtains, incense, dim lighting and your favourite relaxing music playing in the background. In the library, you could have bookcases full of huge old books with different subjects inscribed on their spines, such as universal wisdom. Each room should have a particular and unique purpose to it. For example, every time you want to receive a healing treatment you can go straight to the healing room. On arriving you can ask for sound or colour healing, bathe in a healing hot-water pool or sit under rays of bright, healing light. If you have recurring nightmares, you can go into your dream room and imagine it as a video-editing suite. You play your nightmare out on a large screen and then, with the help of your adviser, edit and transform it to something positive.

Step 5 • enjoy the experience

Once you have created your sanctuary, you can then start using its facilities. Spend as much time as you want here. Try out a healing meditation or some relaxation therapy – allow yourself to really benefit from what you have created. If at any time you feel uncomfortable or come across something that upsets you, just ask your inner adviser to blast it with white light and it will disappear.

Step 6 • leaving the healing sanctuary

Once you are ready to leave the healing sanctuary, simply state that you are ready and the golden heart will instantly appear before you. Say thanks to your inner adviser and open your eyes.

Obviously you can use this visualisation as often as you want. Every time you revisit the sanctuary, continue to refine its details and enjoy the experience. Some of my patients with cancer, enter their sanctuary while undergoing treatment and have found it very helpful in reducing the stress of the experience, and also reducing any adverse effects.

MIND–BODY ESSENTIALS

- Images are the language of the mind. Your experience of reality is heavily influenced by the way your mind interprets reality and the subsequent images and commentary that is generated.

- Visualisation is a powerful and proven skill that allows you consciously to select images that promote health and help you achieve your goals.

- To modify an image that is distressing or holding you back, disassociate from it, make it smaller, further away, duller and out of focus, and make the sounds quieter and muffled.

- To positively transform an image or rehearse a desired outcome, associate with the image, make it bigger, brighter, bolder, nearer, sharper, clearer and in focus, and the sounds louder and crisper.

- For recommended reading see Resources, page 429.

chapter 5

Emotional freedom technique

I came across the emotional freedom technique (EFT) after reading about it on the website of the American physician, Dr Mercola.[1] He claimed that EFT had helped many of his patients overcome various health problems including addictions, anxiety, food cravings and phobias. Four years later, after using it with over 200 of my own patients, I can confirm he is right. The great thing about EFT, and the reason for dedicating a whole chapter to it, is that it can be safely used by anyone in the comfort of their own home. Not only that, it provides a very effective, quick and simple-to-use tool that you can try on virtually any challenge or health problem. My advice, which echoes that of EFT's founder Gary Craig, is to try it on everything.[2]

What is EFT?

The best description of EFT that I have read is one that describes it as psychological acupressure. The basic procedure of EFT is to combine tapping on various parts of the body (which correspond to acupuncture points), while saying specific phrases and affirmations that describe the problem that you wish to address and release. Although this sounds all too simple and unbelievable, the real test is, of course, in trying it.

Fortunately, it doesn't require you to believe in it for it to work. If you would like to go into some detail about how it works, I would encourage you to visit the website of Gary Craig (see Resources, page 421).

What conditions might it help?

Although there isn't (yet) the research to prove it, EFT may help with various health challenge that you are facing. You have nothing to lose by trying it. The areas that I have most experience with, and the ones that I have seen greatest success with, are:

Addictions	Eating disorders
Allergies	Fatigue
Anger	Insomnia
Anxiety	Pain
Compulsions	Panic attacks
Cravings	Phobias
Depression	Stress

How to use EFT

I am going to share with you my adapted version of the emotional freedom technique that I use with my own patients. It is not the original version, and I would encourage you to visit Gary Craig's website to find out more about this. Before attempting to use EFT you should spend some time reading through and familiarising yourself with its different steps, so that when you do start using it you can do so effortlessly and without much thought.

EFT is divided into four steps:

Step 1 Preparation

Step 2 The first sequence

Step 3 The second sequence

Step 4 Repetition

Step 1 • Preparation

Prepare yourself

Find somewhere quiet where you won't be disturbed. Turn your mobile phone off, unplug your house phone and remove any glasses or jewellery that you might be wearing.

Create your short problem statement

Identify the specific problem that you would like to resolve, and create a short problem statement that describes the issue you wish to work with. This should be as personalised as possible and reflect exactly how you feel – don't hold back! Some example short problem statements include:

- I have this deep anger and resentment towards Joseph

- Sarah is driving my crazy

- I can't stand being near Steven

- I am oversensitive to criticism

- I am useless

- I feel unlovable

- I hate myself

- I am uptight about money and finances

- I am terrified of spiders

- I feel scared to death about my job interview

This short problem statement will be used with the 'tapping' part of EFT.

Create your long problem statement

Create your long problem statement by placing your short problem statement into the template as follows:

- Even though [*whatever problem it is you are working on*], I deeply and completely accept and forgive myself, without judgement.

For example: the short statement 'I have this deep anger and resentment towards Joseph' becomes, 'Even though I have this deep anger and resentment towards Joseph, I deeply and completely accept and forgive myself, without judgement.'

Other examples include:

- Even though I hate myself, I deeply and completely accept and forgive myself, without judgement.

- Even though my back is killing me I deeply and completely accept and forgive myself, without judgement.

- Even though I have this feeling of helplessness I deeply and completely accept and forgive myself, without judgement.

This long problem statement will be used with the 'patting the chest' part of EFT.

Rate the problem

Before you start, and to help you keep track of your progress with EFT, it's a good idea to rate the intensity and importance of the problem that you are working with: 10 = the highest intensity level, a major issue for you, 1 = no longer an issue for you.

Bring your attention into your body

Once you have created your EFT problem statements, sit down on a comfortable seat and put both feet flat on the floor. Close your eyes and place your awareness in your feet. Slowly allow your awareness to rise up the entire length of your body until you reach the top of your head. Keep breathing deeply throughout.

Energise your body

This is not part of the original EFT, but something that I have found to be useful with my own patients:

EXERCISE: priming the body

1. Clench both of your fists, bring them to your chest and place them either side of the mid-line, just below the collarbone. Tap firmly for ten seconds.

2. Then, using your left or right hand tap firmly in the centre of your chest, at an area 5cm (2in) below the U-shaped groove where your collarbone meets. Tap firmly for ten seconds.

Step 2 • The first sequence

Patting the chest

Place your full attention on the issue you wish to resolve and say your long problem statement slowly and out loud while patting the upper left portion of your chest (just below your collarbone) with the flat of your hand. Repeat this three times. Keep focused on the issue, breathe deeply throughout and allow yourself to make contact with any emotions, if you can. Once you have finished, move on to the next step.

Tapping the eight points

Using all of your fingertips (unless you have long nails) and with a relaxed, slightly curved hand, tap firmly on both sides of the body at each point in sequence (as illustrated opposite) for the duration it takes to say the short declaration statement. Each tap should be firm, but not painful (although the acupressure points tend to be more sensitive than the surrounding areas). On average you should tap seven times at each point.

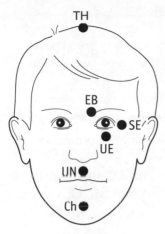

Facial tapping points
(see key)

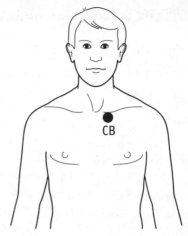

Tapping point on the chest
(see key)

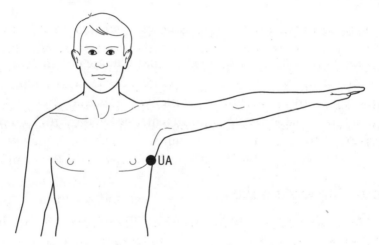

Tapping point under the arm (see key)

Key:

Tapping point	Location
Top of head (TH)	Top of the head
Eyebrow (EB)	Inside aspect of the eyebrow
Side of the eye (SE)	Corner of the eye socket

Tapping point	Location
Under the eye (UE)	Centre of the bone below the eye
Under the nose (UN)	Midline between mid nose and lip
Chin (Ch)	In the groove of the chin
Collarbone (CB)	Just below your left collarbone
Underarm (UA)	On the torso about 10cm (4in) below the armpit

Once finished, place both hands on the centre of your chest (the place you would point to if you were pointing to yourself), close your eyes and take three deep breaths. The first cycle is now complete.

Step 3 • The second sequence

Reassessment and adjustment of your statement

Take a moment to tune into the issue that you are dealing with, and, using the same scoring system as before, reassess the intensity and importance of the issue. Most people will find that their score has dropped by at least a couple of points, maybe even more. Your goal is always to get the score to zero. If your score is above 0, make a slight adjustment to your problem statement to reflect this. For example:

'Even though I *still* feel this deep anger and resentment towards my father, I deeply and completely accept and forgive myself, without judgement.'

'Even though I *still* have this loathing towards myself, I deeply and completely accept and forgive myself, without judgement.'

Now repeat the steps one and two of the EFT procedure again, but this time using your adjusted statement. So, for the patting the chest part, you will say something like, 'Even though I *still* feel this deep anger and resentment towards my father, I deeply and completely accept and forgive myself, without judgement.' And for the tapping the eight points 'I *still* feel this deep anger and resentment towards my father.'

Once you've completed another cycle, one of three things tends to happen. Firstly, you get down to zero, which is great because that means you are finished. Secondly, there is no change in the score. If this is the case, choose a statement that most accurately reflects the issue. Alternatively, you might find that a deeper issue has revealed itself. Don't be afraid to chase the issues as they come. Thirdly, you might get your score down to 1 or 2. If this is the case, repeat the cycle one final time using the following statement:

'This problem is now resolved completely and I deeply and completely accept and forgive myself, without judgement.'

Doing this will usually bring the score down to zero, and indicates that you have successfully resolved the issue that you were working with.

Step 4 • Repetition

Some problems, particularly those that are more complicated and long standing, will require a number of EFT repetitions. Under these circumstances you should use EFT up to a maximum of ten times a day. If there is no obvious improvement within 48 hours, it probably means EFT is not suitable to your circumstances or that you might need some assistance from a professional EFT practitioner. See Resources, page 421 for more information.

Using EFT at home

As you become familiar with EFT, you will find that it is very easy to use and that it rarely takes more than 20 minutes to address a specific issue. If you get stuck or are unsure about the tapping, I suggest that you buy the EFT course or purchase one of the many books that goes into some detail about how to use EFT (see Resources, page 421).

When thinking of issues that might be appropriate to use with EFT, a number of my patients have found the following series of questions to be useful in focusing on issues that might be affecting them in some way. I invite you to spend ten minutes or so answering the questions. My advice would then be to address one issue a day. Because many issues are interconnecting, you will almost certainly find that once you have successfully cleared an issue, the intensity and importance of other issues will also change. So keep reassessing whether an issue is important for you or not.

Use a notebook to record your answers to these questions:

1. What are my five worst mistakes?

2. What are my five greatest fears or things that are holding me back?

3. What five areas of my life am I not facing up to at the moment?

4. What are my five worst memories?

5. What are five factors/issues undermine my self-belief?

MIND–BODY ESSENTIALS

- EFT is a powerful and effective self-help tool that can help to deal with many different issues and problems.

- Being clear about the issue you wish to address, formulating specific statements that describe the problem and giving yourself plenty of time are the keys to successful EFT.

- Try to get into the habit of using EFT every day, at least for the first two weeks.

- If you get stuck or are unclear about some aspect of EFT, you can download a free EFT protocol (see Resources, page 421).

- EFT can also be used for making positive choices; see Dr Patricia Carrington's website (see Resources, page 421).

- For recommended reading see Resources, page 429.

chapter 6

Emotional trauma release

If you have suffered emotional trauma of any kind, then I want to offer you some realistic hope for setting yourself permanently free from the emotional upset surrounding it. I'm really excited by what I'm about to share with you, as I believe the two techniques in this chapter have the potential to benefit and help transform the lives of thousands, if not millions, of people.

What is emotional trauma?

Emotional trauma means different things to different people, but for the purpose of this chapter we're going to take it to mean abuse, psychological bullying, assaults, heartbreak, accidents, muggings, phobias, or witnessing a disturbing incident. The damage and trauma that follows results not just from the specifics of the event itself, but even more importantly from the way your bodymind responded and continues to respond to the event. If your body-mind goes into denial, shock or is simply overwhelmed and therefore unable to handle what has happened, the painful emotional charge generated in response to the event gets lodged and trapped inside of you. Someone who has experienced this kind of trauma will tell you – and see if this is true for you – that some fundamental aspect of them changed that day, and that they have never been the same since.

The consequences

Just as each person's experience of an emotionally traumatic event can be different, so can the way that the emotional trauma impacts on his or her life. Here are just some of the many effects and consequences of having experienced emotional trauma:

Addictions	Low self-esteem
Anxiety	Nightmares
Depression	Obsessive–compulsive behaviour
Flashbacks	Phobias
Insomnia	Relationship problems
Loss of confidence	Work problems

Overall, emotional trauma impacts most greatly on the quality of life that a person is experiencing, with health, relationships, work and confidence being the most badly affected.

How can you recognise it?

One of the easiest ways to assess whether you are being affected by an experience from the past is to think about a specific person or event and to become aware of what you are feeling in your body. A feeling of heaviness, distress, upset, anger, irritability, numbness or any negative emotional state suggests that at some level you are still being affected by that event. If you have a moment, try this exercise.

EXERCISE: events from the past

1. In a notebook, make a list of five emotionally traumatic and stressful events or experiences with people that you would like to be free of.

2. Once you have written them down, spend a few moments with each, close your eyes, breathe deeply and become aware of what you are feeling. You can stop getting caught up in the emotions by commenting, silently or out loud, on what you are experiencing. For example, 'When thinking about Peter, I feel heaviness in my stomach, I feel nauseous and upset.'

3. Once you've finished (it need only take a couple of seconds), turn your attention to the next one and repeat the exercise. The list that you create now is going to be the basis of the work that you do at the end of this chapter.

Deactivating emotional trauma

One of the breakthroughs in my own treatment of patients with emotional trauma was the regular success that two techniques – EmoTrance developed by Silvia Hartmann,[1] and The Fast Trauma and Rewind Technique, developed by Richard Bandler and refined by the Human Givens Institute[2] – had on deactivating emotional trauma. What really appealed to me most about these approaches was that they were not only extremely effective but they also worked quickly (taking on average 30 minutes); they don't involve us talking about the problem, or even me knowing what the problem was, and they were painless – it wasn't necessary for the patient to relive any of the trauma again.

However, my sharing with you the details of these two techniques does come with a caveat. The first and most important is that I strongly urge you to consult with a practitioner who is trained in either of these approaches; it is much more effective and much safer if they are used under supervision and with the support of someone who is trained in them. However, I know of many people who have used them on themselves, particularly EmoTrance, and achieved excellent, lasting results. The second caveat is that you shouldn't use these if you don't feel it is right to do so, and you should stop using them if you start becoming overwhelmed. Both are clear signs from the bodymind that you need to do this work with a practitioner. So, bearing this in mind, here are the two techniques that I believe have the potential to revolutionise the field of counselling and psychotherapy.

1 EmoTrance

This is the simplest of the two approaches that I am going to share with you and the one I use most with my patients. In a nutshell it's designed to help trapped emotional charge leave your bodymind. It is particularly effective, in my own experience, for:

Anxiety	Resentment
Grief	Sadness
Heartbreak	Fear

The best way to understand EmoTrance is to try it on yourself:

EXERCISE: EmoTrance

1. Think of a statement, fact, thought or criticism that causes you to feel upset or to feel 'negative' emotions. This could be a person or a phrase that upsets you such as 'You are fat', 'You are useless', 'You disappoint me'.

2. Write this issue down on a piece of paper, turn it face down, take a deep breath, then turn it back over and allow yourself to feel any emotions. (If you don't feel anything choose another issue.)

3. Pay close attention to where you feel it in your body. If there is more than one site, choose the one that feels the strongest. What you are feeling is just trapped energy (emotion) that wants to move.

4. If you can, gently place your hands on that area and get a sense of which direction the energy wants to go. If you don't get an immediate indication, start massaging the area with your hands – holding the intention of softening it as you do so.

5. When the energy starts to move (which it will do), get a feel for which part of your body it wants to exit. This can be any location – the top of the head, mouth, nose, hands, feet, anything goes! If it's not obvious which exit route it wants to take, just be patient and continue softening until it starts exiting your body.

6. Allow all of the energy to exit your body. If it appears to get stuck, gently rub that area or trace the route you feel it wants to take with one of your hands – that often helps.

7. More often than not, there will be residual energy (emotion) in your body, so to make sure that all of the emotional charge has been deactivated, repeat the whole procedure again, starting from step 3.

8. Keep repeating (on average it takes two to three cycles) until you feel no unpleasant sensation at all.

9. Now breathe in the issue deeply, breathe it all the way up the length of your body and out through the top of your head. If you feel lighter, more energised and much clearer around the issue, then you have successfully deactivated that emotional trauma – well done!

10. Take a moment to consider how this experience will change your behaviour and the way you feel about the issue.

This might appear to be a little complicated, but once you've tried it you'll see how straightforward it is. The key is to be patient with yourself. Part of your mind will try to rush you and persuade you that it isn't working for you. If this happens to you, just slow down, breathe deeply and continue.

EmoTrance in action

To demonstrate how EmoTrance works in practice, I'm going to share with you a real-life example of an EmoTrance session that I did with a woman called Erica who had depression. In her own words she told me that the greatest source of upset in her life was the relationship with her husband. Here's the dialogue that took place:

Me: Tell me about your husband

Erica: He frustrates the hell out of me, he's lazy, he won't do any work around the house and he spends more time with his mates than he does with me. He makes me feel worthless and so angry.

Me: Where do you feel that worthlessness and anger?

Erica: I feel it in the centre of my chest right here [*points to the area*].

Me: OK, what you are feeling is energy that wants to flow out of your body, breathe through this area, massage it gently and ask yourself, where does this energy want to go? All energy wants to flow out of the body, where does it want to flow to?

Erica: It seems to want to go up into my throat?

Me: That's great. Gently tell that energy to soften and flow, allow it to flow, remember all energy wants to move. What are you feeling now?

Erica: It's strange, I can feel this tightness in my throat, and now I feel it moving into my mouth – it wants to come out of my mouth! [*Three minutes later*] It's all moved out!

Me: Great, you're doing really well. How do you feel now?

Erica: I feel much better, much calmer.

Me: Fantastic. Now think about your husband again, where do you feel him in your body? [*Then Erica points to her stomach area. We then spend the next five minutes softening and allowing that energy to flow down and fully out of her legs*.] How do you feel now?

Erica: I feel as though a heavy weight has been lifted [*tears in her eyes*]. Wow, this is amazing; I can feel much more connected to him. I don't feel any anger, I just feel – more at peace.

Me: That's great, now breathe in deeply and spend a few moments with these new feelings that you have towards your husband. Get a real sense of how this is going to improve your relationship positively and how you will now be different towards him.

This is the beauty of EmoTrance, it requires no lengthy discussions, no interpretations and no need to talk about the problem, just the ability to feel where the problem is, soften it and allow it to flow out. The other interesting thing was that because Erica was no longer finding her husband irritating and pressurising him to clean the house, he, of his own accord, started to do more around the house. Erica went on to use EmoTrance on a number of issues that were causing her upset. This included the beliefs 'I am not good enough' and 'I am unlovable', her grievances against two of her ex-partners and, most importantly for her, the anger she held towards her father. In addition to this she was able to start enjoying the very positive benefits that result from using EmoTrance on a daily basis, which included enhanced energy levels, improved self-esteem, self-love and self-awareness, and the confidence that whenever she feel stuck or upset she could manage it by using EmoTrance.

Using EmoTrance in your own life

As I mentioned before, it is preferable for you to see an EmoTrance practitioner; the website has a list (see Resources, page 422). However, because of its simplicity you can try it by yourself. My suggestion is to use EmoTrance to discharge the emotional trauma relating to the stressful events that you identified early on. Stick to one a day, give yourself at least 30 minutes, and, at least in the early days, do it where you know you won't be disturbed. As you get more experienced with using EmoTrance, it will be much quicker (taking just a few minutes, or even seconds). I often encourage my patients to spend five minutes or so in the evening, going over the events of the day, and discharging any emotional upset that they might have accumulated. This emotional housekeeping is a great way to keep your bodymind in good shape, plus an essential part of helping you achieve your total-health potential.

2 The fast trauma and phobia cure

This technique needs to be done either with the assistance of a trained practitioner, or with 'The Effective Anxiety Management – Without Drugs' CD, from the Human Givens Foundation (see Resources, page 422). The CD is great, because you can use it at home and it will be like having a therapist in the room with you. In a nutshell, the technique converts a memory with a high emotional charge into one that no longer causes emotional upset. It is particularly effective for:

Obsessive behaviour	Post-traumatic stress disorder
Phobias	Traumatic memories

Although I'm not going to provide the exact details of how to use this technique I will provide an overview so that you can get an idea of what to expect.

The process

The CD or practitioner will help you enter a deep state of relaxation. Once relaxed, you are asked to imagine yourself in a special place in which you feel totally safe and at peace. Once you are calm you will be asked to think of the traumatic event or incident that you would like to deactivate. Having aroused those emotions you will then be encouraged to refocus on your surroundings and relax further.

Within your safe place are a television set and video recorder, and a remote control will magically materialise. You will be asked to imagine yourself floating to one side of your body, so that you are able to watch yourself watching the TV screen. Using the remote control you will be invited to switch on the TV and press fast forward on the video recorder. The film that plays starts at the time when the trauma occurred and ends at a point in time when you felt safe again. As you continue to watch yourself watching the film, the video will fast forward from start to finish. When it has finished you will be invited to get back in your body and imagine pressing the rewind button, so that you can see yourself going backwards through the trauma. Then you will watch the same film going forward quickly and then backwards, until you feel no further emotion. Once this is achieved you will then be guided out of the relaxation. The technique is complete.

Like EmoTrance this technique sounds too good to be true, but it is very effective. I highly recommend that you contact a Human Givens practitioner or buy the CD (see Resources, page 422).

MIND–BODY ESSENTIALS

- Experiencing an emotional, traumatic event can significantly affect an individual's quality of life and trigger a number of health problems ranging from anxiety and depression to phobias and panic attacks.

- The key to recovering from emotional trauma is not to cover up the symptoms with drugs, but to deactivate the trauma. Two of the best techniques for doing that are EmoTrance and the fast trauma and phobia cure.

- EmoTrance involves placing your full attention on the issue you wish to let go of: locate it in your body; breath in and out of that area and tell the energy to 'soften and flow'; allow it to move and sense where it wants to exit your body. Once it starts flowing, allow it to exit completely from your body. Once moved out, revisit the issue and repeat EmoTrance a couple of times, until you no longer feel any negative emotions, but feel energised and light. Other tips: massage the area; stroke the route it wishes to take with your hands; take deep breaths; have loving patience!

- If you are interested in using the fast trauma and phobia cure contact the Human Givens Foundation (see Resources, page 422).

- For recommended reading see Resources, page 429.

chapter 7

Exercise

What's your immediate gut response when you hear the word exercise? Does it lift and excite you? Or do you feel heavy and profoundly uncomfortable? If you are anything like the rest of the population then the chances are it's the latter! In fact, in the UK so many people associate exercise with hardship, pain and effort, that 32 per cent of the British population are completely sedentary; that is, they participate in no regular exercise.[1] One study of 17,000 Australians found that 30 per cent could be classified as sedentary.[2]

So why should you exercise? Well, first up, committing to a programme of exercise greatly increases your chances of taking care of your body. People who exercise tend to be more in tune with their body and more sensitive to its needs. They are more aware of what they put into their body, more aware of how the structure of their body feels, more likely to supplement and more likely to sleep and relax more. Of course I am generalising, and there are plenty of exceptions, but I have seen it with my own patients: those who start exercising make a quicker and longer-lasting positive change to their health and life than those who don't.

What are the health benefits?

A study published in the November 2002 issue of the *Annals of Epidemiology* found that physical activity levels were more important than body weight in determining a person's risk of death. They also found that moderate levels of physical activity were sufficient to lower the risk of death from all causes.[3]

Other studies have shown that regular exercise reduces stress levels, helps shift perspective on problems, increases energy, builds muscle and reduces body fat.[4]

What is the best type of exercise?

There is no one definitive type of exercise. The key really is to find a couple of different types of exercise that you enjoy and to rotate around those. Generally a good exercise programme should include:

- **Aerobic training** This helps to improve the health of the heart and circulation system, and to maintain optimum weight. Examples include jogging, brisk walking, cycling, swimming or rebounding (using a mini-trampoline).

- **Weight-training or strength-training** This increases metabolic rate (therefore helping with weight loss), improves muscle strength and co-ordination, and prevents osteoporosis. Examples include weight training, climbing stairs, push-ups, sit-ups, using resistance bands and cycling.

- **Flexibility or stretching exercises** These improve overall range of movement, mobility and co-ordination. Examples include yoga and Pilates.

How long should you exercise for?

The UK government recommends a minimum of 30 minutes for adults, and 60 minutes for children, of moderate-intensity physical activity on at least 5 days of the week.[5] Moderate-intensity exercise is activity that causes a noticeable increase in breathing and heart rate. One way to gauge moderate activity is with the 'talk test': exercising hard enough to break into a sweat but not so hard that you can't carry on a conversation.

Creating your exercise programme

Make exercise a priority

The number-one reason people don't exercise is because they haven't got enough time, which is another way of saying, 'I don't prioritise and value exercise.' I mentioned in my introduction to this book about identifying reasons to change, reasons so compelling that they motivate you and bring you through the most difficult of times – such as when it rains! If you are struggling to find a reason to do exercise for yourself then why don't you train to run on behalf of a charity in a fun run or half-marathon? My advice is to be clear about why it is you want to exercise, choose a couple of types of exercise that are enjoyable, and then commit to exercising five days a week – most people find first thing in the morning the best. If this means starting your day 40 minutes earlier, and going to bed earlier, so be it – remember, this is your health and life we are talking about!

Address the barriers to you exercising

Write down all of the possible scenarios that would stop you from exercising and then use the emotional freedom technique on page 332 to address them one by one. This technique helps to reprogramme self-limiting beliefs and fears, and to transform them into beliefs that will support and empower you. If it helps, tell everyone you know that you are starting an exercise programme and ask for their support.

If you are new to exercise, go slow

If it's been a while since you exercised regularly, or this is the first time for you, my advice would be to see your GP – to check your heart out – particularly if you smoke, have any risk factors for heart disease, are aged over 40 or get short of breath easily. Once you get the green light, start with walking. It's the most natural and safest way to start exercising. As you get used to it, start increasing the intensity so that you eventually work up to a brisk walk. Use the talk test to guide you. Once you can manage brisk walking, you are ready to graduate to something more intensive such as jogging or cycling.

Consider interval training

Once you are in an established routine of aerobic exercise, for example you comfortably run for 30 minutes five times a week, the next stage is to change the way you train so that you continue to challenge your body. For example, you can increase the duration of the exercise, say from 30 to 45 minutes, five times a week, or change the way you exercise, by exercising in bouts of increasing intensity and shortened duration. The latter is particularly good at training your heart to adapt rapidly to a change in physical demand. A typical interval-training programme would look something like this:

1. Once you are established on 30 minutes five times a week, change each of those individual sessions so that they become two ten-minute sessions of greater intensity, with a five-minute break in between.

2. After a few more weeks, and once you feel ready, break the session into four five-minute sessions with one to two minutes of rest in between.

Continue with this approach until you find your optimum level of duration and intensity. This approach to training is very effective in reducing body fat and gaining muscle tone and/or mass.

Be creative with your exercise choices

Gardening, weeding, mowing, raking, vacuuming, climbing stairs, dancing, playing golf, brisk walking, painting, decorating and sex all count as exercise. If you find it really difficult to take time out in the morning to exercise, then build it into your day. For example, you could park 15 minutes' walk away from your place of work: a brisk walk there and back in the evening is your 30 minutes. Other ideas include: taking the stairs rather than the escalator or lift, going for a brisk 30-minute walk at lunchtime, walking rather than driving, buying a bicycle and cycling to work.

Stretch during and after exercise

A University of Sydney study found that stretching prior to exercises can increase the risk of injury, so keep your stretches to between and after exercise.[6] Make the stretching movement to the point at which the muscle feels tight but not painful. Hold it at that point to allow for the muscle fibres to relax and strengthen, without bouncing. Breathing out through the area that you're stretching can help with the relaxation. Between 10 and 30 seconds is usually enough. Repeat your stretches up to three or four times.

An alternative to using weights

If you don't have access to weight-training equipment try the following. To strengthen a certain muscle group, tighten the muscle gently until it feels comfortably taut. Hold the contraction then relax the muscle completely for a few seconds before tightening again. You then progress with that strengthening process by (a) increasing the length of time of the hold; (b) increasing the number of repetitions; and (c) adding a small weight.

Get someone to motivate and support you

Most people find it much easier to stick with an exercise programme if they have someone motivating them. But don't fall into the trap of partnering with a friend or family member who isn't motivated, because there is a high chance you'll both stop exercising at the first sign of wet weather! My advice, if you can afford it, is to employ the services of a certified personal trainer, someone you get on well with, but, more importantly, someone who has the skill and knowledge to help you achieve your exercise goals. See Resources, page 422, to find about finding a personal trainer.

MIND–BODY ESSENTIALS

- Exercise should be at the heart of any health programme.

- Thirty minutes of moderate-intensity exercise, five times a week is associated with numerous health benefits. These range from improving mood and self-esteem to reducing the risk of cancer and heart disease.

- Try to combine different forms of exercise into your routine – you are aiming to include aerobic, weight training and flexibility training.

- By prioritising exercise, finding a compelling reason to exercise, and getting personal and even professional support, you will greatly increase the likelihood of sticking to a programme.

- For recommended reading see Resources, page 429.

chapter 8

Focusing

The skill of focusing, when learnt and used effectively, could turn out to be one of the most useful approaches that you take from this book. It's a simple process of noticing how your body feels about something and then listening to what your body wisdom has to say to you. By entering into a caring relationship with your feelings and accepting them as they are, the doors to change and insight open wide, and relief from tension follows. What's more, and perhaps most importantly, you will experience the wholeness, peace and respect that comes from honouring the wisdom of the body.[1]

The guidance I have provided below is enough to give you an experience of focusing. However, my advice is to contact the Focusing Institute[2] for details of a practitioner who lives near to you. It's a lot easier using focusing under the guidance of someone who is trained to use it.

When to use focusing

Here are just a few suggestions as to when and how you can use it:

- Whenever you feel uncomfortable or distressing emotions

- If you sense you are stuck or unsure of something

- To gain greater self-acceptance and to let go of self-limiting beliefs and thoughts

- If you are procrastinating

- To help alleviate emotional trauma

- To help develop body awareness and access body wisdom

- To gain greater insight and clarity around a subject

- If you want to achieve total health!

How to use focusing

There isn't a fixed approach or formula to using focusing, and what you do will, no doubt, vary to a degree each time you use it. The following, therefore, is one of many suggested ways of using the focusing skill. My suggestion is that you read through the instructions slowly and then try it out for yourself. Some people find it useful to write down their insights and experiences in a journal after each session; if that appeals, I'd encourage you to do so.

Step 1 • Preparation

In the early stages of working with focusing, try to give yourself plenty of time to get used to it. Twenty, or preferably 30 minutes, is ideal. Find somewhere quiet, where you won't be disturbed, sit yourself down and get comfortable.

Step 2 • Focus

If you have a particular issue in mind that you would like to work with, such as a habit or problem, that's great, if not, see what comes up for you in the moment.

Step 3 • Sense your body

EXERCISE: body scan

1. Take a couple of deep breaths, close your eyes and then turn your attention to your body. Become aware of how your back is supported by the chair you are sitting on and your feet supported by the floor.

2. Breathe deeply. Now turn your attention to the area of your feet. Do you feel any tightness, heaviness, constriction, calmness, or nothing? If you do, just notice it for the moment.

3. Next, bring your attention up into your legs and repeat – what do you sense? And continue this up through the body: the pelvic area, the abdomen, chest, throat and then head area. When you reach the top, take a few more deep breaths.

The idea of this exercise is to get you used to feeling bodily sensations. With practice you should be able to do this body scan very quickly. For the moment go slowly.

Step 4 • Invite your body to communicate

If you have an issue that you would like to work with, say to yourself or out loud, 'How am I about [the issue]?' For example, 'How I am about Susan?', 'How am I about public speaking?' Alternatively, if you have no issue, say, 'What sensation would like my awareness?' In both cases just notice when you feel something and its location. If you sense nothing at first, don't worry, something will arise, although it might be subtle and vague. If you are unsure whether you are feeling something or not, the chances are that you are, so go with that. The most common locations for the body to communicate with you are the throat, chest and solar plexus area (just below your chest bone). When you feel something, describe what it is you are feeling. For example, 'I am feeling sadness in my chest'; 'I am feeling a knot in my stomach area.' What you are feeling is a 'felt sense': a bodily sensation that has meaning.

Step 5 • Say hello and describe it

Once you have located a felt sense, gently and directly say, 'Hello, I know you are there.' Then notice what happens. Does it get stronger, weaker, disappear, or is there no change? Now describe it as precisely as you can to yourself. Give yourself time to do this and keep your attention on the felt sense. If your mind wanders, take a breath and bring your attention back. The idea is to find a description that matches what it is you are feeling. When you have a description, offer it to the feeling and wait for feedback. For example, say your description was 'panic', say to the feeling, 'Is panic right?' One of three things will happen next. Firstly, you've hit the jackpot, so to speak, and your description feels right. This might cause the feeling to disappear and you to experience a release, or the feeling might get stronger and you receive an insight or feel a shift in your energy, towards lightness, peace or happiness. If so you need not go any further. Secondly, you might sense you are heading in the right direction, but that it's not quite right. If so, choose something else and re-offer it – in this case, an alternative might be 'fear'. Or thirdly, there's no sense of the description being correct – if so try another description and see how your body responds.

Step 6 • Describe it from its point of view

Up until now you've been describing it from your point of view, now you are going to describe it from the point of view of the feeling. For example, you might think it feels sad, whereas from its point of view it 'feels like grief'. Once you have a response, re-offer your insight and sense whether it is right or not.

Step 7 • Ask some questions

This is a very interesting part of the process. By adopting a friendly rapport and open attitude towards the felt sense, your body can (but not always) provide answers to questions that you might have. When doing this, treat the felt sense with respect and sensitivity. By accepting it as it is, it is much more likely to enter into a relationship with you. Breathe deeply as you ask these questions and be patient. Here are some suggested questions:

- What's caused you to feel this way?

- What do you need?

- What actions need to be taken?

- What would my body feel like if the issues underlying you were resolved?

- What's in the way of it all being OK?

Having asked any of these questions it's important to continue breathing and to wait for answers. You won't necessarily want to use all of the questions, and you might, for example, want to use you own questions; either way allow yourself to be open to different ideas. The felt sense needs to trust you before it will reveal itself to you. With each answer, read it back and check your response.

Step 8 • Bring the conversation to a close

Once you've been in a dialogue for a while, and you are nearing the finish, ask the felt sense, 'Is it OK to stop in a minute? Is there anything you want to tell me before I do?' Quite often it's in the last few moments that the felt sense will reveal something of importance to you, so do wait to hear it. Once you have finished, give thanks and say that you will be back sometime. Take some time to reflect on what you have learnt and, more importantly, allow yourself to become aware of any bodily shift that has taken place. Most people report feeling more calm, grounded and at peace.

So that's the basic structure of the focusing approach. It is not the only way of focusing and, once you start using it, you'll find that it's much better to be flexible in your approach, rather than sticking to a particular way. Like all things, the more you practise the better and more confident you will become.

MIND–BODY ESSENTIALS

• Focusing is a skill that can be used to access your body's wisdom and bring insight to issues that require clarity.

• You can use it to let go of tension, overcome addictions, experience peace and access your body's wisdom.

• The eight steps of focusing can be summarised as: preparation, focus, sense your body, invite your body to communicate, say hello and describe it, describe it from its point of view, ask some questions, bring the conversation to a close.

• For recommended reading see Resources, page 429.

chapter 9

Goal setting

Imagine being out at sea in a boat and not knowing where it is you want to be sailing to. The chances are you'd soon be frustrated, despondent and exhausted; your energy and focus would be on reacting to what the ocean throws at you in the moment – it's a very disempowering place to be. In this scenario your attention is on coping with what is happening to you, rather than being focused on where you would like to be and using the moment-to-moment experiences as a means to get you there. Contrast this with having a goal. Goals change your relationship to the moment and bring new meaning to the situation. They help you tap into a stream of energy that can carry you forward, even when times seem dark and despairing. Think back to a time when you overcame physical or psychological difficulties by focusing on the goal. Notice how much more difficult the situation would have been if that goal hadn't been there. Now think back to a time in your life when you didn't have any goals, and didn't know which direction you were heading in. Notice the big difference in the way each feels. Having a goal really can be the difference between hope and hopelessness, depression and fulfilment.[1]

Creating goals

Not too long ago, I used to be a big believer in setting goals. I had goals for pretty much every aspect of my life – money, relationships, health, work and so on – but, despite my enthusiasm and regular visualisation sessions, they rarely came true. It took me a lot of time, and reading and workshops to find out why! Essentially, I discovered that the most important factor in being able to manifest goals is the level of consciousness from which the goal was made. If the goal is about self-glorification or ego, or if it involves hurt or harm to another, it doesn't seem to happen. However, when the goal comes from a place of self-acceptance and gratitude and is infused with emotion and absolute belief, it happens – often in more meaningful ways than expected. Here are a few insights that I've had and taught to people I work with on the factors that make goals appear to be much more likely to become a reality:

The goal is realistic and is in alignment with your skills and talents
It's all very well having a goal of being the next X-factor winner, but if you don't have the talent to sing and perform, then it's not going to happen.

The goal is focused on what you really need, rather than what you think you need
A classic example of this was a workshop attendant of mine who said she wanted to have a million pounds in her bank account, live in a beautiful house and be married to someone rich. This, of course, sounds great, but when we explored this further, by repeatedly asking the question, 'Why do you want this?' (we did this 8 times), it turned out that she simply wanted to feel safe and secure (this related back to an incident when she was a child). So her real need in this case was not to have a million pounds in her bank account, but to address her insecurity. After further discussion, her goal became to use emotional freedom technique to dissolve her fear of insecurity. When you set your goals ask yourself, 'Am I choosing this goal because of some underlying fear, belief or worry?' In my experience, dealing with the underlying issues is a much more powerful tool for change.

The goal is placed in the background of your awareness

Most people tend to think of a goal and then forget about it. One way to overcome this is to think of your goal as being like a picture frame and your day-to-day experiences as the content of the picture. This allows you to deal with the events of the day, without losing sight of your goal. You can also use this to sense whether what you are doing is in alignment with your goal. Does it feel right?

The goal is specific, positively stated, legal, challenging, ethical, realistic, measurable, and time-specific

For example, 'I want to lose weight' is not a great goal – it's focused on the negative, it's non-specific and provides no indicator of a time frame. A much better goal would be 'I will achieve a weight of 10 stone by October 10th.'

The goal is in harmony with your intuition

Accessing your intuition – the aspect of you that holds wisdom and insight – is a very useful barometer, both in formulating a goal and in helping you decide which actions will help you fulfil that goal. It takes time and practice to access intuition, but breathing deeply and noticing subtle insights, thoughts and feelings is a good place to start.

How to manifest your goals

The following is a framework that I provide at my workshops for manifesting goals. Commit yourself to using it for the next three months. Use a notebook as you work through the following:

1. Decide on the specific goal/outcome that you would like (write it down).

2. How desirable and challenging is this goal – score between 1 (not challenging) and 10 (extremely challenging)? Your goal should score at least 5.

3. Think about your goal, breathe deeply and turn your attention to your body. Do you feel harmony or resistance/conflict?

Signs of conflict	Signs of harmony
Feel contracted, uneasy or uncomfortable	Feel expanded, light and at peace
Confusion	Clarity and alertness
Heavy, sleepy and/or tired	Uplifted, energised and/or content
Doubt	Knowing
Boredom	Enthusiasm and motivation

4. If you feel conflict, which aspect of your goal is causing the conflict (look at each part of your goal in turn and tune into the feedback from your body)?

5. Modify and rewrite your goal until you feel signs of harmony (write down your new goal).

6. Now close your eyes, breathe deeply and create a movie of what your life would look like and how you would feel once this goal has been accomplished. Give yourself plenty of time to do this. If it helps, use the questions below to help inspire you. It's important that you associate with the image of yourself – that is, you experience yourself as the person in the movie. If you get stuck on this have a look at the creative visualisation mind–body tool for help.

    What do you see that shows you have solved the problem or achieved the goal?

    What are other people doing or saying that tells you that you have succeeded?

    What does it feel like?

    When do you realistically want to be in this position – the one that you see in your mind's eye?

    How will you know that you have achieved your goal? Is there a measure you can use?

    How much control or influence do you have with regard to this goal?

7. Now I want you to turn your attention to the past. Try to identify a moment or experience from the past when you successfully completed a goal. Relive it and allow yourself to become energised by it. Once you feel that energy running through, let go of the old memory and animate your new movie with this energy. Infuse it with life and make it as real as possible.

8. Repeat this process three more times. You will know when it's complete, because when you think of your goal, you will see and feel it as an energised reality. It will feel real.

9. If you get disorientated, confused or become unsure of what you are doing, just open your eyes, take a deep breath, or have a glass of water and start again.

10. Once you have completed this process, my advice is to tune into it for at least a couple of seconds at the start of each day. This will help you refocus and keep on track. If you start to experience signs of resistance (see above), use this as an opportunity to ask yourself the question, 'What do I really need?' Life's experiences can often lead to a change in our values and aspirations, so be open to the idea that your goal may, or may not, evolve with time.

11. My final piece of advice would be for you to recognise and acknowledge the great mystery of the universe that we live in.

Once you've achieved a goal

Have you ever achieved a goal and then been disappointed by the way it made you feel? Or do you move from one goal to the next without really allowing yourself to enjoy the experience of having achieved a goal? If the answer is yes to either of these, it probably indicates that the goals you are setting yourself aren't focused on what you really need, but on what you think you need. Many people are caught up in the idea that they need to achieve something or be someone. Where do those ideas come from? What do you really need? These are questions that are worth asking yourself. What's more, when you achieve your goals do you allow yourself time to enjoy the moment? Are you giving thanks to yourself, to every one else involved, and to consciousness for helping your goal come true? Taking time to give thanks is important, as is enjoying the rewards of achieving your goal. Finally, when following your goals, don't lose sight of what is right in your life, of all the things that you have to be grateful for. It appears – and I speak from my own experience here – that a dominant attitude of gratitude provides the fertiliser for making dreams and goals come true.

MIND–BODY ESSENTIALS

- Goals are creative requests for how we would like ourselves and the world to be in the future.

- An absence of goals is associated with lack of meaning and is experienced as hopelessness and helplessness.

- Creating realistic and achievable goals brings renewed purpose and meaning, and can help you move through difficult times and circumstances. Goals carry you forward.

- Making goals that are based on real needs, self-acceptance, gratitude and guided by intuitive impulses can increase the probability of that goal becoming an actuality.

- Use the goal manifestation structure to help you make your goals come true. When they do materialise, allow yourself to enjoy the rewards and give thanks at every level to everyone who helped you on the way.

- For recommended reading see Resources, page 429.

chapter 10

Instant stress release

Here are a few quick, simple and effective techniques for defusing stress and clearing tension from the bodymind. Whenever you find yourself feeling slightly rushed or overwhelmed with what you are doing, simply STOP and use one of the following.

De-stress points

1. Lightly place the fingers of both hands over the frontal eminence points on your forehead (the raised areas) and stretch your skin slightly. These are the points halfway between your normal hair-line and your eyes. Now place your thumbs on your temples next to your eyes and take a deep breath.

2. Keep your fingers on these places for at least five minutes – just keep breathing deeply. Notice how the emotional intensity starts to fade. Continue until you feel calm and at peace.

Feet breathing

1. Close your eyes and become aware of your feet on the floor. Start breathing in and out of your feet.

2. Keep your full attention here, just breathe and notice how much calmer you feel. When you feel better open your eyes.

Soft eyes

1. Take a couple of deep breaths in and out through your stomach area.

2. Now focus on a spot slightly above the level of your head. Keeping your eyes open, begin to widen your field of vision and become aware of what you can see in the corner of each of your eyes.

3. Keeping your field of vision soft, just notice what you see.

4. Breathe deeply and notice how relaxed you now feel.

The A, B, C approach

A = Awareness
Notice that you are caught up in a whirlwind of stressful thoughts or emotions. (This helps you to start separating yourself from your thoughts.)

B = Breathing
Take three deep breaths – breathing in and out through your solar plexus/belly area. Straighten your spine, relax your shoulders and raise the corners of your mouth. (This helps you to feel calm and more centred.)

C = Choose
This is when you take conscious control of the situation by switching your focus. Choose one of the following options:

Change the questions that you are asking yourself
The type of question you ask yourself has a dramatic effect on your well-being and response to the situation you are in.

Whenever you hear yourself asking questions that start with 'who', 'why', and 'when', such as 'Why did he do that do me?', 'Who is responsible for this?', 'When will they get back to me?', immediately *choose* a question that starts with 'how' or 'what', and which includes the word 'I' and involves taking action. For example: 'What can I do?', 'How can I improve the situation?' (This swaps a disempowering question, over which you have no control, to an empowering question that is geared to finding a solution.)

Change your focus to appreciation

By choosing to focus on, and experience the emotion of, appreciation, you instantly access 'heart intelligence', the source of intelligent awareness and insight from which creativity and personal power come.

1. Take 3 further deep breaths, as though breathing through the heart area.

2. Now focus on a memory from the past, during which you experienced the emotion of appreciation. Make the memory brighter, bigger and bolder. Animate it; turn up the volume. What can you smell, what can you hear, how do you feel?

3. Allow yourself to experience the emotion of appreciation, breathe it in and out. If your mind gets distracted or you lose attention, just bring back your focus to the image.

4. Allow yourself to now enjoy the feeling of appreciation. Keep breathing in and out of the heart area for at least a couple of minutes. Notice how much calmer you are.

All of these choices are giving you the opportunity to transform the way you feel, think and behave. Try them all and see which suits you best.

MIND–BODY ESSENTIALS

- Having a few simple and effective stress-management techniques to hand will help you to manage stressful encounters.

- The key to using these is to become aware that you are stressed in the first place! When you notice that you are stressed, take a couple of deep breaths, and then use your favourite instant stress release tool.

- For recommended reading see Resources, page 429.

chapter 11

Journaling

One of the most useful ways of off-loading worries, gaining insight into challenges and processing ideas and things that happen to you is to keep a dedicated diary or journal. This might not sound that appealing, particularly if you haven't done this before, but my experience is that when people start using one they get a lot of benefit from it.

How to journal

There is no right or wrong way to keep a journal, and with time you'll find what works for you. In the meantime here are a few suggestions to get you started:

- Most people find that a personal diary dedicated to journaling is ideal. It should be for your own eyes only, and kept with you wherever you go. This allows you to record insights as they come up.

- It doesn't matter what you write, how you write it, whether it's grammatically correct or punctuated – anything you write is an expression of your reality. Try not to judge what you write. If you find yourself judging yourself, read Tame the inner critic mind–body tool (page 395).

- Try writing in your journal at least once a day. This might be on waking up, or just before bed – whatever works for you.

- There are no strict guidelines for what you do and don't write, but in the early days it's a good idea to stick to some kind of format, until you've found out what works for you. The things you can include are:

The key events of the day
How you feel about a certain issue that has affected you
Any thoughts, insights or new perspectives that you have had

Emotional housekeeping

Journaling is a useful way of identifying whether there is emotional housekeeping to be done. It can offer you an opportunity to tune into your day and check in with yourself as to whether you are still carrying any negative emotional charge. If you are, you can write about it, or use a technique like the emotional freedom technique.

Setting intentions

Getting a felt sense of how you want tomorrow to go and writing it down is a very useful way of stating how you would like your day to look. You've got nothing to lose in trying this, and you might just surprise yourself. I started using this and was really quite impressed with how it appeared to make my days much better. I also spend a few moments visualising what my day might look and feel like after writing it down.

Off-loading worries

If you suffer from mind chatter or excessive amounts of worry, you might find it quite useful to write those thoughts and feelings into your journal. This can help to stop thoughts from circulating around your mind and help create the mental space for insights to come through. For this you can either write down the thoughts exactly as you have them, or you can list the problems as you see them. If you are extremely upset, write quickly and constantly until you exhaust yourself; it's a very effective way of discharging the energy of emotion – try it. Once you've finished, spend a few moments identifying any action that needs to take place, or whether there are any lessons to be learnt here. It is rarely enough to write about problems, there must also be some kind of resolution as well.

Getting insight

If you are feeling stuck or blocked on a certain issue or area of your life, take a few deep breaths and write down what the issue is in your journal. Now go into a state of relaxation or meditation, ask for insight into the issue, and then (and this is important) return your attention to your breathing and allow an insight or solution to reveal itself to you. More often than not, thinking about a problem rarely provides a solution, whereas relaxing allows ourselves to be open to moments of creative insight.

Focusing on gratitude

It's the easiest thing in the world to take for granted and fail to acknowledge the many wonderful things that we have to be grateful for. The whirlwind of life can be so consuming and absorbing it's rare to hear of someone who takes a moment each day to give thanks for the various things and moments that they have experienced. Whether it's the sun shining brightly, the old lady who smiled at you or the fact that you have a roof over your head – everything presents an opportunity to practise gratitude. In your journal write down at least five things you are grateful about. Then, taking each one in turn, breathe deeply and allow yourself to experience the gratitude in your body.

MIND–BODY ESSENTIALS

- Journaling is a useful and empowering way to access creative insight, offload worries and take stock of your life and life situations.

- Try to get into the routine of using a journal. Writing at the same time each day can help.

- There is no right or wrong way to keep a journal, it really depends on you and what you want to gain from using it.

- If you vent your frustrations and emotions in your diary, remember to take some action to examine those feelings and resolve the underlying factors, otherwise you won't receive any benefit.

- Finish off your session with the gratitude exercise. It's a lovely way of giving thanks for the things we tend to take for granted. It also helps to switch our attention from what is wrong with our world to what is right.

- For recommended reading see Resources, page 430.

chapter 12

Meditation

Learning to meditate can change your life. When used regularly, meditation can help you overcome health challenges ranging from addictions and depression to cancer and heart disease. It can help quieten a chattering mind, calm distressing emotions, and help relax a tense body. It can even lower blood pressure and relieve insomnia. But for me its true function and original purpose is in opening the door to a whole other dimension, in which we experience our deep connectedness to everything. For me this experiencing of connection has been the catalyst for some of the most enlightening and meaningful experiences of my life. The warmth and feeling of being nurtured that comes from deep meditation is truly incredible.

Different approaches to meditation

There are many styles of meditation, which differ slightly in their approach and focus, but in essence they are all bringing you to a state of acceptance and oneness with the moment. The method by which you reach this state varies from focusing on something – for example an image or object such as a candle – to the exclusion of everything else, or repeating a mantra (a word with no meaning), or by becoming the witness (observer) of whatever arises in the moment. It's worth trying all of these to get an idea of which suits you most. I'd recommend that you contact your local meditation class, or get yourself a meditation CD or try one of the styles of meditation, called mindfulness, which is described below.

Meditation research

Of the many various forms of meditation, transcendental meditation (TM) has the most impressive research database behind it: 600 scientific studies and 108 publications in scientific journals. Here are just a few of the studies showing the benefits from meditation:

- A analysis of 198 independent treatment outcomes found that transcendental meditation produced a significantly larger reduction in tobacco, alcohol and illicit drug use than either standard substance-abuse treatments (including counselling, pharmacological treatments and relaxation training) or prevention programmes (such as programmes to counteract peer-pressure and promote personal development). Whereas the effects of conventional programmes typically decrease sharply by three months, the effects of transcendental meditation on total abstinence from tobacco, alcohol, and illicit drug ranged from 51 to 89 per cent over an 18–22 month period.[1]

- A study of patients seeking treatment for post-traumatic stress problems found that those who learned transcendental meditation showed a significant reduction in insomnia after four months.[2]

- The effects of transcendental meditation were compared to those of progressive muscle relaxation and the usual medical care offered to patients with high blood pressure. For those using TM, the decreases in systolic and diastolic blood pressure were twice as great as those for the subjects in the two other groups.[3]

Mindfulness meditation

To be mindful of something is to become aware of something. Mindfulness meditation is a wonderfully enlightening way of bringing awareness to whatever is happening in the moment.[4] It involves witnessing (noticing) what is happening as it is happening, without mental resistance. As you practise it you might be shocked by the degree to which you have previously been unconscious (not aware of) your thoughts, your feelings, actions and what is going on around you. For example, when you last went for a walk, can you remember what you saw, felt and thought? Here are some tips to get you started with mindfulness meditation:

1. Decide when you want to practise mindfulness. I usually recommend using it when brushing teeth, washing and walking. Then, as you get better at it, using it whenever you meet someone.

2. Starting tonight, when you brush your teeth, rather than brushing your teeth and thinking about something completely unrelated, become aware of the experience of brushing your teeth. Notice your thoughts, your feelings and sensations, allow yourself to become aware of the total experience without judgement or analysis. This is mindfulness – well done!

3. Try this again when you have a shower or bath and when you go for a walk. Most people will be caught up in their thinking when they go for a walk; when you walk mindfully, allow yourself to pay attention to the experience of walking. Start by paying attention to what you are feeling, then what you are thinking, then what you are seeing, then what you are hearing. Rotate around these. With time and practice you will eventually become aware of all of these at the same time.

As your awareness grows, you will start to notice how you feel uncomfortable in certain situations, or that your body feels heavy after eating certain foods. Furthermore, you might start to notice patterns of predictable behaviour, of yourself and other people. For example, you might notice that feelings of anxiety always precede you getting the urge to eat chocolate or smoke a cigarette. Sometimes the light of awareness will result in the spontaneous change of these behaviours – more often than not it lessens the hold they have over us. What's more, as your awareness expands and deepens, your ability to see and acknowledge the reality of each moment deepens, and with that comes a greater connection and appreciation of life.

MIND–BODY ESSENTIALS

- Meditation is a spiritual practice that can help to drop away the barriers to experiencing our state of connectedness to everything and everyone.

- Meditation, when practised regularly, has been shown to help manage stress, reduce blood pressure, treat depression and anxiety, overcome addictions, develop awareness and advance spiritual, emotional and psychological development.

- If you want to learn to meditate, you can join a class, start yoga, follow the instructions on a CD, or practise the mindfulness meditation offered in this section.

- For recommended reading see Resources, page 430.

chapter 13

Relaxation

The most popular mind–body therapy by far is relaxation. Learning how to relax deeply, and allowing accumulated stress and tension to dissolve not only feels great but it's also an essential part of keeping healthy. Regular relaxation can help you manage stress, reduce levels of pain and discomfort, increase wound healing, and even help you access greater creativity.[1]

But what is relaxation? When I talk to my patients about relaxation there appears to be quite a lot of confusion surrounding what counts as relaxation and what doesn't. So here are my guidelines to help you out. These are the four criteria that need to be fulfilled for something to count as relaxation. Two relate to the 'event' and two to your mindset:

Event

1. It should have no adverse effects on your health. So smoking, drugs and alcohol do not count!

2. It should trigger the relaxation response. Your body has an inbuilt physiological mechanism called the relaxation response. Essentially, it's designed to return the body to a place of balance. Signs to watch out for indicating that it has been triggered include: feeling calm and relaxed, and more connected to your

surroundings; a decrease in your heart rate; the relaxation of your muscles; and a deepening and slowing of your breathing.

Your Mindset

3. Being able to surrender, enjoy and be present to the experience is a key component of relaxing. If your mind is distracted or you are not able to enjoy the experience then it doesn't count as relaxation. For example, having a massage is relaxing only if you allow yourself to dissolve into the experience of the massage.

4. Everyone has different tastes and preferences, so finding a relaxation practice that fits in with you is important. Going for a walk in the countryside could be deeply relaxing for one person, but boring or unpleasant for another.

OK, so those are the rules. The next thing is for you to find a couple of relaxation practices that you can realistically use each day. Here are some suggestions: meditation, yoga, chi kung, walking, massage, music, self-hypnosis, deep breathing, biofeedback and visualisation. Whatever you choose, make sure it fulfils the four criteria above.

A relaxation exercise that I teach in my workshops is what I call the bodymind relaxation visualisation. I often use it in conjunction with relaxing music. I encourage you to try it.

EXERCISE: the bodymind relaxation visualisation

1. Find a quiet, warm place where you will be undisturbed. Put on some soft relaxation music if you feel that might help you.

2. Sit relaxed, close your eyes lightly and, while keeping your eyes closed, focus on the area between your eyebrows.

3. Imagine yourself in a place that you associate with being deeply relaxed. It could be somewhere you've been before, or you can make somewhere up. Take a deep breath and allow yourself to sense the calmness of that place.

4. Now, turn your attention to your breathing, place your hand on your stomach area and breathe as though you are drawing air in

and out of the stomach area. This will help you to breathe deeply and effectively.

5. Touch the tip of your tongue on the point where the roof of the mouth meets the upper front teeth, when you breathe in. Traditional Chinese Medicine practitioners believe that this creates a connection between the governing vessel meridian and the conception vessel, thus allowing you to bring in vital energy to balance the whole of the body. When you breathe out, open your mouth slightly, gently dropping the tip of the tongue.

6. Continue with your deep abdominal breathing – just be aware of your breath going in and then out.

7. Say out loud, 'I am physically relaxed' on the in-breath, and, 'I let go of all tension' on the out-breath. Continue this for one minute.

8. Now turn your attention to your feet. Imagine and feel your feet filling up with a white, rejuvenating energy. Feel its warmth as it circulates around your feet – and as it does so, dissolving all stress, all tension and all discomfort.

9. See and feel that bright, white energy slowly rise in a spiralling fashion up into both ankles. As you breathe in, allow this relaxing energy to rise up higher on into your calves, your knees and on up into the thighs. When it reaches the base of your spine, also feel and see it in your fingertips, ascending slowly into the fingers, the wrists, the forearms, the elbows, the upper arms and, finally, into the shoulders themselves. All the while, the warm energy continues rising up the spine, abdomen and chest, until it meets the energy from your shoulders at your neck. Allow it to continue up the front, back and side of the head and all the way to the top. Wait a moment, return your attention to your breathing and enjoy the peace that follows.

10. Wait a moment, then return your attention to your breathing and enjoy the peace that follows.

11. Now mentally scan your body for tension. If you locate any tension, deliberately increase that tension, bring it to its maximum intensity and then let it go suddenly and completely.

Repeat this, paying particular attention to areas of the face and shoulders that carry most of the body's tension. This process takes just a few minutes and will greatly enhance your ability to relax.

12. Once all tension has been dissolved, imagine a shower of bright, white energy pouring down from the top of your head, descending to the neck, the shoulders and to the area of the heart, and from the heart spilling out into and around the body. Picture yourself sitting within a sea of bright, white light. Allow yourself as much time as you wish to enjoy this relaxed state.

MIND–BODY ESSENTIALS

- For the body to heal and the bodymind to progress towards total health, relaxation needs to be part of your daily routine.

- Relaxation, through the use of visualisation, breathing or meditation stimulates the relaxation response, an in-built programme in which the parasympathetic nervous system is activated. This balances the state of arousal generated by the sympathetic nervous system in response to prolonged stress.

- To qualify as a relaxing experience, four criteria need to be fulfilled: no adverse effects on your health, it triggers the relaxation response, you are present and able to enjoy and surrender to the experience, and it fits in with your own preferences.

- Choose a daily relaxation practice and make it become a habit, so that it's as natural to you as eating or going to sleep.

- For recommended reading see Resources, page 430.

chapter 14

Sleep

Getting a good night's sleep is every bit as important as eating a healthy diet and exercising regularly. Sleep researchers, medical doctors and numerous health-and-safety organisations have been voicing their concerns about the link between sleep deprivation and ill health for quite some time. The Institute of Medicine in America, for example, published a report highlighting the association between sleep deprivation and heart disease, obesity, diabetes, high blood pressure, stroke and depression. Other researchers have found links between insufficient sleep and immune suppression, breast cancer, irritability, fatigue, poor concentration and deteriorating memory.[1]

While scientists are yet to grasp the full complexity and function of sleep, they do know that sleep represents a critical period during which the bodymind rejuvenates, repairs and recharges itself. Failing to get a minimum of seven, and preferably eight, hours of sleep a night on a regular and consistent basis leads to sleep deprivation. And sleep deprivation represents a major barrier to total health.

Sleep deprivation

A 2005 survey carried out by the American National Sleep Foundation revealed how serious and widespread a problem sleep deprivation is.[2]

About 40 per cent of people get fewer than seven hours sleep on week-days, 70 per cent get fewer than eight hours. Sleep deprivation is a way of life for most people. Those most likely to be at risk include commuters, those who work long hours and/or spend a long time in their car, parents with small children, and insomniacs. (Someone with insomnia has a problem getting to sleep and/or staying asleep.) Here's a taste of just some of the detailed research linking sleep deprivation to ill health and even death:

- The less you sleep, the more likely you are to eat the following day, and the higher the risk of obesity. Researchers at the University of Bristol, found that people who habitually slept for just five hours a night had 15 per cent more ghrelin, a hormone which increases feelings of hunger, than those who slept for eight hours, and 15 per cent less leptin, a hormone that suppresses appetite.[3]

- Wakefulness for 24 hours is equivalent to a blood alcohol level of 0.10 per cent, which is above the legal driving limit. Surgeons awake all night made 20 per cent more errors and took 14 per cent longer to complete the tasks than those who had had a full night's sleep.[4]

- A modest amount of sleep deprivation can increase levels of inflammatory chemicals within the body by 40 to 60 per cent. This will not only exacerbate pre-existing inflammation, such as arthritis and back pain, but also increase the risk of developing chronic health problems.[5]

- According to the UK's department for transport about 20 per cent of vehicle accidents are related to falling asleep at the wheel while driving on long journeys on trunk roads and motorways.[6] In America the National Highway Traffic Safety Administration estimates that 100,000 accidents and 1,500 traffic fatalities annually are caused by drowsy driving.[7]

Are you sleep deprived?

I use this questionnaire to identify patients of mine who might be sleep deprived. A score of 5 or more suggests that you might be suffering from sleep deprivation.

QUESTIONNAIRE: sleep deprivation

For each question score 0 for no; 1 for occasionally; 3 for yes, then total up the section.

Do you:

1. Think you are sleep deprived? (score 5) □
2. Feel tired most of the time? □
3. Ever nod off while driving? □
4. Work long hours? □
5. Spend more than two hours in the car each day? □
6. Sleep less than eight hours more than five times a week? □
7. Have depression? □
8. Drink alcohol most evenings? □
9. Have insomnia? (score 5) □

Total score □

How to improve your sleep

If sleep deprivation or insomnia is a problem for you, give the following a try:

Step 1 • What is the underlying problem?

The first and most important step in helping yourself is to work out the underlying reason for your sleep problem. Take a few moments to answer the following questions:

1. Is there any part of your life that you are dissatisfied with?

2. How are your relationships, work, money or health?

3. Do you need to get some exercise?

4. Are you overweight?

5. Are you eating or drinking any stimulants or taking any alcohol in the evening?

6. What are you not facing up to?

7. Are you in pain?

8. Are you depressed, anxious or worried?

9. Are you taking medications – could it be them?

10. Do you drink alcohol before going to bed?

11. Is it something to do with your environment – for example, too much noise, heat, cold or light?

12. Is it related to hormones – are you leading up to, or going through, the menopause?

A yes answer to any of these, suggests that these areas might be contributing to your sleep problem. If you haven't done so already, use the total-health questionnaire on page 21 to help you work out which of the chapters of this book will help you to address the issues. If you struggle to do this, consider asking a friend for help. Alternatively, find yourself a healthcare professional or life coach who you intuitively trust. Getting some objective input can illuminate issues that are staring us in the face.

Step 2 • Take a supplement to help you sleep

As an alternative to using sleeping tablets, you might want to consider taking a natural supplement to help your bodymind re-establish its natural sleep rhythm. Here are the ones that I use most often with my patients:

5-HTP

The supplement 5-HTP (5-hydroxytryptophan) is an amino acid that becomes converted in the body to serotonin, the good mood hormone, and then into melatonin, the sleep hormone. Although the body produces its own melatonin throughout the day and maximally in the early hours of the morning, levels can drop by 50 per cent by the time someone reaches the age of 50. By taking 50 to 100mg 5-HTP just before bedtime you not only induce sleep but also help to stimulate your immune system, neutralise free radicals and even help to reduce high blood pressure and high cholesterol. Please note that 5-HTP shouldn't be taken if you are on antidepressants, unless you are being supervised by a doctor or a nutritional therapist.

Valerian

The most popular herbal supplement for insomnia is valerian. Valerian root makes getting to sleep easier and increases deep sleep and dreaming. As with all of the other supplements that I recommend, valerian does not cause a morning 'hangover', a side effect common to prescription sleep drugs.

Passion flower extract

Passion flower extract (*Passiflora incarnata*) has been used by Native American Indians as a sedative and sleep aid for hundreds of years. Today, it is revered by herbalists the world over for its sedative and tranquillising abilities and is approved by the German Commission E in the treatment of insomnia and nervousness.

Hops

The plant hops has been used traditionally, usually as a tea, for treating insomnia, particularly for those whose insomnia results from an upset stomach.

Step 3 • Try these sleep-promoting tips

Here are some ideas to help you get to sleep and stay asleep:

- Get into a routine whereby you go to bed and get up at the same times each day.

- Avoid eating heavy meals at least two hours prior to going to sleep.

- Avoid caffeine, nicotine and alcohol late in the day or at night.

- Give the emotional freedom technique a try (page 332).

- Listen to a sleep self-hypnosis tape before going to bed.

- Try a relaxation technique (see page 380).

- Avoid naps after 3 pm.

- Get regular exercise, but make sure you don't exercise within three hours of sleeping – morning is generally best for most people.

- If light is a problem use a sleeping mask; if noise is a problem use ear plugs.

- Follow a routine to help you relax and wind down before sleep, such as taking a warm bath, having a hot drink, reading a book or listening to music.

- Take a warm bath with lavender oil to unwind before bedtime.

- Keep your bedroom for sleep and intimacy, not for watching television and lying around.

- Keep your bedroom in complete darkness while you sleep.

- Keep a slightly cool temperature in the room, as this helps one to get to sleep and to achieve a deeper level of sleep: 18–21°C (65–70°F) is the ideal temperature.

- If you have things on your mind, try off-loading them into a journal, talking about them or trying some relaxation.

- If you are still awake after 20 minutes of attempting to sleep, get up and do something relaxing such as drinking a cup of chamomile tea.

MIND–BODY ESSENTIALS

- Sleep is as important as a healthy diet and regular exercise when it comes to maintaining health and reducing the risk of disease.

- Getting less than seven to eight hours of sleep a night is associated with numerous health problems, including obesity, heart disease, diabetes, depression, immune suppression and cancer.

- Natural sleep support supplements are preferable to sleeping tablets, which can be addictive and can cause a hangover effect; 5-HTP, valerian, passion flower and hops are just some of the supplements that you could consider taking.

- If these sleep recommendations don't work after four weeks, you should consult with an integrated medical doctor or your GP.

- For recommended reading see Resources, page 430.

chapter 15

Symptom dialogue

Is it possible that your bodymind is trying to speak to you through your symptoms? Is there something to be learnt? Are there upsides to having your illness? There is no doubt in my mind that switching the focus from 'how can I treat this disease/symptom' to 'what is this disease/symptom trying to communicate to me' is an essential part of creating total health. Most of us have been conditioned to view a symptom as the enemy, as something that needs to be removed or eradicated, without giving any thought as to what the symptom might by trying to communicate to us.

While I appreciate this is not for everyone, embracing symptoms for what they are – a wake-up call and invitation to redesign the way you live your life – can be a liberating and highly empowering experience. The following process – one I call symptom dialogue – is similar to the one that I use in my workshop. It takes about an hour to do, and is best done in a quiet place where you won't be disturbed.

Step 1

The first thing to do once a symptom or condition arises is to acknowledge it for what it is: a message from your bodymind, attempting to bring your awareness to something that needs addressing. Think, feel and say out loud, 'I thank my body for giving me this opportunity to know myself better.'

Step 2

Ask yourself, 'Am I fighting my symptoms or disease?' The more you resist your symptoms, the more hostility, frustration or anger you show to them, the more stressed your body becomes and the greater the degree of bodymind imbalance. Acceptance of the reality of your experience as it is in the moment helps to relieve some of the mental anguish and emotional suffering attached to it. It also frees up energy to support your healing.

Step 3

Now we want to find out what is at the heart of the problem. We start by setting an intention to discover the core issues that underlie the symptom or life situation and the lessons to be learnt. At this stage you might find it useful to use a relaxation process – this will help you get into the right state of mind.

Step 4

Make your disease/symptom/situation into an object, something that you can imagine or sense. You can do this by closing your eyes and seeing what image, word or object is revealed to you. The object can be absolutely anything – from a wooden cross to a tangerine. Accept the first thing that comes up. This will make it easier for you to explore and find out more information about it.

Step 5

Take a blank piece of paper (or use your journal) and at the top write, 'If this disease/symptom/situation could speak to me what would it say?' Without stopping to think, write down whatever you start to see, feel or think. Try not to analyse it, think about it, judge it or correct it, just keep writing. It doesn't matter how far fetched it might be, and it certainly doesn't matter if it doesn't make sense, just allow it to spill out. If the same idea, thought or feeling keeps recurring, write it down as many times as you have it. When you stop, ask yourself, is there more? Then keep writing. This process often reveals important information about your symptoms.

Step 6

Using a new piece of paper (or using your journal), create two columns. Title the left one 'downsides of having this problem' and the right side 'upsides of this problem'. Take your time over this, and, while breathing deeply, write down your answers. Try to take as many different perspectives on it as you can. Most people find it easy to list the downsides. However, the key is to find an equal number of downsides and upsides. Whereas at first glance this might sound impossible, I assure you it's not, they do exist – you have to change your perspective on it.

Step 7

Having completed the first six steps you can conclude this exercise by writing on another piece of paper, 'What action needs to take place?' Most people by now will have much greater clarity and insight surrounding a particular illness or situation. Identifying what action needs to be taken provides an empowering path forward.

MIND–BODY ESSENTIALS

- Symptoms are messages from the bodymind, alerting you to a state of imbalance. They are not the enemy but an opportunity to learn something about yourself.

- Changing your relationship to your symptoms can be healing in itself. Fighting and resisting symptoms, such as pains or aches, leads to a vicious circle in which the emotional and psychological component of the experience makes the physical problem worse, and vice versa. Accepting the reality of the symptoms and embracing their message instantly relieves some of the suffering attached to it.

- Taking time out to explore your symptoms either through focusing or symptom dialogue can bring clarity and insight that was previously obscured.

- For recommended reading see Resources, page 430.

chapter 16

Tame the inner critic

'I'm fat', 'No one loves me', 'There's no hope for me', 'I'm useless', 'I'm never going to be better', 'I'm a bad person', ' I hate myself'. These are just some of the censored thoughts that a patient of mine called Josephine had about herself. She believed completely that each was true, and because of that she was depressed. One of the first steps I take when working with a patient like Josephine is to explain and help her understand the origin of these voices.

The world of subpersonalities

Inside each and everyone one of us is not just one personality but tens of personalities called subpersonalities.[1] Each is in effect a different person with unique beliefs, perspectives, dislikes, likes, opinions and feelings. Here are some of the more common ones:

- **The Pleaser** This subpersonality is very sensitive to meeting the needs of others, so that it can be praised and feel good about itself. It is kind, caring and agreeable, but pretty bad at taking care of its own needs. The pleaser does what it thinks it should do, rather than what is best for you.

- **The Rule Maker** This is the subpersonality who needs to be in control and have as little disruption to their life as possible. It writes all of the rules and instructs you to behave in a way that covers up and protects your vulnerability.

- **The Rebel** This subpersonality loves to break rules. If you've got a rebel running your life, you will feel antagonistic to pretty much everything. If someone tells you what to do, it will make you do the opposite.

- **The Perfectionist** This subpersonality has exceedingly high standards. It drives you to perform, achieve goals and keep you ahead of the game. It is relentless in its pursuit of recognition and success – and it is impossible to satisfy!

- **The Victim** This subpersonality manipulates situations so that in some way they can get some sympathy or attention. A victim is very good at spinning stories to 'bend the truth'. They suck energy in, by trapping other people's attention.

- **The Performer** This subpersonality loves to be seen and to entertain others. It gets its kick out of meeting and even exceeding other people's expectations.

- **The Exaggerator** This subpersonality is a drama queen, it exaggerates and distorts the truth in order, and for fear of, being found out as a liar. It tells imaginative stories but will be defensive and secretive when challenged.

- **The Spiritual One** This subpersonality aspires to live life according to higher principles and seeks to experience a connection with a greater intelligence or God.

Even though all of these subpersonalities exist within you, some of them will dominate your life more than others. These core subpersonalities are the ones that we identify with and what we believe ourselves to be. The remainder – usually those that hold the opposite characteristic of the main subpersonalities – tend to get suppressed. So, for example, someone who strongly identifies with The Pleaser will suppress The Rebel. Interestingly, we tend to most harshly judge those people who display the characteristics that we suppress. There are also occasions when these hidden selves reveal themselves. For example, the 'extrovert' or 'the flirt' coming out at a party (usually under the influence of alcohol)!

How subpersonalities are formed

There seems to be no doubt that we come into this world with a certain temperament – a genetically inherited tendency to certain behaviours. However, a considerable part of our personality is shaped by the environment within which we were raised. We arrive in the world vulnerable and exquisitely sensitive to our environment. In order to survive and protect this vulnerability our mind creates psychological strategies – otherwise known as subpersonalities – to defend ourselves. Their role is to provide a protective shield around our vulnerability, keep us safe and do their best to get us attention and acceptance by those within our environment. So, fundamentally, these subpersonalities are formed for our benefit. One of the most important 'protectors' and the one I want to discuss in some detail is the inner critic:

The inner critic

We each have an inner critic inside of us, but, for some people, the voice of the inner critic and the power it holds over them is immense.[2] In these people the inner critic can be a potent cause of depression and anxiety. The original function of the inner critic was to protect you from emotional pain, embarrassment and shame, by pre-empting situations that might bring this about. By intervening before the outside world can get you through its own criticisms, it is attempting to protect you – although it definitely doesn't feel like it's protecting you at the time! So while the intentions of the inner critic are fundamentally well meaning, it can be a significant source of emotional distress. The following are just some of the ways in which the inner critic influences your life, it:

- Points out your weaknesses and flaws

- Verbally attacks and suppresses you

- Judges others and finds in them what it hates in you

- Prevents you from growing and developing as a human being

- Diminishes your self-confidence and self-esteem

- Cannot be pleased by you

- Gives you a hard time for being the way you are

- Tells you that you deserve to be in the situation that you are in

- Contributes significantly to, and perpetuates, depression, anxiety, self-harming behaviours and worry

- Keeps you frightened, fearful and ineffective

Although the content of what the inner critic says tends to be similar among people with strong inner critics, it is heavily influenced by childhood experiences. As small children we tend to internalise our parents' judgements of us and take them on board as truth. For example, if you were regularly told by your father that 'you are worthless and will never amount to anything' that will probably become your truth. Your inner critic will replay that message to you and your life might well reflect that message, unless you decide to rebel against it – which, thankfully, many people do. The inner critic is also extremely smart and very cunning, and because it knows you inside out, it will push your buttons in those places that hurt most. But it's not all bad news with the inner critic, because most inner critics can be turned around and befriended so that they become highly perceptive partners in life. So if you've got a strong inner critic, here's what to do:

How to tame the inner critic

Step 1 • Become aware that you are not the inner critic

Just realising that those critical comments and thoughts that you have are not from the real you but from the inner critic can be a breath of fresh air in itself. If it helps, imagine the inner critic as a gremlin that follows you around. It genuinely wants to protect you from harm, but because of its emotional immaturity it doesn't know how to help and protect you effectively. From now on, when you hear the inner critic, say to yourself, 'That's the inner critic speaking.'

Step 2 • Make sure you've resolved any body-based imbalances

We've already explored the powerful influence our body's hormones, biochemistry and even posture can have on the way you feel. It's important to make sure that all of these areas are being addressed as you follow the advice in this chapter. Just switching to a healthy diet, exercising a couple of times a week, taking a few supplements such as fish oil and 5-HTP and correcting any hormone imbalances can turn down the hold that the inner critic has on you.

Step 3 • Reclaim your power from the inner critic

I've used the following visualisation with a number of patients who have strong inner critics and found it to be particularly useful in shifting the power from the inner critic to the real, authentic you. This takes about five minutes to do and is best done at a time of day when you know you won't be disturbed.

EXERCISE: inner critic

1. Close your eyes. What image comes to mind when you think of the inner critic? How big does it feel? Is it the size of an apple, you, a car, a house, the planet?

2. Keeping your eyes closed, turn your attention to yourself. How big or small in comparison to this image do you feel?

3. Now alternate your attention between the image of the inner critic and yourself, and notice how the image starts to change its size; although it might get slightly larger initially, it will start to get smaller and you will start to feel bigger. Just breathe deeply and give yourself plenty of time – there's no rush.

4. Continue alternating between yourself and the image, until the image reduces to a size that you feel comfortable with – the equivalent size of a small child seems to be what most people prefer. Having reached this stage, breathe in deeply and allow yourself to experience your own power. You should feel stronger, more expansive and calmer.

Some people need only to do this exercise once; others every day for a couple of weeks. Try it out and see how you get on. The more you do it the easier you'll find it.

Step 4 • Embrace the inner critic

Following on from the above visualisation, you could try the next step, which is to switch from resisting and being angry towards the inner critic, to accepting and embracing it, just as a loving parent would do to a child.

EXERCISE: embracing the inner critic

1. Take a couple of deep breaths and close your eyes. See the image of your inner critic (if you have followed Step 3, you should be feeling much larger than it). Now, very gently, tell the inner critic in your own words that you understand that it is trying to help you and that you are thankful for that. Continue breathing deeply.

2. Now imagine a golden sphere of light in the area of your heart. This is a safe and loving place in which your inner critic can stay and experience the love and acceptance that you have for him or her. Don't worry if you don't feel loving and accepting, just imagining it will work.

3. Gently imagine picking up the inner critic in your hands and holding it to your heart area. Now invite him or her into your heart. Don't force or rush it, just allow it to happen in its own time.

4. Once the inner critic is sitting in your heart, just allow it to be. Watch it and tell it, in your own words, that you value it but that you are now in charge and you are going to take care of it from now

on. Spend however long feels comfortable doing this – one to ten minutes is the norm.

5. When it feels right, tell the inner critic that it can come back into your heart whenever you want. Place both hands over your heart area and take a few moments to give thanks and appreciation for the experience.

Using this exercise for at least seven days in a row and then once weekly thereafter works well for most people.

Step 5 • Tone down the inner critic

In this exercise you are going to catch the inner critic at work and turn down the power of the inner critic using your voice. This is a good exercise to use with almost immediate effect when your inner critic plays up.

EXERCISE: toning down

1. When you notice the inner critic speaking to you, repeat the exact same words in the exact same tone, but say them out loud.

2. Now locate the area of your body from where the voice is coming. For example, it could be the throat, head or solar plexus.

3. Tell the inner critic to move down to your little finger of either your right or left hand. Breathe deeply as you do so and feel it move down – this can feel a little unusual when it happens, but it works!

4. Now continue verbalising what the inner critic is saying, but deliberately change the tone of what is being said. You want to make the energy lighter, so speak with a softer, quieter voice, as though whispering, or pretend you are speaking to someone that you care about. Say the exact same words but say them with love and care. Alternatively, make the voice sound like Mickey Mouse! Use whatever works for you.

The idea of this exercise is to take the 'sting out of the tail' of the inner critic. Some people find it very effective, but as with all of these exercises, the real challenge is in actually using them.

MIND–BODY ESSENTIALS

- Each of us has numerous subpersonalities, which are designed to protect us and help us survive and thrive in the world.

- We tend to identify with three or four main subpersonalities and suppress those that display the opposite characteristics.

- The inner critic is the voice that criticises us. While wanting to protect us from shame and emotional pain, it can be a potent contributor to depression and anxiety.

- Freedom from the harmful effects of the inner critic, or any of the subpersonalities, starts by becoming aware that you are not your subpersonalities, the real you is the awareness in which these subpersonalities arise.

- Using visualisations can help to reduce the power that the inner critic has over you and switch the relationship that you have to it from being parented by it to parenting it.

- For recommended reading see Resources, page 430.

The mind–body connection

One of the most fascinating parts of my own investigation into the subject of holistic health and healing has been exploring the mind and body, and how the two communicate. For thousands of years many of the ancient health systems, including those of traditional Chinese medicine and Ayurvedic medicine, recognised the pervasive influence of mind on body and body on mind. In fact, from the perspective of Hindu monism, a philosophy that has significantly influenced and shaped Ayurvedic medicine, everything is ultimately one, and the entire universe and every single being in it is an expression of this oneness. Therefore, our body and mind are not just communicating, they are 'one' appearing as two – they are the two sides of the same coin.

When I first came across this idea I struggled to understand it. How could the mind and body be the same thing? Where is the evidence to support this?

The mind–body pioneers

The roots of evidence go back to the 1920s. A researcher called Walter Cannon discovered that psychological and physical stress alters our body's physiology via activation of a branch of the nervous system called the sympathetic nervous system, and by stimulating the release of chemicals from the adrenal glands.[1] Both of these are the means by which the body prepares for 'fight or flight'. The 'father of stress', Hans Selye, then went on to elaborate how this stress response was responsible for contributing to ill health in people who were chronically stressed. For example, stress has been associated with heart disease, high blood pressure and depression.[2] In the 1970s, Dr Herbert Benson reported on the benefits of using meditation, yoga and biofeedback to trigger the 'relaxation response', a physiological mechanism designed to return the stressed state to balance.[3] About the same time, scientists working within the field of psychoneuroimmunology (the scientific study of the mind–nervous-system–immune-system interactions), were also starting to get to the nuts and bolts of the mind–body connection.

The molecules of emotion

The breakthrough in mind–body research came with the discovery of the naturally occurring mood-altering substances called neuropeptides. The first neuropeptide to be discovered was beta-endorphin. A chemical consisting of a short chain of amino acids, beta-endorphin was found to produce high levels of pain relief and tranquillisation, as well as a wide range of other emotional, behavioural, and physiological effects by binding on to matching receptor sites of the body's cells. According to the psycho-pharmacologist and author of *Molecules of Emotion*, Candace Pert, beta-endorphins, along with the other 100 or so neuropeptides that have been discovered to date, don't just influence the way we feel they are also the physical correlates of our emotions.[4] Put another way, these small and rather unassuming peptide molecules are the bridge between body and mind: they are the means by which our mind speaks to our body, and our body to our mind.

In the late 1970s it was initially thought that it was just the brain and nervous system that could produce and receive these neuropeptides. Now it's been shown that every tissue in the body can; this includes your immune system, skin, muscles, endocrine system, and even digestive system. Every part of your body knows what every other part is up to. For example, the cells of your immune system are listening to your thoughts right now. Not only that, your immune cells are speaking back by producing their own messenger neuropeptides, which in turn affects what you think and how you feel and behave. Your emotions are literally directing your physiology and your thoughts.

So when we talk about the body and mind, what are we really talking about? The truth is we can no longer distinguish between the physiology of the body and the psychology of the mind – they are one and the same, just as the Hindu philosophers believed.

Evidence for the mind–body connection

It's one thing for me to tell you how the mind and body are connected, but what is much more compelling is for me to share with you some of the research that supports it, and even more compelling still are the exercises that allow you to experience the mind–body connection for yourself. I've arranged this into two parts, the first looks at how factors primarily influencing the body, such as exercise and nutrition, affect the mind. The second looks at how psychological factors, such as emotions and attitude, affect the body.

Part one: influencing the body through the mind

I use the following exercise in my workshops to demonstrate how our emotions influence the physical body. It takes just a couple of minutes to do.

EXERCISE: the mind influencing the body

1. Find somewhere to sit and then close your eyes.

2. Think back to an event in which you were upset, sad or anxious about something.

3. Breathe in deeply and allow yourself to feel those emotions.

4. Once you feel them fully, become aware of your body. How is your body responding to these emotions?

5. See if you are aware of any of the following: facial flushing, tension and tightness in the muscles, rapid heart beat, quick and shallow breathing, shaking, sweating, dry mouth, sighing, grinding of teeth, lump in the throat, lightness or heaviness.

6. Now repeat the same procedure, but this time think of a memory that makes you feel happy.

7. What can you feel in your body now?

Most people, having done this exercise, will get a real sense of the impact that their emotional state had on their body. Indeed, our bodies are constantly expressing our emotions. Take the face for example. According to Paul Ekman, a psychology professor emeritus at the University of California, it is possible to read other people's true feelings by watching out for fleeting involuntary changes, called micro-expressions in their face. His research has found that there are over 10,000 different combinations of facial-muscle movements relating to the different feelings that we can have inside. Ekman and his colleague Friesen were able to demonstrate that the co-ordinated tightening of certain facial muscles not only triggered the corresponding emotion but could also affect blood pressure and pulse rate.[5] Yet further proof of the mind–body connection.

Research evidence

Here is just a handful of the studies that demonstrate the impact of emotional/psychological factors on physical health:

- A study of 518,240 older couples found that if one of the partners died the stress experienced by the remaining partner increased the likelihood of them dying as well. The greatest risk was within 30 days of a spouse entering the hospital or dying, and the risk remained elevated for up to two years.[6]

- A study in the journal *Circulation* in 1997 found people who were assessed as mild worriers had almost twice the average risk of developing heart problems, compared to non-worriers. People with high levels of worry experienced more than 2.5 times the risk.[7]

- Medical students who became angry quickly when under stress were three times more likely to develop premature heart disease and five times more likely to have an early heart attack than their calmer colleagues in a 2002 study. The authors pointed out that this predicted heart disease even before such traditional risk factors as diabetes and hypertension became apparent.[8]

- A UK study found men who had depression were three times more likely to develop heart disease than those without depression.[9]

- Your perception of ageing may also impact how long you live. A 2002 study reported that older individuals who viewed ageing in a positive light lived on average $7^1/_2$ years longer than those who had a negative view of ageing.[10]

These studies look at how specific mind–body approaches can influence the health of the physical body:

- A controlled study of women with premenstrual syndrome (PMS) were taught to trigger the relaxation response twice daily for three months. At the end of the study period they experienced a 58 per cent reduction in the severity of their symptoms, compared with those who had not received the training.[11]

- A 1998 study divided patients who were receiving light therapy for treatment of their moderate-to-severe psoriasis into two groups. The first were taught a guided imagery process, which involved visualising the light slowing the growth and dividing rate of the skin cells. The second group did not receive any instruction. The results from the first group, the guided imagery group, found that they were able to arrive at the 'halfway improvement mark' 50 per cent sooner than the control group.[12]

- A study by David Spiegel, a psychiatrist at Stanford University followed 86 women with metastatic breast cancer over a period of ten years. The researchers found that those who participated in supportive/expressive therapy, which involving sharing and processing the emotional states of having their condition, lived twice as long (an average of 36.6 versus 18.9 months) when compared to the control subjects who did not participate.[13]

Part two: influencing the mind through the body

The following exercise is designed to demonstrate how your body influences your emotional and mental states:

EXERCISE: the body influencing the mind

1. Find somewhere to sit and close your eyes.

2. Think back to an event in which you were upset or sad about something.

3. Breathe in deeply and allow yourself to feel those emotions.

4. Once you feel sad and upset, make a mental note of how you are feeling and the positioning of your body.

5. Now, keeping your focus on the same event, adjust your spine so that you are now sitting upright.

6. Consciously relax your shoulders, look slightly upwards and deliberately raise the corners of your mouth, as though you are smiling.

7. Notice how you are feeling now.

This is a nice simple exercise to demonstrate the powerful influence that posture has on our emotional state. Most people having done this exercise would have found that the feelings of upset or sadness lifted considerably just by making some small adjustments to their posture. Some other ideas for showing how the body influences the mind include noting how your mood changes when you:

- Take a couple of deep breaths

- Are touched lovingly by someone

- Have a massage

- Go for a run

- Exclude foods from your diet to which you are intolerant

- Exclude sugar, alcohol and/or caffeine from your diet for two weeks

More evidence for the mind–body connection!

Research evidence

Here are just a handful of the studies that demonstrate the relationship between physiology and emotional/psychological health:

- Exercise is a potent antidepressant. A 1990 meta-analysis (an analysis that statistically summarised 80 studies of exercise and depression), concluded that exercise is as beneficial as antidepressants in the short and long term. The greater the length of the exercise programme and the larger the total number of exercise sessions, the more significant the decrease in depression.[14]

- A double-blind study conducted at the Veterans' Administration New York Harbor Healthcare System in Brooklyn found that 3g of fish oil per day significantly reduced the levels of anger in patients known to exhibit aggressive behaviour. No change was observed in the patients who did not receive the fish oil.[15]

- A study carried out by the Department of Social and Criminal Justice at California State University monitored the behaviour of over a thousand young offenders. They found that making positive changes to their diet improved their behaviour by between 40 and 60 per cent. Those with the lowest levels of vitamins and minerals as determined by blood tests at the start of the trial experienced the greatest benefit. Their behaviour improved by up to 90 per cent.[16]

- Thirty patients with diagnoses ranging from depression and anxiety to confusion and difficulty concentrating were investigated to see if food allergies were contributing to their mental and emotional symptoms. The results concluded that allergies to food, particularly wheat, milk, sugar and eggs, were a significant contributor to these symptoms.[17]

- A team of researchers recruited 106 middle-aged men and women who had high cholesterol levels but were otherwise healthy. The results showed that participants with lower blood levels of omega-3 fatty acids (EPA and DHA), as measured through blood sampling, were most likely to display mild or moderate symptoms of depression, a more negative outlook, and have less control over impulses. In contrast, the study participants with higher blood levels of omega-3s were less likely to experience depression, and more likely to exhibit a positive outlook and have better control of their impulses.[18]

Meals and snacks for your metabolic type

Once you know your metabolic type (Barrier 1), you can start using the suggested foods to create your healthy eating plan. By planning a couple of meals ahead and buying in the ingredients beforehad, the likelihood of you sticking to the healthy eating plan is greatly increased. If you are a 'mixed-type', use suggestions from both menus.

Protein-types

Breakfast	Snacks	Lunch/Dinner
Almond or organic soya milk blended with flax oil, whey protein powder, handful of berries and chopped apple or pear	Oatcakes with hummus (chickpeas), almond, peanut or hazelnut butter (sugar-free), mackerel pâté, guacamole (avocado) or tahini (sesame seeds)	Baked sweet potato with hummus, and a side salad with avocado, celery, and olive oil dressing
Organic sausages, bacon and poached eggs on rye toast with butter	Apple with a handful of nuts and/or seeds	Roast beef, with spinach, carrots and green beans with butter

Breakfast	Snacks	Lunch/Dinner
Sugar-free muesli with whole milk, coconut and ground mixed seeds	Nut and seed bar or a handful of olives	Lamb chops with cauliflower cheese and steamed spinach with butter

Carb-types

Breakfast	Snacks	Lunch/Dinner
Organic, live natural yogurt, with berries and/or chopped fruit	Rye crackers with hummus or taramsalata	Vegetable soup, with soda bread, + /- ham, chicken or salad sandwich using wholegrain bread
Oat porridge made up with rice, oat or almond milk and sweetened with a handful of raisins and/or chopped apple/pear	Apple with four almonds or four walnuts	Buckwheat pasta, with pesto, and chopped tomatoes, broccoli and chilli beans
Sugar-free muesli with oat/rice milk or natural yogurt	Raw broccoli and peppers with hummus	Vegetable stir-fry with brown basmati rice

Resources

Health practitioners (UK)

If you need some help and advice in overcoming a health challenge, I recommend that you contact one or more of the following organisations:

The Integrated Medical Practice
This is my own clinic.
W: www.drmarkatkinson.com
T: 0845 094 6450

British Society for Ecological Medicine
For doctors who practise allergy, environmental and nutritional medicine.
W: www.bsaenm.org
T: 01547 550339

British Society of Integrated Medicine
For doctors who practise integrated medicine.
W: www.bsim.org.uk
T: 01962 718000

Human Givens Institute
For practitioners trained in the Human Givens approach to mental health.
W: www.humangivens.com
T: 01323 811662

Complementary Medical Association
The world's largest professional organisation for complementary therapists.
W: www.the-cma.org.uk
T: 0845 1298434

The British Naturopathic Association
The professional body for naturopaths.
W: www.naturopaths.org.uk
T: 0870 745 6984

The British Association of Nutritional Therapists
The professional body for nutritional therapists.
W: www.bant.org.uk
T: 08706 061284

Health practitioners in other countries

Australasian Integrative Medical Association
Provides a list of general practitioners and/or specialists who are members of the AIMA and practising some form of integrative medicine.
W: www.aima.net.au
T: (03) 8699 0582

New Zealand Natural Medicine Association
Provides a list of health professionals dedicated to the promotion of integrative healthcare.
W: www.nznma.com
T: 64 9 4432 066

South African Society of Integrated Medicine
Provides a list of registered health practitioners, who practise, or have
an interest in, integrative medicine.
W: www.integrativemedicine.co.za
T: 27-21-885 1010

The American Association of Integrative Medicine
Provides a list of health professionals dedicated to the promotion of
integrative healthcare.
W: www.aaimedicine.com
T: 417.881.9995

American Holistic Medical Association
Provides a list of health professionals dedicated to the promotion of
holistic healthcare.
W: www.holisticmedicine.org
T: 425/967-0737

Supplement companies

UK

Higher Nature
One of the UK's leading supplement companies.
W: www.highernature.co.uk
T: 0800 458 4747

Revital
Mail order and retail company selling high-quality supplements,
foods, books and CDs.
W: www.revital.com
T: 0800 252875

Worldwide

Higher Nature deliver products worldwide, you can order them via
their website www.highernature.com. Other more country-specific
suppliers include:

Australia

Blackmores: www.blackmores.com.au / 61 2 9951 0111
Solgar: www.solgar.com.au / 1-877-SOLGAR-4

South Africa

Bioharmony: www.bioharmony.co.za / (021) 762 8803

New Zealand

Aurora Natural Therapies: www.aurora.org.nz / (03) 578-1236

USA

Nature's Plus: www.naturesplus.com / (800) 645-9500
Solgar: www.solgar.com / 1-877-SOLGAR-4

Organic food (UK)

All of these deliver fresh, organic food and drink direct to your home:

Abel & Cole
W: www.abel-cole.co.uk
T: 08452 62 62 62

Planet Organic
W: www.planetorganic.com
T: 020 7221 1345

Riverford
W: www.riverford.co.uk
T: 0845 600 2311

Allergy-free food (UK)

Goodness Direct
One of my favourite companies, stocks everything from organic and allergy-free foods, to non-toxic toiletries/cleaning products, vitamins and herbal remedies.
W: www.goodnessdirect.co.uk
T: 0871 871 6611

The Village Bakery
Wheat-free breads, biscuits and cakes.
W: www.village-bakery.com
T: 01768 881811

Organic/allergy-free food outside the UK

Australia

Sunnybrooks Gluten Free Shop
W: www.glutenfreeshop.com.au
T: 03 9578 6400

New Zealand

Huckleberry Farms
W: www.huckleberryfarms.co.nz
T: 09 6308857

South Africa

Organics Online
Tel.: 27 (0)83 407 3931
Website: http://www.organicsonline.co.za

USA

Diamond Organics
W: www.diamondorganics.com
T: 888-674-2642

Diagnostic testing (UK)

Both offer food allergy testing, as well as other tests such as hormonal analysis, and candida/parasite testing:

Individual Wellbeing Diagnostic Laboratories
W: www.iwdl.net
T: 020 8336 7750

Cambridge Nutritional Sciences
W: www.cambridge-nutritional.com
T: 01353 863279

Australia

Nutritional Laboratory Services
W: www.nlabs.com.au
T: +613 9663 1554

New Zealand

Ideal Health
W: www.healthyonline.co.nz
T: +649 4432 584

South Africa

Molecular Diagnostic Services
W: www.mdsafrica.net
T: +27 31 267 7000

Allergies (UK)

Allergy testing: Individual Wellbeing Diagnostic Laboratories on 020 8336 7750 and Cambridge Nutritional Sciences on 01353 863279
Food Allergen Cellular Test (FACT), for IgG and IgA immune responses: Individual Wellbeing Diagnostic Laboratories on 020 8336 7750
The IgG Elisa allergy blood test: Cambridge Nutritional Sciences on 01353 863279

Australia

Nutritional Laboratory Services
W: www.nlabs.com.au
T: +613 9663 1554

New Zealand

Ideal Health
W: www.healthyonline.co.nz
T: +649 4432 584

South Africa

Molecular Diagnostic Services
W: www.mdsafrica.net
T: +27 31 267 7000 or

USA

Optimum Health Resource Labs
W: www.yorkallergyusa.com
T: (888) 751-3388

Bach Flower Remedies (UK)

Crystal Herbs
W: www.crystalherbs.com
T: 01379 642374

USA

Herbal Remedies
W: www.herbalremedies.com
T: 1-307-577-6444

Australia

The Organic House
W: www.organichouse.com.au
T: (07) 5564 2753

New Zealand

Weleda
W: www.weleda.co.nz
T: (06) 872 8700

South Africa

Vital
W: www.vital.co.za
T: 27 21 900 2600

Candida and parasites (UK)

Candida

You can buy oxygenated magnesium products from Higher Nature or Dulwich Health on 020 86705883
Comprehensive parasitology: for more information contact Individual Wellbeing Diagnostic Laboratories on 020 8336 7750

Diet (UK)

Alkaline salts

One recommended product is: Higher Nature's AlkaClear
Green powders: recommended products are Progreens (from Nutrilink on 08704 054 002), Kiki Nature's Living Superfoods, Healthy & Essential Barleans Greens, Nature's Plus Source of Life Green Lightening, Allergy Research Group Progreens, Savant Beyond Greens, and Dr Robert O. Young's own greens powder, Innerlight SuperGreens
Liquid chlorophyll: recommended products include NOW liquid chlorophyll, Jason Winter Liquid Chlorophyll, Nature's Plus Chlorophyll

Mineral test kit: For more information visit www.mineraltestkit.co.uk or www.bodybio.com

USA

Dr Robert O. Young's Innerlight SuperGreens
W: www.innerlightinc.com
T: 800-677-0997

South Africa

Natrodale High Potency Spirulina with Chlorella, from Vital
W: www.vital.co.za
T: 27 21 900 2600

Australia

Vital Greens from Vital Greens
W: www.vitalgreens.com
T: 02 9918 7077

New Zealand

Pure Green from Go Green
W: www.gogreen.net.nz
T: 64 6 7511163

Emotional freedom technique (EFT)

For information about how EFT works, visit the website of Gary Craig, www.emofree.com. For the EFT course on DVD go to www.emofree.com. EFT books: *Adventures in EFT* by Silvia Hartmann (available from www.dragonrising.com) and *The Healing Power of EFT and Energy Psychology* by David Feinstein, Donna Eden and Gary Craig, Piatkus Books, (2006). You can also download a free EFT protocol from www.mercola.com or www.emofree.com. See also Dr Patricia Carrington's website www.eftupdate.com
To find a qualified EFT therapist, please visit www.theamt.com.

Emotional trauma release (UK)

EmoTrance

For a qualified trainer, see website www.emotrance.com which has a list. *For details of practitioners and to purchase the CD* contact The Human Givens Institute on 01323 811662 or visit humangivens.com

Exercise (UK)

Personal trainer

Go to www.nrpt.co.uk to find a personal trainer near to you.

Hormonal imbalances (UK)

Adrenal stress index (ASI) saliva test: for more information about this test visit the website of Individual Wellbeing Diagnostic Laboratories www.iwdl.net or phone 020 8336 7750

Hormone saliva test: from Individual Wellbeing Diagnostic Laboratories on 020 8336 7750

Natural progesterone: for more information and ordering progesterone cream see www.npis.info or phone 07000 784849

Testosterone saliva test: contact Individual Wellbeing Diagnostic Laboratories on 020 8336 7750

Thyroid: you can arrange a total thyroid screen test by contacting the website of Individual Wellbeing Diagnostic Laboratories www.iwdl.net or phone 020 8336 7750

Australia

Nutritional Laboratory Services
W: www.nlabs.com.au
T: +613 9663 1554

New Zealand

Ideal Health
W: www.healthyonline.co.nz
T: +649 4432 584

USA

Test Medical Symptoms
W: www.testsymptomsathome.com
T: 888-595-3136

Saliva tests

If you contact Individual Wellbeing Diagnostic Laboratories on 020 8336 7750 they will send out the kit, you provide a saliva sample and return it to them.

Stress avoidance

Relaxation/mind training CDs: some recommended sites are www.selfhelpproducts.co.uk and www.mindbodyspiritdirect.co.uk

Australia

Jack Lim Productions
W: www.relaxationmusic.com.au
T: +61 3 9836 6961

USA

Serenity Music
W: www.serenitymusic.com
T: 1 800 869 1684

New Zealand

Bliss Music
W: www.bliss-music.com
T: 09-812 8329

South Africa

Mind Frame www.mindframe.co.za

Toxicity (UK)

Electromagnetic fields

To strengthen the body's own electromagnetic fields and help protect normal brain function in users of mobile phones: see Qlink www.qlinkworld.co.uk. Or www.q-linkproducts.com (USA)

For safe household cleaning products: www.ecover.com and www.spiritofnature.co.uk.

Mercury test: Kelmer test can be ordered from Biolab in London www.biolab.co.uk / telephone: 020 7636 5959

Negative air ioniser device: For more information see www.elanra.co.uk

Removal of heavy metals: to read more about NDF visit the website www.healthydetox.org. You can get NDF from Higher Nature (www.highernature.co.uk)

Reverse osmosis systems: contact Freshly Squeezed Water on 01276 600 870 or visit www.freshlysqueezedwater.com

Shower filter: to reduce chlorine contact Healthy House www.healthy-house.co.uk

Toxic shock from tampons: for more information see www.tamponalert.org.uk.

For personal care products: tampons Absolutely Pure (www.absolutelypure.com), Neways (www.neways.com) and Goodness Direct (www.goodnessdirect.co.uk). Natracare www.natracare.com produce a range of 100 per cent cotton tampons that do not produce the toxin associated with toxic shock

Water filters: wellness filter system (www.highernature.co.uk) or a reverse osmosis system (www.freshlysqueezedwater.com) will provide you with clean water, free from contaminants

For more information on electromagnetic fields, see also *The Powerwatch Handbook* by Alasdair and Jean Philips, Piatkus Books (2006)

Natural products (rest of the world)

USA

Yves Rocher
W: www.yvesrocherusa.com
T: 1-888-909-0771

Australia

Biome
W: www.biome.com.au
T: 1300 301767

New Zealand

Shop New Zealand
W: www.shopnewzealand.co.nz
T: 64-9-373-3733

South Africa

W: www.vital.co.za
T: 27 21 900 2600 or

Recommended reading

Part 2: The 14 barriers to total health

Barrier 1: Unhealthy diet

Elson Haas, *Staying Healthy with Nutrition*, Celestial Arts (rev. edn), 2006
Patrick Holford, *The Optimum Nutrition Bible*, Piatkus Books, 2004
Harold Kristal and James Haig, *The Nutrition Solution: A Guide To Your Metabolic Type*, North Atlantic Books, 2003
William Wolcott and Trish Fahey, *The Metabolic Typing Diet*, Broadway Books, 2002

Barrier 2: Body acidification

Christopher Vasey, *The Acid–Alkaline Diet for Optimum Health: Restore Your Balance by Creating pH Balance in Your Diet*, Healing Arts Press (rev. edn), 2006
Robert Young, *The pH Miracle: Balance Your Diet, Reclaim Your Health*, Time Warner Paperbacks, 2003

Barrier 3: Digestive health imbalance

Darina Allen, *Healthy Gluten-Free Eating: The Ultimate Wheat-free Recipe Book*, Kyle Cathie, 2004

Patrick Holford, *Improve Your Digestion*, Piatkus Books, 2000

Elizabeth Lipski, *Digestive Wellness*, McGraw-Hill Education (rev. edn), 2004

Rick Marx, Nancy T. Marr, *The Everything Gluten-free Cookbook: 300 Appetizing Recipes Tailored to Your Needs*, Adams Media Corporation, 2006

Barrier 4: Toxicity

Paula Baillie-Hamilton, *Stop the 21st Century Killing You: Toxic Chemicals Have Invaded Our Life. Fight Back! Eliminate Toxins, Tackle Illness, Get Healthy and Live Longer*, Vermilion, 2005

Doris Rapp, *Our Toxic World: A Wake-up Call*, Practical Allergy Research Foundation, 2003

Barrier 5: Chronic inflammation

Floyd Chilton, *Inflammation Nation: The First Clinically Proven Eating Plan to End the Secret Epidemic*, Simon & Schuster Ltd (repr.) 2006

Barry Sears, *The Anti-inflammation Zone: Reversing the Silent Epidemic That's Destroying Our Health*, HarperCollins (repr.) 2006

Barrier 6: Hormonal imbalances

Jesse Hanley, *Tired of Being Tired*, Penguin Books (new edn), 2004

Byron Katie, *Loving What Is*, Ryder & Co, 2002

Jacob Teitelbaum, *From Fatigued to Fantastic*, Avery Publishing Group (rev. edn), 2001

Sex hormonal imbalance:

Kate Neil, Patrick Holford, *Balancing Hormones Naturally*, Piatkus Books (new edn), 1998

Christiane Northrup, *Women's Bodies, Women's Wisdom: The Complete Guide to Women's Health and Well-being*, Piatkus Books; (rev. edn), 1998

Ann Rushton, Shirley Bond, *Natural Progesterone: The Natural Way to Alleviate Symptoms of Menopause, PMS, Endometriosis and Other Hormone-related Problems*, HarperCollins, 2003

Insulin imbalance (metabolic syndrome):

Antony Haynes, *The Insulin Factor*, HarperCollins, 2004

Karlene Karst, *The Metabolic Syndrome Program: How to Lose Weight, Beat Heart Disease, Stop Insulin Resistance and More*, John Wiley and Sons, 2006

Barrier 7: Candida and parasites

Leon Chaitow, *Candida Albicans: The Non-drug Approach to the Treatment of Candida Infection*, HarperCollins (new edn), 2003

Ann Louise Gittleman, *Guess What Came to Dinner?: Parasites and Your Health*, Avery Publishing Group (rev. edn), 2001

Candida cookbooks:

Pat Connolly, *The Candida Albicans Yeast-free Cookbook: How Good Nutrition Can Help Fight the Epidemic of Candida*, Keats Pub Inc (rev. edn), 2000

Erica White, *Beat Candida Cookbook: Over 250 Recipes with a 4-point Plan for Attacking Candidiasis*, HarperCollins (rev. edn), 1999

Barrier 8: Unmet emotional needs

Joe Griffin and Ivan Tyrrell, *Human Givens: A New Approach to Emotional Health and Clear Thinking*, Human Givens Publishing, 2004

Barrier 9: Psychological stress

David Allen, *Getting Things Done*, Piatkus Books, 2002

Robert L. Leahy, *The Worry Cure*, Piatkus Books, 2006

Barrier 10: Addictions

Joe Griffin and Ivan Tyrrell, *Freedom from Addiction: The Secret Behind Successful Addiction Busting*, Human Givens Publishing, 2005

Barrier 11: Disconnection

Harville Hendrix, *Getting the Love You Want*, Pocket Books (new edn), 2005

Pia Mellody, *Intimacy Factor: The Ground Rules for Overcoming the Obstacles to Truth, Respect, and Lasting Love*, HarperCollins (repr.), 2003

Barrier 12: Denial of reality

Patricia A. Farrell, *How to Be Your Own Therapist: A Step-by-step Guide to Building a Competent, Confident Life*, McGraw-Hill Contemporary (new edn), 2004

Barrier 13: Emotional mismanagement

Dr Darlene Mininni, *The Emotional Tool Kit*, Piatkus Books, 2006
Candace Pert, *Molecules of Emotion*, Pocket Books (new edn), 1999
Candace Pert, *Everything You Need to Know to Feel Go(o)d*, Hay House, Oct 2007

Barrier 14: Low self-esteem

Cheri Huber, *There is Nothing Wrong with You: Going Beyond Self-Hate, A Compassionate Process for Learning to Accept Yourself Exactly as You Are*, Keep it Simple Books, 2001
Byron Katie, *Loving What Is*, Ryder & Co, 2002
Dr Maxwell Maltz, *Psycho-Cybernetics*, Simon and Schuster, 1994
Hal and Sidra Stone, *Embracing Your Inner Critic*, Harper San Francisco, 1993

Part 3: The mind–body toolbox

Chapter 1 Appreciation

Noelle Nelson, *The Power of Appreciation in Everyday Life*, Insomniac Press, 2006

Chapter 2 Bach Flower Remedies

Mechthild Scheffer, *Bach Flower Therapy: the Complete Approach*, HarperCollins, 1998
Edward Bach, *Heal Thyself*, C. W. Daniel Co. Ltd (new edn), 1996

Chapter 3 Conscious breathing

Donna Farhi, *The Breathing Book: Vitality and Good Health Through Essential Breath Work*, Holt (Henry) & Co., 1996
Gay Hendricks, *Conscious Breathing*, Bantam Doubleday Dell Publishing Group, 1995

Chapter 4 Creative visualisation

Shakti Gawain, *Creative Visualization*, New World Library (new edn), 2002

Ronald Shone, *Creative Visualization*, Inner Traditions Bear and Company, 1998

Chapter 5 Emotional freedom technique

David Feinstein, Donna Eden and Gary Craig, *The Healing Power of EFT and Energy Psychology: Revolutionary Methods for Dramatic Personal Change*, Piatkus Books, 2006

Silvia Hartmann, *Adventures in EFT: The Essential Field Guide to Emotional Freedom Techniques*, Dragon Rising (rev. edn), 2000

Chapter 6 Emotional trauma release

Joe Griffin and Ivan Tyrrell, *Human Givens: A New Approach to Emotional Health and Clear Thinking*, Human Givens Publishing, 2004

Silvia Hartmann, *Oceans of Energy*, Dragon Rising, 2003

Chapter 7 Exercise

Paul Chek, *How to Eat, Move and Be Healthy*, C.H.E.K Institute, 2004

Bob Greene, *Bob Greene's Total Body Makeover*, Simon & Schuster Australia, 2005

Chapter 8 Focusing

Ann Weiser Cornell, *The Power of Focusing*, New Harbinger Publications, 1996

Eugene Gendlin, *Focusing: How to Open Up Your Deeper Feelings & Intuition*, Rider & Co., 2003

Chapter 9 Goal setting

Napoleon Hill, *Think and Grow Rich*, Vermilion (rev. edn), 2004

Maxwell Maltz, *The New Psycho-cybernetics*, Souvenir Press Ltd (rev. edn), 2002

Chapter 10 Instant stress release

Dale Carnegie, *How to Stop Worrying and Start Living*, Vermilion (new edn), 2007

Don, Colbert, M.D., *Stress Less*, Siloam Press, 2005

Chapter 11 Journaling

Louise DeSalvo, *Writing as a Way of Healing: How Telling Stories Transforms Our Lives*, Beacon Press, 2000

Chapter 12 Meditation

Madonna Gauding, *The Meditation Bible: A Definitive Guide to Meditations for Every Purpose*, Godsfield Press Ltd, 2005

Maharishi Mahesh Yogi, *Science of Being and Art of Living: Transcendental Meditation*, Plume Books, 2001

Chapter 13 Relaxation

Sarah Brewer, *Simply Relax: The Beginner's Guide to Relaxation*, Duncan Baird Publishers, 2000

Mike George, *1001 Ways to Relax: How to Beat Stress and Find Perfect Calm*, Duncan Baird Publishers, 2003

Chapter 14 Sleep

Deepak Chopra, *Restful Sleep: Complete Mind–body Programme for Overcoming Insomnia*, Rider & Co. (new edn), 2000

Paul Glovinsky, *The Insomnia Answer: A Personalized Drug-free Program for Identifying and Overcoming the Three Types of Insomnia*, Perigee Books, 2006

Chapter 15 Symptom dialogue

Arnold Mindell, *The Quantum Mind and Healing: How to Listen and Respond to Your Body's Symptoms*, Hampton Roads Publishing Co., 2004

Chapter 16 Tame the inner critic

Richard David Carson, *Taming Your Gremlin*, HarperCollins Publishers, 2003

Hal and Sidra Stone, *Embracing Your Inner Critic*, HarperSanFrancisco, 1993

References

Introduction

1. Mental Health Foundation, *Mental illness: The Fundamental Facts*, 1993.
2. Department of Health Policy and Guidance on Coronary Heart Disease, www.dh.gov.uk
3. National Audit Office, *Tackling Obesity in England*, The Stationery Office, 2001.
4. Eaton, S.B., Konner, M., Shostak, M., 'Stone agers in the fast lane: chronic degenerative diseases in evolutionary perspective', *American Journal of Medicine*, 84 (1988), pp. 739–49.

Part 1

Chapter 1: Taking charge of your health

1. Murray, W.H., *The Story of Everest*, Dent, 1953.

Chapter 2: What are your barriers to total health?

1. Pert, C., *Molecules of Emotion*, Pocket Books, 1999.
2. Sarno, J., *The MindBody Prescription*, Warner Books, 1998.
3. King, D., 'Can allergic exposure provoke psychological symptoms? A double-blind test', *Biolological Psychiatry*, Vol. 16(1) (1981), pp. 3–19.
4. O'Reilly, et al., 'Childhood Schizophrenia', *Psychiatric Quarterly*, Vol. 27 (1953), pp. 3–81.

Part 2

Barrier 1: Unhealthy diet

1. Allergy UK. www.allergyuk.org

2. Benton, B., 'The impact of the supply of glucose to the brain on mood and memory', *Nutrition Reviews*, Vol. 59(1 Pt 2) (2001), pp. S20–1.

3. Smith, K., et al., 'Relapse of depression after rapid depletion of tryptophan', *Lancet*, Vol. 349 (1997), pp. 915–19.

4. Rudin, D., 'The major psychoses and neuroses as omega-3 essential fatty acid deficiency syndrome: substrate pellagra', *Biological Psychiatry*, Vol. 16(9) (1981), pp. 837–50.

5. Benton, D., Roberts, G., 'Effect of vitamin and mineral supplementation on cognitive functioning', *Psychopharmacology* (Berl), Vol. 117(3) (1995), pp. 298–305.

6. Canty, D., Zeisel, S., 'Lecithin and choline in human health and disease', *Nutrition Reviews*, Vol. 52(10) (1994), pp. 327–39.

7. Philpott, W., Kalita, D., *Brain Allergies*, Keats Publishing, 1980.

8. Healthxxcel. www.healthexcel.com

9. Oomen, C., et al., 'Association between trans fatty acid intake and 10-year risk of coronary heart disease in the Zutphen Elderly Study: a prospective population-based study', *Lancet*, Vol. 357 (9258), pp. 746–51.

10. Watkins, B. A., and Seifert, M. F., 'Food Lipids and Bone Health', in R. E. McDonald and D. B. Min (eds), *Food Lipids and Health*, Marcel Dekker, Inc. (1996), p. 101.

11. Meyer, K., et al., 'Carbohydrates, dietary fibre, and incident type 2 diabetes in older women', *American Journal of Clinical Nutrition*, Vol. 71(4) (April 2000), pp. 921–30.

12. Larsson, S., et al., 'Consumption of sugar and sugar-sweetened foods and the risk of pancreatic cancer in a prospective study', *American Journal of Clinical Nutrition*, Vol. 84(5) (November 2006), pp. 1171–6.

13. Walton, et al., 'Adverse reactions to aspartame: double blind challenge in patients from a vulnerable population', *Journal of Biological Psychiatry*, Vol. 34(1–2), (1993), pp. 13–17.

14. Joosens, J. V., Hill, M. J., Elliot, P. et al., 'Dietary salt, nitrate and stomach cancer mortality in 24 countries', European Cancer Prevention (ECP) and the INTERSALT Cooperative Research Group, *International Journal of Epidemiology*, Vol. 3 (1996), pp. 494–504.

15. US Environmental Protection Agency. www.epa.gov/mercury/advisories

16. Worthington, V., 'Effect of agricultural methods on nutritional quality: a comparison of organic with conventional crops', *Alternative Therapies*, Vol. 4(1) pp. 58–69.

17. Barclay, G.R., 'Effect of psychosocial stress on salt and water transport in the human jejunum', *Gastroenterology*, Vol. 93 (1987) pp. 91–7.

18. Giduck, S.A., 'Cephalic reflexes: their role in digestion and possible roles in absorption and metabolism', *Journal of Nutrition*, 117(7) (July 1987).

19. Food Standards Agency, 'National Diet & Nutrition Survey: Adults aged 19 to 64', Vol. 5 (2004).

20. ibid.

21. Elia, M., 'The Malnutrition Advisory Group consensus guidelines for the detection and management of malnutrition in the community', *Nutrition Bulletin* Vol. 26(1) (2001), pp. 81–3.

22. 'Meat and dairy, where have the minerals gone?', *Food Magazine*, 72 (Jan/March 2006), p. 10.

23. Benefits of Supplements. Council for Responsible Nutrition. www.crnusa.org

24. Holmquist, C., et al., 'Multivitamin supplements are inversely associated with risk of myocardial infarction in men and women: Stockholm Heart Epidemiology Program (SHEEP)', The American Society for Nutritional Sciences, *Journal of Nutrition*, 133 (August 2003), pp. 2650–54.
25. Munger, K.L., et al., 'Vitamin D intake and incidence of multiple sclerosis', *Neurology*, 62 (13 January 2004), pp. 60–65.
26. Mills, J., 'Food fortification to prevent neural tube defects: is it working?', *Journal of the American Medical Association*, 285 (2001), pp. 3022–3.
27. Julie, A., et al., 'Vitamin supplement use and incident cataracts in a population-based study', *Archives of Ophthalmology*, 118 (2000), pp. 1556–63.
28. Jacobs, E., et al., 'Multivitamin Use and Colorectal Cancer Incidence in a US Cohort. Does Timing Matter?', *American Journal of Epidemiology*, 158 (2003), pp. 621–8.
29. The Mental Health Foundation, The Feeding Minds Report (p. 10), www.mentalhealth.org.uk
30. Garg, H. K., Singal, K. C., Arshad, Z., 'Zinc taste test in pregnant women and its correlation with serum zinc level', *Indian Journal of Physiology and Pharmacology*, Vol. 37(4) (1993), pp. 318–22.

Barrier 2: Body acidification

1. Young, R., *The pH Miracle: Balance Your Diet, Reclaim Your Health*, Time Warner Books, 2003.
2. Sahlin, K., Alvestrand, A., Bergstrom, J., Hultman, E., 'Human intracellular pH and bicarbonate concentration as determined in biopsy samples from the quadriceps muscle of man at rest', *Clinical Science and Molecular Medicine*, 53 (1977), pp. 459–66.
3. Kurtz, I., Maher, T., Hulter, H.N., Schambelan, M., Sebastian, A., 'Effect of diet on plasma acid-base composition in normal humans', *Kidney International*, 24 (1983), pp. 670–80.
4. Frassetto, L., Todd, K., Morris, R., Sebastian, A., 'Estimation of net endogenous non-carbonic acid production in humans from diet potassium and protein contents', *American Journal of Clinical Nutrition*, 68 (1998), pp. 576–83.
5. Frassetto, L., Sebastian, A.. 'Age and systemic acid-base equilibrium: analysis of published data', *Journals of Gerontolology* (1996), 51A:B pp. 91–9.
6. Crooks, W., *The Yeast Connection: A Medical Breakthrough*, Random House, 1986.
7. Maughan, R.J., and Greenhaff, P.L., 'High intensity exercise performance and acid-base balance: the influence of diet and induced metabolic alkalosis', in F. Brouns (ed.), *Advances in Nutrition and Top Sport*, Karger, 1991, pp. 147–65.
8. Bobkov, V.A., 'Acid-base balance parameters of the synovial fluid in patients with early-stage rheumatoid arthritis', *Terapevticheski Arkhiv*, 72 (12) (2000), pp. 35–8.
9. Philpott, W., *Magnet Therapy: Alternative Medicine Definitive Guide*, Future Medicine Publishing, 2000.
10. Santiago, E., Lopez-Moratalla, N., Lopez-Zabaza, M.J., Iriate, A.J., Campo, M.L., 'Effect of pH on the sensitivity of mitochondrial ATPase to free ATP, ADP and anions', *Revista española de fisiología*, Vol. 36(4) (December 1980), pp. 413–20.
11. Choi, H., Atkinson, K., Karlson, E., Willett, W., Curhan, G., 'Purine-rich foods, dairy and protein intake, and the risk of gout in men', *New England Journal of Medicine*, Vol. 350(11) (2004), pp. 1093–103.

12. Tucker, K.L., Morita, K., Qiao, N., Hannan, M.T., Cupples, A., Kiel, D.P., 'Colas, but not other carbonated beverages, are associated with low bone mineral density in older women: The Framingham Osteoporosis Study', *American Journal of Clinical Nutrition*, Vol. 84(4) (October 2006).

13. Young R., *The pH Miracle: Balance Your Diet, Reclaim Your Health*, Time Warner Books, 2003.

14. Remer, T., and Manz, F., 'Potential renal acid load of foods and its influence on urine pH', *Journal of the American Dietetic Association*, 95 (1995), pp.791–797

15. Frassetto, L., Morris, R.C. Jr, Sebastian, A., 'Potassium bicarbonate reduces urinary nitrogen excretion in postmenopausal women', *Journal of Clinical Endocrinology & Metabolism*, 82 (1997), pp. 254–9. Frassetto, L., Morris, R.C. Jr, Sebastian, A., 'Potassium bicarbonate increases serum growth hormone concentrations in postmenopausal women', *Journal of the American Society of Nephrology*, 10 (1996), p. 1349 (abstr.).

Barrier 3: Digestive health imbalance

1. Holford, P., *Improve Your Digestion*, Piatkus, 2000. Lipski, E., *Digestive Wellness*, McGraw-Hill Education, 2004.

2. ibid.

3. ibid.

4. ibid.

5. Gershon, M., *The Second Brain*, HarperCollins, 1998.

6. Esplugues, J., Barrachina, M., Beltrán, B., Calatayud, S., Whittle, B., Moncada, S., 'Inhibition of gastric acid secretion by stress: a protective reflex mediated by cerebral nitric oxide', *Proceedings of The National Academy of Sciences*, USA. Vol. 93 (December 1996), pp. 14839–44.

7. Goodwin, R. D., and Stein, M.B., 'Generalized Anxiety Disorder and Peptic Ulcer Disease Among Adults in the United States', *Psychosomatic Medicine*, 64 (2002), pp. 862–6.

8. Mayer, E.A., Naliboff, B.D., and Chang, L., 'Basic pathophysiologic mechanisms in irritable bowel syndrome', *Digestive Disorders*, 19 (2001), pp. 212–18.

9. Salt, W., Neimark, N., *Irritable Bowel Syndrome and the Mind–Body–Spirit Connection: Seven Steps for Living a Healthy Life with a Functional Bowel Disorder, Crohn's Disease*, ebrandedbooks.com, 2002.

10. Holford, *Improve Your Digestion*, and Lipski, *Digestive Wellness*.

11. ibid.

12. ibid.

13. ibid.

14. *US News and World Report*, Vol. 106, 1989, p. 777.

Barrier 4: Toxicity

1. (EEA) European Environmental Agency and (UNEP) United Nations Environment Programme, 1998 'Chemicals in Europe: low doses, high stakes?' Annual message 2 on the state of Europe's environment.

2. Baillie-Hamilton, P., *Stop the 21st Century Killing You*, Vermilion, 2005.

3. ibid.

4. World Resources Institute, www.wri.org

5. 'Our planet, our health: report of the WHO commission on health and environment', World Health Organization, Geneva, 1992.
6. 'Mothers' milk: Record levels of toxic fire retardants found in American mothers' breast milk', EWG (Environmental Working Group), Washington, DC, 2003. Available online at http://www.ewg.org/reports/mothersmilk/
7. 'Body burden: the pollution in people', EWG (Environmental Working Group), Washington, DC, 2003. Available online at http://www.ewg.org/reports/bodyburden/
8. Talska, G., et al., 'Genetically based n-acetyltransferase metabolic polymorphism and low-level environmental exposure to carcinogens', *Nature*, 369 (1994), pp. 154–6.
9. Pizzorno, J., *Total Wellness*, Prima Health, 1998
10. Weinhold, B., 'Epigenetics', *Environmental Health Perspectives*, Vol. 14 (March 2006).
11. Anway, M.D., Cupp, A.S., Uzumcu, M., Skinner, M.K., 'Epigenetic transgenerational actions of endocrine disruptors and male fertility', *Science*, Vol. 308 (5727) (3 June 2005), pp. 1466–9.
12. Campbell, M., et al., 'Biotransformation of caffeine, paraxanthine, theophylline, and theobromine by polycyclic aromatic hydrocarbon-inducable cytochrome P-450 in human liver microsomes', *Drug Metabolism and Disposition*, 15 (1987), pp. 237–49.
13. Environmental Protection Agency, www.epa.gov/airnow.
14. Kaiser, J., 'Air pollution: evidence mounts that tiny particles can kill', *Science*, Vol. 289(54767) (7 July 2000), pp. 22–3.
15. Pope, A., et al., 'Cardiovascular Mortality and Long-Term Exposure to Particulate Air Pollution', *Circulation*, 109 (2004), pp. 71–7.
16. Coghill, R., *Electropollution: How to Protect Yourself Against It*, HarperCollins, 1990.
17. Cragle, D. L., Shy, C. M., Struba, R. J., Siff, E. J., 'A case-control study of colon cancer and water chlorination in North Carolina', in Jolley, R. L., Bull, R. J. and Davis, W. P. (eds), *Water Chlorination: Chemistry, Environmental Impact and Health Effects*, Lewis Publishers, 1985, pp. 153–9. Cantor, K. P., Lynch, C. F., Hildesheim, M., Dosemeci, M., Lubin, J., Alavanja, M., and Craun, G. F., 'Drinking water source and chlorination by-products: I. In risk of bladder cancer', *Epidemiology*, 9 (1998), pp. 21–8.
18. Groves, B., *The Fluoride Deception*, Seven Stories Press, US, 2006.
19. Rapp, D., *Our Toxic World: A Wake-up Call*, Practical Allergy Research Foundation, 2003.
20. Robbins, R., et al., 'Production of toxic shock syndrome toxin 1 by Staphylococcus aureus as determined by tampon disk-membrane-agar method', *Journal of Clinical Microbiology*, Vol. 25(8) (August 1987), pp. 1446–9.
21. Huggins, H., *Uninformed Consent: Hidden Dangers in Dental Care*, Hampton Roads Publishing Co., 1999.
22. Wenstrup, D., Ehmann, W., Markesbery, W., 'Trace element imbalances in isolated subcellular fractions of Alzheimer's disease brains', *Brain Research*, 533 (1990), pp. 125–30.
23. Lorscheider, F., Vimy, M., 'Evaluation of the safety issue of mercury release from dental fillings', *FASEB Journal*, Vol. 7 (December 1993), pp. 1432–3.
24. Food Standards Agency, www.food.gov.uk. 'Fact sheet on Pregnancy'.
25. Agency for Toxic Substances and Disease Registry, www.atsdr.cdc.gov. 'Fact sheet on Cadmium'.

26. Agency for Toxic Substances and Disease Registry, www.atsdr.cdc.gov. 'Fact sheet on Lead'.
27. Thurnell-Read, J., *Geopathic Stress & Subtle Energy*, Life-Work Potential, 2006.

Barrier 5: Chronic inflammation

1. Challem, J., *The Inflammation Syndrome: The Complete Nutritional Program to Prevent and Reverse Heart Disease, Arthritis, Diabetes, Allergies and Asthma*, John Wiley & Sons Inc., 2004.
2. Ridker, P.M., Cushman, M., Stampfer, M.J., Tracy, R..P, Hennekens, C.H., 'Inflammation, aspirin, and the risk of cardiovascular disease in apparently healthy men', *New England Journal of Medicine*, 336 (1997), pp. 973–9.
3. Shacter, E., 'Chronic Inflammation and Cancer', *Oncology*, 16 (2002), pp. 217–32.
4. Akiyama, H., et al., 'Inflammation and Alzheimer's disease', *Neurobiology of Aging*, 21 (2000), pp. 383–421.
5. Ridker, P.M., Cushman, M., Stampfer, M.J., Tracy, R.P., Hennekens, C.H., 'Plasma concentration of C-reactive protein and risk of developing peripheral vascular disease', *Circulation*, 97 (1998) pp. 425–8.
6. Koenig, W., Sund, M., Frohlich, M., Fischer, H.G., Lowel, H., Doring, A., et al., 'C-reactive protein, a sensitive marker of inflammation, predicts future risk of coronary heart disease in initially healthy middle-aged men. Results from the MONICA (Monitoring Trends and Determinants in Cardiovascular Disease) Augsburg Cohort Study, 1984 to 1992', *Circulation* 99 (1999), pp. 237–42.
7. Ridker, P.M., Hennekens, C.H., Buring, J.E., et al., 'C-reactive protein and other markers of inflammation in the prediction of cardiovascular disease in women', *New England Journal of Medicine*, 342 (2000), pp. 836–43.
8. Wang, S., Zheng Wei, 'Antioxidant activity and phenolic compounds in selected herbs', *Journal of Agricultural and Food Chemistry*, Vol. 49 (11) (2001), pp. 5165–70.

Barrier 6: Hormonal imbalances

1. Koukkari, W.L., Sothern, R.B., *Introducing Biological Rhythms*, Springer, 2006.
2. Neil, K., Holford, P., *Balancing Hormones Naturally*, Piatkus, 1998.
3. Cherniske, S., *The DHEA Breakthrough*, Ballantine Books, 1998.
4. Hollowell, J.G., Staehling, N.W., Flanders, W.D., et al., 'Serum thyrotropin, thyroxine and thyroid antibodies in the United States population (1988 to 1994): National Health and Nutrition Examination Survey (NHANES III)', *Journal of Clinical Endocrinology and Metabolism*, Vol. 87(2) (Feb 2002), pp. 489–99.
5. Blanchard, K., *What Your Doctor May Not Tell You About Hypothyroidism*, Little, Brown & Company, 2004.
6. Broda Barnes Research Foundation, www.brodabarnes.org
7. Degen, G.H., Bolt, H.M., 'Endocrine disruptors: update on xenoestrogens', *International Archives of Occupational and Environmental Health*, 73 (2000), pp. 433–41.
8. Lee, J., *Dr John Lee's Hormone Balance Made Simple: The Essential How-to Guide to Symptoms, Dosage, Timing, and More*, Little, Brown & Company, 2006.
9. Stein, D.G., 'The case for progesterone', *Annals of the New York Academy of Sciences*, 1052 (June 2005), pp. 152–69.

10. Bone, K., 'Vitex agnus-castus: scientific studies and clinical applications', *European Journal of Herbal Medicine*, 1 (1994), pp. 12–15.

11. Gruenwald, J., 'Standardised black cohosh (Cimicifuga) extract clinical monograph', *Quarterly Review of Natural Medicine*, (Summer 1998), pp. 117–25.

12. Hirata, J.D., Swiersz, L.M., Zell, B., et al., 'Does dong quai have estrogenic effects in postmenopausal women? A double-blind, placebo-controlled trial', *Fertility & Sterility*, 68 (1997), pp. 981–6.

13. Shippen, E., *The Testosterone Syndrome: The Critical Factor for Energy, Health and Sexuality: Reversing the Male Menopause*, M. Evans & Co. Inc., 2001.

14. Muti, P., Westerlind, K., Wu, T., et al., 'Urinary estrogen metabolites and prostate cancer: a case-control study in the United States', *Cancer Causes and Control*, Vol. 13(10) (December 2002), pp. 947–55.

15. Hryb, D.J., Khan, M.S., Romas, N.A., Rosner, W., 'The effect of extracts of the roots of the stinging nettle (Urtica dioica) on the interaction of SHBG with its receptor on human prostatic membranes', *Planta Medica*, Vol. 61(1) (Feb 1995), pp. 31–2.

16. Netter, A., Hartoma, R., Nahoul, K., 'Effect of zinc administration on plasma testosterone, dihydrotestosterone and sperm count', *Archives of Andrology*, Vol. 7(1) (August 1981), pp. 69–73.

17. Wilt, T.J., Ishani, A., Stark, G., et al., 'Saw palmetto extracts for treatment of benign prostatic hyperplasia', *JAMA*, 280 (1998), pp. 160–9.

18. British Nutrition Foundation, BNF in Europe, 'Ob-Age, Report 2: The metabolic syndrome', available at http://www.nutrition.org.uk. Eckel, R.H., Grundy, S.M., Zimmet, P.Z., 'The metabolic syndrome', *Lancet*, Vol. 16, 365(9468) (April 2005), pp. 1415–28. Lakka, H.M., Laaksonen, D.E., Lakka, T.A., et al., 'The metabolic syndrome and total and cardiovascular disease mortality in middle-aged men', *JAMA*, Vol. 288(21) (4 December 2002), pp. 2709–16.

19. Galland, L., *The Fat Resistance Diet*, Broadway Books, 2005.

20. Savage, D.B., Petersen, K.F., Shulman, G.I., 'Mechanisms of insulin resistance in humans and possible links with inflammation', *Hypertension*, Vol. 45(5) (May 2005), pp. 828–33.

21. 'Third Report of the National Cholesterol Education Program (NCEP) Expert Panel on Detection, Evaluation, and Treatment of High Blood Cholesterol in Adults (Adult Treatment Panel III) final report', *Circulation*, Vol. 106(25) (17 December 2002), pp. 3143–421.

22. Anderson, R.A., Cheng, N., Bryden, N.A., et al., 'Elevated intakes of supplemental chromium improve glucose and insulin variables in individuals with type 2 diabetes', *Diabetes* Vol. 46(11), (November 1997), pp. 1786–91. Bahijri, S.M., Mufti, A.M., 'Beneficial effects of chromium in people with type 2 diabetes, and urinary chromium response to glucose load as a possible indicator of status', *Biological Trace Element Research*, Vol. 85(2) (February 2002), pp. 97–109.

23. Ebbesson, S.O., Risica, P.M., et al., 'Omega-3 fatty acids improve glucose tolerance and components of the metabolic syndrome in Alaskan Eskimos: the Alaska Siberia project', *The International Journal of Circumpolar Health*, Vol. 64(4) (September 2005), pp. 396–408.

24. Liu, J., et al., 'Memory loss in old rats is associated with brain mitochondrial decay and RNA/DNA oxidation: partial reversal by feeding aceyl-l-carnitine and/or R-alpha-lipoic acid', *Proceedings of the National Academy of Sciences*, Vol. 99(4) (19 February 2002), pp. 2356–61.

25. Hodgson, J.M., Watts, G.F., et al., 'Coenzyme Q10 improves blood pressure and glycaemic control: a controlled trial in subjects with type 2 diabetes', *European Journal of Clinical Nutrition*, Vol. 56(11) (November 2002), pp. 1137–42.
26. Neu, J., et al., 'Glutamine: clinical applications and mechanisms of action', *Current Opinion in Clinical Nutrition and Metabolic Care*, Vol. 5(1) (January 2002), pp. 69–75.

Barrier 7: Candida and parasites

1. Crooks, W., *The Yeast Connection: A Medical Breakthrough*, Random House, 1986.
2. Chaitrow, L., *Candida Albicans: The Non-drug Approach to the Treatment of Candida Infection*, HarperCollins, 2003.
3. Gittleman, A., *Guess What Came to Dinner?: Parasites and Your Health*, Avery Publishing Group, 1994.
4. Lee, M. J., Johanson, J. F., Baskin, W. N., Barrie, S. 'Trends in intestinal parasitology part II: commonly reported parasites and therapeutics', *Practical Gastroenterology*, Vol. 16 (1992), pp. 38–46.

Barrier 8: Unmet emotional needs

1. Griffin, J., Tyrrell, I., *Human Givens: A New Approach to Emotional Health and Clear Thinking*, HG Publishing, 2004.

Barrier 9: Psychological stress

1. Health & Safety Executive, www.hse.gov.uk/stress
2. Cooper, C., Palmer, S., *Conquer Your Stress*, Chartered Institute of Personnel & Development, 2000.
3. Sapolsky, R., *Why Zebras Don't Get Ulcers*, Saint Martin's Press, 2004. Selye, H., *The Stress of Life*, McGraw-Hill Publishing Co., 1978.
4. Merali, Z., 'Why childhood trauma brings ill health later on', *New Scientist*, 2587 (2007), p. 8.

Barrier 10: Addictions

1. Noble, E., 'The gene that rewards alcoholism', *Scientific American, Science and Medicine* (March/April 1996), pp. 52–61.
2. Werbach, M., *Nutritional Influences on Mental Illness: A Sourcebook of Clinical Research*, Third Line Press, 1999.
3. DiClemente, C., *Addiction and Change: How Addictions Develop and Addicted People Recover*, Guilford Press, 2003.
4. Guenther, R., 'Role of nutritional therapy in alcoholism treatment', *International Journal of Biosocial Research*, Vol. 4(1), 1983, pp. 5–18.

Barrier 11: Disconnection

1. Waite, L. J., 'Does Marriage Matter?', Presidential Address to the American Population Association of America, 8 April 1995; Waite, L. J., 'Does Marriage Matter?', *Demography*, 32 (1995), pp. 483–507.

2. Morowitz, H., 'Hiding in the Hammond Report', *Hospital Practice* (August 1975), p. 39.
3. Caspi, A., Harrington, H., Moffitt, T., Milne, B., Poulton, R., 'Socially isolated children 20 years later: risk of cardiovascular disease', *Archives of Pediatrics & Adolescent Medicine*, 160 (2006), pp. 805–11.
4. Berkman, L., Leo-Summers, L., Horwitz, R., 'Emotional support and survival after myocardial infarction: a prospective, population-based study of the elderly', *Annals of Internal Medicine*, 117 (1992), pp. 1003–9.
5. Albrecht, K., *Social Intelligence: The New Science of Success*, Jossey-Bass, 2006.

Barrier 13: Emotional mismanagement

1. Mininni, D., *The Emotional Toolkit*, Piatkus, 2006.
2. Chess, S., *Temperament: Theory and Practice*, Brunner-Mazel, 1996.
3. Pert, C., *Molecules of Emotion*, Pocket Books, 1999.

Part 3

Chapter 1: Appreciation

1. Institute of HeartMath, www.heartmath.com
2. Childre, Doc, *The Heartmath Solution*, HarperSanFrancisco, 2000.

Chapter 2: Bach Flower Remedies

1. Bach, E., *The Essential Writings of Dr Edward Bach*, Vermilion, 2005.
2. Howard, J., *The Bach Flower Remedies Step by Step: A Complete Guide to Selecting and Using the Remedies*, Vermilion, 2005. Ball, S., *The Bach Remedies Workbook*, Vermilion, 2005.

Chapter 3: Conscious breathing

1. Hendricks, G., *Conscious Breathing*, Bantam Doubleday Dell Publishing Group, 1995. Farhi, D., *The Breathing Book: Vitality and Good Health Through Essential Breath Work*, Holt (Henry) & Co., 1996.

Chapter 4: Creative visualisation

1. Shone, R., *Creative Visualisation*, Inner Traditions, Bear and Company, 1998. Gawain, S., *Creative Visualization*, New World Library 2002.
2. Hartmann, S., Project Sanctuary III, www.sidereus.org

Chapter 5: Emotional freedom technique

1. Mercola, J., www.mercola.com
2. Craig, G., www.emofree.com

Chapter 6: Emotional trauma release

1. Hartmann, S., *Oceans of Energy*, Dragon Rising, 2003.
2. Griffin, J., Tyrrell, I., *Human Givens: A New Approach to Emotional Health and Clear Thinking*, HG Publishing, 2004.

Chapter 7: Exercise

1. British Heart Foundation Statistics, 2006, www.bhf.org.uk
2. Owen, N., Bauman, A., 'The descriptive epidemiology of a sedentary lifestyle in adult Australians', *International Journal of Epidemiology*, Vol. 21(2) (April 1992), pp. 305–10.
3. Crespo, C.J., et al., 'The relationship of physical activity and body weight with all-cause mortality: results from The Puerto Rico Heart Health Program', *Annals of Epidemiology*, Vol. 12(8) (November 2002), pp. 543–52 (10).
4. 'Medical aspects of exercise: benefits and risks', Summary of a Report of the Royal College of Physicians, *Journal of the College of Physicians*, London, Vol. 25(3) (1991 July), pp. 193–6.
5. Department of Health Exercise Recommendations, www.dh.gov.uk
6. 'A randomised trial of pre-exercise stretching for prevention of lower-limb injury', *Medicine and Science in Sports and Exercise*, Vol. 32(2), pp. 271–7, 2000.

Chapter 8: Focusing

1. Cornell, A., *The Power of Focusing: Finding Your Inner Voice*, New Harbinger Publications, 1996.
2. The Focusing Institute, www.focusing.org

Chapter 9: Goal Setting

1. King, L., 'The health benefits of writing about life goals', *Personality and Social Psychology Bulletin*, Vol. 27(7) (2001), pp. 798–807.

Chapter 12: Meditation

1. Maharishi Vedic Education Development Corporation, www.tm.org
2. ibid.
3. ibid.
4. Kabat-Zinn, J., 'Mindfulness meditation: what it is, what it isn't, and its role in health care and medicine', in Haruki, Y., Suzuki, M. (eds), *Comparative and Psychological Study on Meditation*, Eburon, 1996. Kabat-Zinn, J., *Wherever You Go, There You Are: Mindfulness Meditation in Everyday Life*, Hyperion Books, 2005.

Chapter 13: Relaxation

1. Benson, H., *The Relaxation Response*, Avon Books, 2000.

Chapter 14: Sleep

1. Institute of Medicine, www.ion.edu/sleep
2. Lauderdale et al., 'Respond to "How Much Do We Really Sleep?"', *American Journal of Epidemiology*, Vol. 164(1) (1 July 2006), pp. 19–20.
3. Taheri, S., Lin, L., Mignot, E., Austin, D., Young, T., 'Short sleep duration is associated with reduced leptin, elevated ghrelin, and increased Body Mass Index', Public Library of Science (PLoS), 7 December 2004, DOI: 10.1371/journal.pmed.0010062.
4. Taffinder, N. J., et al., 'Effect of sleep deprivation on surgeons' dexterity on laparoscopy simulator', *Lancet*, 352 (1998), p. 1191.
5. Vgontzas, A.N., Papanicolaou, D.A., Bixler, E.O., et al., 'Circadian interleukin-6 secretion and quantity and depth of sleep', *Journal of Clinical Endocrinology & Metabolism*, Vol. 84(8) (1999), pp. 2603–07.
6. Think, www.thinkroadsafety.gov.uk
7. The National Highway Traffic Safety Administration, www.nhtsa.dot.gov

Chapter 16: Tame the inner critic

1. Stone, H., *Embracing Our Selves: Voice Dialogue Manual*, Nataraj Publishing, 1989.
2. Stone, H., Stone, S., *Embracing Your Inner Critic: Turning Self-Criticism into a Creative Asset*, HarperSanFrancisco, 1993.

Appendix I: The mind–body connection

1. Cannon, W.B., *The Wisdom of the Body*, Norton, 1932.
2. Selye, H., *The Stress of Life*, McGraw-Hill, 1956.
3. Benson, H., *The Relaxation Response*, Morrow, 1976.
4. Pert, C., *Molecules of Emotion*, Pocket Books, 1999.
5. Ekman, P., *Emotions Revealed: Understanding Faces and Feelings*, Phoenix Press, 2004.
6. Berkman, L., Leo-Summers, L., and Horowitz, R.,. 'Emotional support and survival after myocardial infarction: a prospective, population-based study of the elderly', *Annals of Internal Medicine*, 117 (1992), pp. 1003–9.
7. Kubzansky, L.D., Kawachi, I., Spiro, A., Weiss, S.T., Vokonas, P.S., Sparrow, D., 'Is worrying bad for your heart? A prospective study of worry and coronary heart disease in the Normative Aging Study', *Circulation*, Vol. 95(4) (18 February 1997), pp. 818–24.
8. Chang, P., Ford, D., Meoni, L., Wang, N., Klag, M., 'Anger in young men and subsequent premature cardiovascular disease', *Archives of Internal Medicine*, 162 (2002), pp. 901–06.
9. Hippisley-Cox, J., Fielding, K., Pringle, M., 'Depression as a risk factor for ischaemic heart disease in men: population based case-control study', *British Medical Journal*, 316 (1998), pp. 1714–19.
10. Levy, B., Slade, M., Kunkel, S., Stanislav, K., 'Longevity increased by positive self-perceptions of aging', *Journal of Personality and Social Psychology*, Vol. 83(2) (August 2002), pp. 261–70.
11. Goodale, I., Domar, A., and Benson, H., 'Alleviation of premenstrual syndrome symptoms with the relaxation response', *Obstetrics and Gynecology*, Vol. 75(4) (1990), pp. 649–55.

12. Kabat-Zinn, J., Wheeler, E., Light, T., Skillings, A., Scharf, M., Cropley, T.G., Hosmer, D. and Bernhard, J., 'Influence of a mindfulness-based stress reduction intervention on rates of skin clearing in patients with moderate to severe psoriasis undergoing phototherapy (UVB) and photochemotherapy (PUVA)', *Psychosomatic Medicine*, 60 (1998), pp. 625–32.
13. Spiegel D., Bloom, J. R., Kraemer, H. C. and Gottheil, E., 'Effects of psychosocial treatment on survival of patients with metastatic breast cancer', *Lancet* (October 14 1989), pp. 888–91.
14. North, T.C., McCullagh, P. and Tran, Z.V., 'Effect of exercise on depression', *Exercise and Sport Sciences Reviews*, Vol. 18 (1990), pp. 379–415.
15. Buydens, L., Branchey, M., Roy, A., 'N-3 polyunsaturated fatty acids decrease feelings of anger in a population of substance abusers', *Neuropsychopharmacology*, Vol. 30(1) (2005), S87–S88.
16. Schoenthaler, S.J., et al., 'The effect of randomised vitamin-mineral supplementation on violent and non-violent anti-social behaviour among incarcerated juveniles', *Journal of Nutritional & Environmental Medicine*, Vol. 7 (1997), pp. 343–52.
17. King, D. S., 'Can allergic exposure provoke psychological symptoms? A double-blind test', *Biological Psychiatry*, Vol. 16(1) (1981), pp. 3–19.
18. Conklin, S.M., Harris, J.I., Manuck, S.B., Hibbeln, J.R., Muldoon, M.F., 'Plasma fatty acids are associated with normative variation in mood, personality, and behavior', Abstract 1228, American Psychosomatic Society 64th Annual Meeting, 1–4 March 2006, Denver, Colorado, accessed online http://www.psychosomatic.org/events/AbstractsForJournal06.pdf

Meet Dr Mark

Dr Mark offers consultations from his clinic and runs workshops, retreats and training courses throughout the year.
If you could like more information about any of these, then please visit www.drmarkatkinson.com or phone 0845 094 6450.

Index